P9-EDT-112

Arthritis Sourcebook

Basic Consumer Health Information about Specific Forms of Arthritis and Related Disorders, Including Rheumatoid Arthritis, Osteoarthritis, Gout, Polymyalgia Rheumatica, Psoriatic Arthritis, Spondyloarthropathies, Juvenile Rheumatoid Arthritis, and Juvenile Ankylosing Spondylitis; Along with Information about Medical, Surgical, and Alternative Treatment Options, and Including Strategies for Coping with Pain, Fatigue, and Stress

Edited by Allan R. Cook. 575 pages. 1998. 0-7808-0201-2. $78.

Back & Neck Disorders Sourcebook

Basic Information about Disorders and Injuries of the Spinal Cord and Vertebrae, Including Facts on Chiropractic Treatment, Surgical Interventions, Paralysis, and Rehabilitation, Along with Advice for Preventing Back Trouble

Edited by Karen Bellenir. 548 pages. 1997. 0-7808-0202-0. $78.

"The strength of this work is its basic, easy-to-read format. Recommended."
— *Reference and User Services Quarterly, Winter '97*

Blood & Circulatory Disorders Sourcebook

Basic Information about Blood and Its Components, Anemias, Leukemias, Bleeding Disorders, and Circulatory Disorders, Including Aplastic Anemia, Thalassemia, Sickle-Cell Disease, Hemochromatosis, Hemophilia, Von Willebrand Disease, and Vascular Diseases; Along with a Special Section on Blood Transfusions and Blood Supply Safety, a Glossary, and Source Listings for Further Help and Information

Edited by Karen Bellenir and Linda M. Shin. 575 pages. 1998. 0-7808-0203-9. $78.

Brain Disorders Sourcebook

Basic Consumer Health Information about Strokes, Epilepsy, Amyotrophic Lateral Sclerosis (ALS/Lou Gehrig's Disease), Parkinson's Disease, Brain Tumors, Cerebral Palsy, Headache, Tourette Syndrome, and More; Along with Statistical Data, Treatment and Rehabilitation Options, Coping Strategies, Reports on Current Research Initiatives, a Glossary, and Resource Listings for Additional Help and Information

Edited by Karen Bellenir. 600 pages. 1999. 0-7808-0229-2. $78.

Burns Sourcebook

Basic Information about Various Types of Burns and Scalds, Including Flame, Heat, Electrical, Chemical, and Sun; Along with Short- and Long-Term Treatments, Tissue Reconstruction, Plastic Surgery, Prevention Suggestions, and First Aid

Edited by Allan R. Cook. 600 pages. 1999. 0-7808-0204-7. $78.

Cancer Sourcebook, 1st Edition

Basic Information on Cancer Types, Symptoms, Diagnostic Methods, and Treatments, Including Statistics on Cancer Occurrences Worldwide and the Risks Associated with Known Carcinogens and Activities

Edited by Frank E. Bair. 932 pages. 1990. 1-55888-888-8. $78.

"Written in nontechnical language. Useful for patients, their families, medical professionals, and librarians."
— *Guide to Reference Books, '96*

"Designed with the non-medical professional in mind. Libraries and medical facilities interested in patient education should certainly consider adding the *Cancer Sourcebook* to their holdings. This compact collection of reliable information . . . is an invaluable tool for helping patients and patients' families and friends to take the first steps in coping with the many difficulties of cancer."
— *Medical Reference Services Quarterly, Winter '91*

"Specifically created for the nontechnical reader . . . an important resource for the general reader trying to understand the complexities of cancer."
— *American Reference Books Annual, '91*

"This publication's nontechnical nature and very comprehensive format make it useful for both the general public and undergraduate students." — *Choice, Oct '90*

New Cancer Sourcebook, 2nd Edition

Basic Information about Major Forms and Stages of Cancer, Featuring Facts about Primary and Secondary Tumors of the Respiratory, Nervous, Lymphatic, Circulatory, Skeletal, and Gastrointestinal Systems, and Specific Organs; Statistical and Demographic Data; Treatment Options; and Strategies for Coping

Edited by Allan R. Cook. 1,313 pages. 1996. 0-7808-0041-9. $78.

"This book is an excellent resource for patients with newly diagnosed cancer and their families. The dialogue is simple, direct, and comprehensive. Highly recommended for patients and families to aid in their understanding of cancer and its treatment."
— *Booklist Health Sciences Supplement, Oct '97*

"The amount of factual and useful information is extensive. The writing is very clear, geared to general readers. Recommended for all levels." — *Choice, Jan '97*

Continues next page

Cancer Sourcebook, 3rd Edition

Basic Information about Major Forms and Stages of Cancer, Featuring Facts about Primary and Secondary Tumors of the Respiratory, Nervous, Lymphatic, Circulatory, Skeletal, and Gastrointestinal Systems, and Specific Organs, Statistical and Demographic Data, Treatment Options, and Strategies for Coping

Edited by Edward J. Prucha. 800 pages. 1999. 0-7808-0227-6. $78.

Cancer Sourcebook for Women

Basic Information about Specific Forms of Cancer That Affect Women, Featuring Facts about Breast Cancer, Cervical Cancer, Ovarian Cancer, Cancer of the Uterus and Uterine Sarcoma, Cancer of the Vagina, and Cancer of the Vulva; Statistical and Demographic Data; Treatments, Self-Help Management Suggestions, and Current Research Initiatives

Edited by Allan R. Cook and Peter D. Dresser. 524 pages. 1996. 0-7808-0076-1. $78.

". . . written in easily understandable, non-technical language. Recommended for public libraries or hospital and academic libraries that collect patient education or consumer health materials."
— *Medical Reference Services Quarterly, Spring '97*

"Would be of value in a consumer health library. . . . written with the health care consumer in mind. Medical jargon is at a minimum, and medical terms are explained in clear, understandable sentences."
— *Bulletin of the MLA, Oct '96*

"The availability under one cover of all these pertinent publications, grouped under cohesive headings, makes this certainly a most useful sourcebook."
— *Choice, Jun '96*

"Presents a comprehensive knowledge base for general readers. Men and women both benefit from the gold mine of information nestled between the two covers of this book. Recommended."
— *Academic Library Book Review, Summer '96*

"This timely book is highly recommended for consumer health and patient education collections in all libraries."
— *Library Journal, Apr '96*

Cancer Sourcebook for Women, 2nd Edition

Basic Information about Specific Forms of Cancer That Affect Women, Featuring Facts about Breast Cancer, Cervical Cancer, Ovarian Cancer, Cancer of the Uterus and Uterine Sarcoma, Cancer of the Vagina, and Cancer of the Vulva, Statistical and Demographic Data, Treatments, Self-Help Management Suggestions, and Current Research Initiatives

Edited by Edward J. Prucha. 600 pages. 1999. 0-7808-0226-8. $78.

Cardiovascular Diseases & Disorders Sourcebook

Basic Information about Cardiovascular Diseases and Disorders, Featuring Facts about the Cardiovascular System, Demographic and Statistical Data, Descriptions of Pharmacological and Surgical Interventions, Lifestyle Modifications, and a Special Section Focusing on Heart Disorders in Children

Edited by Karen Bellenir and Peter D. Dresser. 683 pages. 1995. 0-7808-0032-X. $78.

". . . comprehensive format provides an extensive overview on this subject."
— *Choice, Jun '96*

". . . an easily understood, complete, up-to-date resource. This well executed public health tool will make valuable information available to those that need it most, patients and their families. The typeface, sturdy non-reflective paper, and library binding add a feel of quality found wanting in other publications. Highly recommended for academic and general libraries. "
— *Academic Library Book Review, Summer '96*

Communication Disorders Sourcebook

Basic Information about Deafness and Hearing Loss, Speech and Language Disorders, Voice Disorders, Balance and Vestibular Disorders, and Disorders of Smell, Taste, and Touch

Edited by Linda M. Ross. 533 pages. 1996. 0-7808-0077-X. $78.

"This is skillfully edited and is a welcome resource for the layperson. It should be found in every public and medical library."
— *Booklist Health Sciences Supplement, Oct '97*

Congenital Disorders Sourcebook

Basic Information about Disorders Acquired during Gestation, Including Spina Bifida, Hydrocephalus, Cerebral Palsy, Heart Defects, Craniofacial Abnormalities, Fetal Alcohol Syndrome, and More, Along with Current Treatment Options and Statistical Data

Edited by Karen Bellenir. 607 pages. 1997. 0-7808-0205-5. $78.

"Recommended reference source." — *Booklist, Oct '97*

Consumer Issues in Health Care Sourcebook

Basic Information about Health Care Fundamentals and Related Consumer Issues, Including Exams and Screening Tests, Physician Specialties, Choosing a Doctor, Using Prescription and Over-the-Counter Medications Safely, Avoiding Health Scams, Managing Common Health Risks in the Home, Care Options for Chronically or Terminally Ill Patients, and a List of Resources for Obtaining Help and Further Information

Edited by Karen Bellenir. 592 pages. 1998. 0-7808-0221-7. $78.

Continues in back end sheets

Healthy
Aging
SOURCEBOOK

Health Reference Series

Health Reference Series

First Edition

Healthy Aging
SOURCEBOOK

Basic Consumer Health Information about Maintaining Health through the Aging Process, Including Advice on Nutrition, Exercise, and Sleep, Help in Making Decisions about Midlife Issues and Retirement, and Guidance Concerning Practical and Informed Choices in Health Consumerism; Along with Data Concerning the Theories of Aging, Different Experiences in Aging by Minority Groups, and Facts about Aging Now and Aging in the Future; and Featuring a Glossary, a Guide to Consumer Help, Additional Suggested Reading, and Practical Resource Directory

Edited by
Jenifer Swanson

Omnigraphics, Inc.

Penobscot Building / Detroit, MI 48226

Bibliographic Note

Because this page cannot legibly accommodate all the copyright notices, the Bibliographic Note portion of the Preface constitutes an extension of the copyright notice.

Beginning with books published in 1999, each new volume of the *Health Reference Series* will be individually titled and called a "First Edition." Subsequent updates will carry sequential edition numbers. To help avoid confusion and to provide maximum flexibility in our ability to respond to informational needs, the practice of consecutively numbering each volume will be discontinued.

Edited by Jenifer Swanson

Health Reference Series

Karen Bellenir, *Series Editor*
Peter D. Dresser, *Managing Editor*
Joan Margeson, *Research Associate*
Dawn Matthews, *Verification Assistant*
Margaret Mary Missar, *Research Coordinator*
Jenifer Swanson, *Research Associate*

Omnigraphics, Inc.

Matthew P. Barbour, *Vice President, Operations*
Laurie Lanzen Harris, *Vice President, Editorial Director*
Thomas J. Murphy, *Vice President, Finance and Comptroller*
Peter E. Ruffner, *Senior Vice President*
Jane J. Steele, *Marketing Consultant*

Frederick G. Ruffner, Jr., Publisher

Library of Congress Cataloging-in-Publication Data

Healthy aging sourcebook : basic consumer health information about maintaining health through the aging process . . . / edited by Jenifer Swanson. — 1st ed.
    p. cm. — (Health reference series ; v. 46)
    Includes bibliographical references and index.
    ISBN 0-7808-0390-6 (lib. bdg.)
    1. Aged—Health and hygiene. 2. Middle aged persons—Health and hygiene. 3. Aging. I. Swanson, Jenifer. II. Series.
RA777.6.H427 1999
613'.0438—dc21
                            99-24387
                            CIP

∞

This book is printed on acid-free paper meeting the ANSI Z39.48 Standard. The infinity symbol that appears above indicates that the paper in this book meets that standard.

Printed in the United States of America

Table of Contents

Part III: Caring for the Aging Body

Part IV: Being a Prudent Medical Customer

Part V: Safety Concerns

Part VI: Preparing for Final Decisions

Part VII: Additional Help and Information

Preface

About This Book

In the twentieth century, the average life span and life expectancy in the United States grew markedly, from 47 years in 1900 to 79 years in 1996. This increase in longevity was attributed to better sanitation and improvements in medical care. The American consumer base is expected to continue aging in the twenty-first century. This will result in an even larger group of elderly people, many of whom will be active and healthy.

This *Sourcebook* provides information to help the elderly, soon-to-be elderly, and others understand the aging process and the choices that must be made and pursued to maintain health. These choices include eating habits, exercise practices, sleeping patterns, living situations, and the ability to discern legitimate medical procedures from fraudulent ones. In addition, this book includes chapters that provide information about the theories of aging, the different experiences of diverse minority groups, safety concerns, and end-of-life decisions. A glossary, suggested reading list, references, and resource directory are also provided.

How to Use This Book

This book is divided into parts and chapters. Parts focus on broad areas of interest. Chapters are devoted to single topics within a part.

Part I: The Aging Process provides basic information about aging. Differing aging theories are discussed. Statistics provide ethnological information on minority groups. Quality of life versus longevity is explored.

Part II: Midlife Issues and the Retirement Years covers choices that may need to be made as one progresses through the lifespan. Topics covered include self esteem, making moving decisions as they become necessary, and ideas for moving into old age with a rich and valued sense of self.

Part III: Caring for the Aging Body gives a detailed overview of some of the most important health-related changes that older Americans can make to improve the quality of their lives such as dietary changes, proper sleep, exercise, and relinquishing tobacco.

Part IV: Being a Prudent Medical Customer provides information on understanding preventative medical needs, health fraud, and choosing medical treatment. This part also includes information about the use of medication and the importance of making sure that medicines are used in correct doses and combinations.

Part V: Safety Concerns describes the need for preventative safety measures. Elderly people are more prone to crime and home accidents. A home safety checklist is provided along with ideas for direct communications with medical personnel.

Part VI: Preparing for Final Decisions addresses concerns of one's last years including housing options, living wills, and death.

Part VII: Additional Help and Information provides a glossary, a list of additional reading matter, references for senior consumers, and resources for further information.

Bibliographic Note

This volume contains documents and excerpts from publications issued by the following U.S. government agencies: Administration on Aging (AoA), Agency for Health Care Policy and Research (AHCPR), Federal Trade Commission (FTC), Health Care Financing Administration, National Association of Attorneys General, National Cancer Institutes (NCI), National Institute on Aging (NIA), National Institutes of Health (NIH), Public Health Service, U.S. Consumer Product Safety Commission (CPSC), U.S. Department of Agriculture (USDA), and the U.S. Food and Drug Administration (FDA).

In addition, this volume contains copyrighted documents from the following organizations and periodicals: Alliance on Aging, *American Behavioral Scientist, American Fitness,* American Society on Aging's *Generations,* Assisted Living Federation of America, Brandeis University, *The Brown University Long-Term Care Quality Letter, Cornell University News, FDA Consumer, The Futurist, Generations,* The National Council on the Aging, National Policy and Resource Center on Women and Aging, Resource Center for Aging, University of California at Berkeley, *Senior Health Advisor,* and *Social Work.*

Full citation information is provided on the first page of each chapter. Every effort has been made to secure all necessary rights to reprint the copyrighted material. If any omissions have been made, please contact Omnigraphics to make corrections for future editions.

Acknowledgements

Thanks as always go to all who contributed to this book and most importantly, Karen Bellenir. Thanks and love to my husband, Matt, and my daughter, Devon, both of whom have always stood by my side no matter what. This book is for my brother, Andy. May you age gracefully.

Note from the Editor

This book is part of Omnigraphics' *Health Reference Series.* The series provides basic information about a broad range of medical concerns. It is not intended to serve as a tool for diagnosing illness, in prescribing treatments, or as a substitute for the physician/patient relationship. All persons concerned about medical symptoms or the possibility of disease are encouraged to seek professional care from an appropriate health care provider.

Our Advisory Board

The *Health Reference Series* is reviewed by an Advisory Board comprised of librarians from public, academic, and medical libraries. We would like to thank the following board members for providing guidance to the development of this series:

Nancy Bulgarelli,
William Beaumont Hospital Library, Royal Oak, MI

Karen Morgan,
Mardigian Library, University of Michigan, Dearborn, MI

Rosemary Orlando,
St. Clair Shores Public Library, St. Clair Shores, MI

Health Reference Series *Update Policy*

The inaugural book in the *Health Reference Series* was the first edition of *Cancer Sourcebook* published in 1992. Since then, the *Series* has been enthusiastically received by librarians and in the medical community. In order to maintain the standard of providing high-quality health information for the lay person, the editorial staff at Omnigraphics felt it was necessary to implement a policy of updating volumes when warranted.

Medical researchers have been making tremendous strides, and the challenge to stay current with the most recent advances is one our editors take seriously. Each decision to update a volume will be made on an individual basis. Some of the considerations will include how much new information is available and the feedback we receive from people who use the books. If there's a topic you would like to see added to the update list, or an area of medical concern you feel has not been adequately addressed, please write to:

Editor
Health Reference Series
Omnigraphics, Inc.
2500 Penobscot Bldg.
Detroit, MI 48226

The commitment to providing on-going coverage of important medical developments has also led to some technical changes in the *Health Reference Series*. Beginning with books published in 1999, each new volume will be individually titled and called a "First Edition." Subsequent updates will carry sequential edition numbers. To help avoid confusion and to provide maximum flexibility in our ability to respond to informational needs, the practice of consecutively numbering each volume will be discontinued.

Part One

The Aging Process

Chapter 1

Theories of Aging

Life Span and Life Expectancy

This chapter—and gerontologists—talk about two kinds of life span. One is maximum life span, the greatest age reached by any member of a species. In humans this is 121 years, we think. The other is average life span, the average age reached by members of a population. Life expectancy, the number of years an individual can expect to live, is based on average life spans.

Average life span and life expectancy in the United States have grown dramatically in this century, from about 47 years in 1900 to about 79 years in 1996. This advance is mostly due to better sanitation, the discovery of antibiotics, and improvements in medical care. Now, as scientists make headway against chronic diseases like cancer and heart disease, some think it can be extended even further.

Maximum human life span seems to be another matter. There is no evidence that it has changed for thousands of years despite fabled fountains of youth and biblical tales of long-lived patriarchs. However, very recently, the dream of extending life span has shifted from legend to laboratory. As gerontologists explore the genes, cells, and organs involved in aging, they are uncovering more and more of the secrets of longevity. As a result, life extension may now be more than the stuff of myth and the retardation of disease and disability, realistic goals.

Excerpted from *In Search of the Secrets of Aging*, National Institute on Aging (NIA), NIH Pub. No. 93-2756, Second Edition 1996.

Aging Theories

Gerontology is often described in terms of its major theories. These fall into two main groups, one emphasizing internal biological clocks or "programs," and the other external or environmental forces that damage cells and organs until they can no longer function adequately.

Most gerontologists now agree that no single theory can account for all the changes that take place as we age. In fact, with the tools of biotechnology and an influx of new knowledge, all-encompassing theories of aging are giving way to another perspective. Aging today is viewed as many processes, interactive and interdependent, that determine life span and health, and gerontologists are studying a multitude of factors that may be involved. These include environmental factors that have an impact on aging cells, tissues, and organs as well as the body's genetic response to such factors.

Aging processes can be divided into three general categories—genetic, biochemical, and physiological. The rest of this chapter describes what we know and don't know in each territory and where we think we are likely to find answers to questions about aging and longevity.

Theories of Aging

Theories of aging fall into two groups. The "programmed" theories hold that aging follows a biological timetable, perhaps a continuation of the one that regulates childhood growth and development. The damage or error theories emphasize environmental assaults to our systems that gradually cause things to go wrong. Many of the theories of aging are not mutually exclusive. Here is a brief and very simplified rundown of the major theories.

Programmed Theories

Programmed Senescence. Aging is the result of the sequential switching on and off of certain genes, with senescence being defined as the time when age-associated deficits are manifested.

Endocrine Theory. Biological clocks act through hormones to control the pace of aging.

Immunological Theory. A programmed decline in immune system functions leads to an increased vulnerability to infectious disease and thus aging and death.

4

Error Theories

Wear and Tear. Cells and tissues have vital parts that wear out.

Rate of Living. The greater an organism's rate of oxygen basal metabolism, the shorter its life span.

Crosslinking. An accumulation of crosslinked proteins damages cells and tissues, slowing down bodily processes.

Free Radicals. Accumulated damage caused by oxygen radicals causes cells and eventually organs to stop functioning.

Error Catastrophe. Damage to mechanisms that synthesize proteins results in faulty proteins which accumulate to a level that causes catastrophic damage to cells, tissues, and organs.

Somatic Mutation. Genetic mutations occur and accumulate with increasing age, causing cells to deteriorate and malfunction.

Questions: Selected Readings

Finch, C.E., *Longevity, Senescence and the Genome*, Chicago: University of Chicago Press,1991.

Institute of Medicine, *Extending Life, Enhancing Life: A National Research Agenda on Aging*, Washington, DC: National Academy Press, 1992.

Martin, G.R., and Baker, G.T., *Aging and the Aged. Theories of Aging and Life Extension*, New York: MacMillan, 1993.

Ricklefs, R.E., and Finch, C.E., *Aging—A Natural History*, Scientific American Library, New York: W.H. Freeman, 1995.

Schneider, E.L., and Reed, J.D., "Life Extension," *New England Journal of Medicine* 313:1159-1168, 1985.

Warner, H., Butler, R.N., Sprott, R.L,, Schneider, E.L., eds., *Modem Biological Theories of Aging*, New York: Raven, 1987.

The Genetic Connection

Humans seem to have a maximum life span of about 121 years, but for tortoises it's 150 and for dogs, about 20. What underlies these differences among species are genes, the coded segments of DNA (deoxyribonucleic acid) strung like beads along the chromosomes of nearly every living cell. In humans, the nucleus of each cell holds 23 pairs of chromosomes, and together these chromosomes contain about 100,000 genes.

The link between genes and life span is unquestioned. The simple observation that some species live longer than others—humans longer than dogs, tortoises longer than mice—is one convincing piece of evidence. Another comes from recent, dramatic laboratory studies in which researchers, through selective breeding or genetic engineering, have been able to raise animals with extended life spans. For example, selective breeding has resulted in fruit flies that live nearly twice as long as average.

Longevity Genes

By demonstrating that genes are linked to life span, the long-lived fruit flies have set the stage for more questions: What specific genes are involved? What activates them? How do they influence aging and longevity? In numerous laboratories, the search for answers is on.

Some leads are coming from yeast cells in which researchers have found evidence of 14 genes that seem to be related to aging. Longevity-related genes have also been found in tiny worms called nematodes and in fruit flies. Like yeast, nematodes and fruit flies have short life spans, and their genes, which are known and do not vary greatly, are relatively easy to study.

Some of the genes found in yeast, fruit flies, and nematodes appear to promote longevity, while others may act to shorten life span. Under normal conditions, some genes limit life span, but when these same genes are mutated, they promote longevity instead.

One such gene, *age-1*, has been identified and studied in several laboratories. Long-lived *age-1* mutants were shown to have enhanced antioxidant defenses, including increased levels of two enzymes linked to aging and longevity, in studies conducted by Thomas Johnson, of the University of Colorado at Boulder; Pamela Larsen, of the University of Southern California; and Donald Riddle, of the University of Missouri.

In several laboratories, researchers have linked longevity to the "dauer" genetic pathway, which regulates the development of nematode larvae. The dauer pathway is a sequence of genes activated by environmental conditions less than optimal for nematode development, such as insufficient food and water or overcrowding. Researchers can induce the dauer pathway in larvae, resulting in a hibernation-like, metabolically altered, non-aging state, until suitable environmental conditions reappear, stimulating the resumption of normal development.

Mutations in three genes in the dauer pathway have been shown to result in increased longevity in adult worms. Mutations in one of them, *daf-2*, were found to double nematode longevity by Cynthia Kenyon and her coworkers at the University of California-San Francisco. Larsen and Riddle discovered that worms containing mutations in both *daf-2* and *daf-12* another dauer-pathway gene, have four times the longevity of nonmutant worms. Meanwhile, Gary Ruvkun and his coworkers at Massachusetts General Hospital/Harvard Medical School have discovered that mutations of yet another gene in the pathway, *daf-23*, increase life span two- to three-fold.

Recent studies reveal that the *age-1* and *daf-23* genes are different forms (alleles) of the same gene that encodes a nematode enzyme involved in cellular communication. A similar enzyme exists in mammals.

Further work by several of the researchers reveals that, in order for the mutants in the dauer pathway to exhibit increased longevity, a functional *daf-16* gene must be present.

The genes isolated so far are only a few of what scientists think may be dozens, perhaps hundreds, of longevity-and aging-related genes. Tracking them down in organisms like nematodes and yeast is just the beginning. The next big question for many gerontologists is whether there are counterparts in people—human homologs—of the genes found in laboratory animals.

Other unanswered questions concern the roles played by these genes. What exactly do they do? On one level, all genes function by transcribing their "codes"—actually DNA base sequences—into another nucleic acid called messenger ribonucleic acid or MRNA. Messenger RNA is then translated into proteins. Transcription and translation together constitute the process known as gene expression.

The proteins expressed by genes carry out a multitude of functions in each cell and tissue in the body, and some of these functions are related to aging. So when we ask what longevity or aging-related genes do, we are actually asking what their protein products do at the cellular and tissue levels. Increasingly, gerontologists are also asking how alterations in the process of gene expression itself may affect aging.

Some proteins, such as anti-oxidants, appear to prevent damage to cells, and others may repair damaged DNA or help cells respond to stress; more about these comes later. Other gene products are thought to control cell senescence, a process that could prove to be a key piece in the puzzle of aging and longevity.

Cell Senescence

Picture a cell: The threadlike pairs of chromosomes inhabit a nucleus that sits in a sea of cytoplasm along with other tiny organelles that do the cell's work, the whole surrounded by a membrane at the surface of which the cell sends and receives messages to and from other cells. Then picture the chromosomes, condensing into rod-like structures that divide in two, the nucleus disappearing, the chromosomes migrating to opposite sides of the cell where two daughter nuclei are formed, and after that the entire cell following the chromosomes' lead, pulling apart and forming two identical daughter cells.

This, the process of mitosis, or asexual cell division, gives rise to the 100 trillion or so cells that make up the human body. But it does not go on indefinitely. About the middle of this century, researchers learned that cells have finite life spans, at least when studied in test tubes—in vitro. After a certain number of divisions, they enter a state of cell senescence, in which they do not divide or proliferate and DNA synthesis is blocked. For example, young human fibroblasts—collagen-producing cells frequently used in this branch of aging research—divide about 50 times and then stop. This phenomenon has become known as the Hayflick limit, after Leonard Hayflick, who with Paul Moorhead first described it while at the Wistar Institute in Philadelphia.

Intrigued by the possibility that the Hayflick limit might help explain some aspects of bodily aging, gerontologists have looked for and found links between senescence and human life spans. Fibroblasts taken from 75-year olds, for example, have fewer divisions remaining than cells from a child. Moreover, the longer a species' life span, the higher its Hayflick limit; human fibroblasts have higher Hayflick limits than mouse fibroblasts.

Proliferative Genes

Searching for explanations of proliferation and senescence, scientists have found certain genes that appear to trigger cell proliferation. One example of such a proliferative gene is *c-fos*, which encodes a short-lived protein that is thought to regulate the expression of other genes important in cell division.

But *c-fos* and others of its kind are countered by anti-proliferative genes, which seem to interfere with division. The first evidence of an anti-proliferative gene came from retinoblastoma, an eye tumor. Most normal cells contain two copies of each of their genes, but in the cells of retinoblastoma tumors, one copy of a gene called RB is missing and the other copy is mutated. As a result, retinoblastoma cells cannot make RB protein. Unlike normal cells, cancer cells can keep on dividing indefinitely. When researchers introduced an intact RB gene into retinoblastoma cells, however, they found that the cells stopped dividing. In other words, the protein made by the RB gene appeared to suppress proliferation.

Senescence is the norm in the world of cells. In some cases, however, a cell somehow escapes this control mechanism and goes on dividing, becoming, in the terms of cell biology, immortal. And because immortal cells eventually form tumors, this is one area in which aging research and cancer research intersect. Investigators theorize that a failure of anti-proliferative genes (also known as tumor suppressor genes) is the first step in a complex process that leads to development of a tumor. Senescence, according to this view, may have evolved because it protected against cancer.

Still a mystery is how these genes' products function to promote and suppress cell proliferation. There are indications that a multi-layer control system is at work, involving probably a host of intricate mechanisms that interact to maintain a balance between the two kinds of genes. Many gerontologists are now involved in unraveling these intricacies, studying both the genes and their products to learn which ones influence senescence and how.

Telomeres

In the meantime, scientists are finding more clues to senescence in the architecture of DNA. Every chromosome, they have discovered, has tails at the ends that get shorter as a cell divides. Named telomeres, the tails all have the same, short sequence of DNA bases repeated thousands of times. The repetitive structure stabilizes the chromosomes, forming a tight bond between the two strands of the DNA.

Each time a cell divides, the telomeres shed a number of bases, so telomere length gives some indication of how many divisions the cell has already undergone and how many remain before it becomes senescent.

This apparent counting mechanism, almost like an abacus keeping track of the cell's age, has led to speculation that telomeres do serve as molecular meters of cell division. But they may play a more active role, and telomere researchers are exploring the possibility that these chromosome ends regulate cellular life span in some way.

Telomere research is another territory where cancer and aging research merge. In immortal cancer cells, telomeres act abnormally— they stop shrinking with each cell division. In the search for clues to this phenomenon, researchers have zeroed in on an enzyme called telomerase. Normally absent in most normal adult cells, telomerase seems to swing into action in advanced cancers, enabling the telomeres to replace lost sequences and divide indefinitely. This finding has led to speculation that if a drug could be developed to block telomerase activity, it might aid in cancer treatment.

Whether cell senescence is explained by abnormal gene products, telomere shortening, or other factors, the question of what senescence has to do with the aging of organisms remains and continues to be the focus of intense study.

In the meantime, gerontologists are also studying proteins in the body that may play a role in aging and longevity. Genes hold the codes to these proteins, but what substances turn the genes on and off? And once activated, how do their products interact with the products of other genes? What is their effect on cells and tissues? The biochemistry of aging holds some of the answers.

The Genetic Connection: Selected Readings

Goldstein, S., "Replicative Senescence: The Human Fibroblast Comes of Age," *Science* 249:1129-1133, 1990.

Harley, C.B., Futcher, A.B., Greider, C.W., "Telomeres Shorten During Aging of Human Fibroblasts," *Nature* 345:458-460, 1990.

Hayflick, L., and Moorhead, P.S., "The Serial Cultivation of Human Diploid Cell Strains," *Experimental Cell Research* 25:585-621, 1961.

Jazwinski, S.M., "Genes of Youth: Genetics of Aging in Baker's Yeast," *ASM News* 59:172-178, 1993.

Jazwinski, S.M., "Longevity, Genes, and Aging," *Science* 273:54-59, 1996.

Johnson, T.E., "Aging Can Be Genetically Dissected Into Component Processes Using Long-Lived Lines of Caenorhabditis elegans," *Proceedings of the National Academy of Sciences* 84:3777-3781, 1987.

Kennedy, B.K., Austriaco, N.R., Zhang, J., Guarente, L., "Mutation in the Silencing Gene SIR4 Can Delay Aging in S. cerevisiae," *Cell* 80:485-496, 1995.

Kenyon, C., Chang, J,, Gensch, E., Rudner, A., and Tabtiang, R., "A C. elegans mutant that lives twice as long as wild-type," *Nature* 366:461-464, 1993.

Larsen, P.L., "Aging and Resistance to Oxidative Damage in C elegans," *Proceedings of the National Academy of Sciences* 90:8905-8909, 1993.

Larsen, P.L., Albert, P.S., Riddle, D.L., "Genes That Regulate Both Development and Longevity in C. elegans," *Genetics* 139:1567-1583, 1995.

McCormick, A.M., and Campisi, J., "Cellular Aging and Senescence," *Current Opinion in Cell Biology* 3:230-234, 1991.

Morris, J.Z., Tissenbaum, H.A., and Ruvkun, G., "A phosphatidylinositol-3-OH Kinase Family Member Regulating Longevity and Diapause in Caenorhabditis elegans," *Nature* 382:536–539, 1996.

Pereira-Smith, O.M., and Smith, J.R., "Genetic Analysis of Indefinite Division in Human Cells: Identification of Four Complementation Groups," *Proceedings of the National Academy of Sciences* 85:6042-6046, 1988.

Rose, M.R., "Laboratory Evolution of Postponed Senescence in Drosophila melanogaster," *Evolution* 38:1004-1010, 1984.

Biochemistry and Aging

Treacherous oxygen molecules, protective enzymes, hormones that seem to turn back the clock, and proteins that may speed it up: The biochemistry of aging is a rich territory with an expanding frontier. Major areas of exploration include oxygen radicals and glucose crosslinking of proteins, both of which damage cells; the substances that help prevent and repair damage; and the role of specific proteins, particularly heat shock proteins, hormones, and growth factors.

Oxygen Radicals

Demolishing proteins and damaging nucleic acids, oxygen radicals are thought to be the villains in the day-to-day life of cells. The free radical theory of aging, first proposed by Denham Harman at the University of Nebraska, holds that damage caused by oxygen radicals is responsible for many of the bodily changes that come with aging. Free radicals have been implicated not only in aging but also in degenerative disorders, including cancer, atherosclerosis, cataracts, and neurodegeneration.

A free radical is a molecule with an unpaired, highly reactive electron. An oxygen free radical is a byproduct of normal metabolism, produced as cells turn food and oxygen into energy.

In need of a mate for its lone electron, the free radical takes an electron from another molecule, which in turn becomes unstable and combines readily with other molecules. A chain reaction can ensue, resulting in a series of compounds, some of which are harmful. They damage proteins, membranes, and nucleic acids, particularly DNA, including the DNA in mitochondria, the organelles within the cell that produce energy.

But free radicals do not go unchecked. Mounted against them is a multilayer defense system manned by antioxidants that react with and disarm these damaging molecules. Under some conditions, the familiar vitamins C and E and beta carotene can function as antioxidants. So can enzymes, such as superoxide dismutase (SOD), catalase, and glutathione peroxidase. They prevent most, but not all, oxidative damage. Little by little the damage mounts and contributes, so the theory goes, to deteriorating tissues and organs.

Support for the free radical theory comes from studies of antioxidants, particularly SOD. SOD converts oxygen radicals into the also harmful hydrogen peroxide, which is then degraded by another enzyme, catalase, to oxygen and water.

At the NIA, Richard Cutler has found that SOD levels are directly related to life span in 20 different species; longer-lived animals have higher levels of SOD, suggesting that the ability to fight free radicals has something to do with longer life spans. Levels of other antioxidants—vitamin E and beta-carotene, for example—have also been correlated with life span.

Other studies have shown that inserting extra copies of the SOD gene into fruit flies extends their average life span. In three different laboratories, researchers have reported that transgenic fruit flies, carrying extra copies of the gene for SOD, live 5 to 10 percent longer than average.

Other experimental evidence lends support to the free radical hypothesis. For example, higher levels of SOD and catalase have been found in long-lived nematodes. And in another important study, giving gerbils a synthetic anti-oxidant has reduced high levels of oxidized protein, a sign of aging, in their brains.

The discovery of anti-oxidants raised hopes that people could retard aging simply by adding them to the diet. Unfortunately taking SOD tablets has no effect on cellular aging; the enzyme is simply broken down in the body during digestion

And when anti-oxidant vitamins are added to cells, they compensate by halting production of their own anti-oxidants, leaving free radical levels unchanged.

Researchers have not abandoned all hope for dietary anti-oxidants, however. Current studies, for example, are exploring the possibility that vitamin C can reduce heart disease by blocking oxidation of low-density lipoproteins. Oxidation of these cholesterol-carrying proteins is thought to be a key element in hardening of the arteries. In addition, there is evidence that vitamin E in the diet may be linked to heart attacks, with low vitamin E intake appearing to increase the risk.

At the same time, studies reveal potential risks associated with antioxidant doses of vitamins and other nutrients. For example, beta-carotene may be linked to a higher risk of lung cancer in smokers, and vitamin E is associated with hemorrhagic stroke.

Glucose Crosslinking

Another suspect in cellular deterioration is blood sugar or glucose. In a process called non-enzymatic glycosylation or glycation, glucose molecules attach themselves to proteins, setting in motion a chain of chemical reactions that ends in the proteins binding together or crosslinking, thus altering their biological and structural roles. The process is slow but increases with time.

Crosslinks, which have been termed advanced glycosylation end products (AGEs), seem to toughen tissues and may cause some of the deterioration associated with aging. AGEs have been linked to stiffening connective tissue (collagen), hardened arteries, cataracts, loss of nerve function, and less efficient kidneys.

These are deficiencies that often accompany aging. They also appear at younger ages in people with diabetes, who have high glucose levels. Diabetes, in fact, is sometimes considered an accelerated model of aging. Not only do its complications mimic the physiologic changes that can accompany old age, but its victims have shorter-than-average life expectancies. As a result, much research on crosslinking has focused on its relationship to diabetes as well as aging.

One finding is that the body has its own defense system against crosslinking. Just as it has antioxidants to fight free-radical damage, it has other guardians, immune system cells called macrophages, that combat glycation. Macrophages with special receptors for AGEs seek them out, engulf them, break them down, and eject them into the blood stream where they are filtered out by the kidneys and eliminated in urine.

The only apparent drawback to this defense system is that it is not complete and levels of AGEs increase steadily with age. One reason is that kidney function tends to decline with advancing age. Another is that macrophages, like certain other components of the immune system, become less active. Why is not known, but immunologists are beginning to learn more about how the immune system affects and is affected by aging. And in the meantime, diabetes researchers are investigating drugs that could supplement the body's natural defenses by blocking AGE formation.

Crosslinking interests gerontologists for several reasons. It is associated with disorders that are common among older people, such as diabetes; it progresses with age, and AGEs are potential targets for anti-aging drugs. In addition, crosslinking may play a role in damage to DNA, which has become another important focus for research on aging.

DNA Repair and Synthesis

In the normal wear and tear of cellular life, DNA undergoes continual damage. Attacked by oxygen radicals, ultraviolet light, and other toxic agents, it suffers damage in the form of deletions, or destroyed sections, and mutations, or changes in the sequence of DNA bases that make up the genetic code. Biologists theorize that this DNA damage, which gradually accumulates, leads to malfunctioning genes, proteins, cells, and, as the years go by, deteriorating tissues and organs.

Not surprisingly, numerous enzyme systems in the cell have evolved to detect and repair damaged DNA. For repair, transcription, and replication to occur, the double-helical structure that makes up DNA must be partially unwound. Enzymes called helicases do the unwinding. Researchers have found that people who have Werner's syndrome, a disease with several features of premature aging, have a defect in one of their helicases.

The repair process interests gerontologists. It is known that an animal's ability to repair certain types of DNA damage is directly related to the life span of its species. Humans repair DNA, for example, more quickly and efficiently than mice or other animals with shorter life spans. This suggests that DNA damage and repair are in some way part of the aging puzzle.

In addition, researchers have found defects in DNA repair in people with a genetic or familial susceptibility to cancer. If DNA repair processes decline with age while damage accumulates, as scientists hypothesize, it could help explain why cancer is so much more common among older people.

Gerontologists who study DNA damage and repair have begun to uncover numerous complexities. Even within a single organism, repair rates can vary among cells, with the most efficient repair going on in germ (sperm and egg) cells. Moreover, certain genes are repaired more quickly than others, including those that regulate cell proliferation.

Especially intriguing is repair to a kind of DNA that resides not in the cell's nucleus but in its mitochondria. These small organelles are the principal sites of metabolism and energy production, and cells can have hundreds of them. Mitochondrial DNA is thought to be injured at a much greater rate than nuclear DNA, possibly because the mitochondria produce a stream of damaging oxygen radicals during metabolism. Adding to its vulnerability, mitochondrial DNA is unprotected by the protein coat that helps shield DNA in the nucleus from damage.

Research has shown that mitochondrial DNA damage increases exponentially with age, and several diseases that appear late in life, including late-onset diabetes, have been traced to defects in mitochondria. While such disorders seem to be linked to metabolism, it is not yet known whether age-associated damage also impairs metabolism.

Researchers are searching for answers to this and other questions. They would like to know, for example, how much mitochondrial DNA damage occurs in specific parts of the body, such as the brain, what causes the damage, and how it could be prevented.

Heat Shock Proteins

Despite their name, heat shock proteins (HSPs) are produced when cells are exposed to various stresses, not only heat. Their expression can be triggered by exposure to toxic substances, such as heavy metals and chemicals, and even by behavioral and psychological stress.

What attracts aging researchers to HSPs is the finding that the levels at which they are produced depend on age. Old animals placed under stress—physical restraint, for example—have lower levels of a heat shock protein designated HSP-70 than young animals under similar stress. Moreover, in laboratory cultures of cells, researchers have found a striking decline in HSP-70 production as cells approach senescence.

Exactly what role HSPs play in the aging process is not yet clear. They are known to help the cell disassemble and dispose of damaged proteins and to facilitate the making and transport of new proteins. But what proteins are involved and how they relate to aging is still the subject of speculation and study.

Nikki Holbrook, of the NIA's Gerontology Research Center in Baltimore, Maryland, and other researchers are investigating the action of HSP-70 in specific sites, such as the adrenal cortex (the outer layer of the adrenal gland). Here, and in blood vessels and possibly other sites, the expression of HSP-70 appears to be closely related to hormones released in response to stress, such as the glucocorticoids and catecholamines. Eventually, answers to the puzzle of heat shock proteins may throw light on some parts of the neuroendocrine system, whose hormones and growth factors also appear to be major factors in the aging process.

Hormones

In 1989, at Veterans Administration hospitals in Milwaukee and Chicago, a small group of men age 60 and over began receiving injections three times a week that dramatically reversed some signs of aging. The injections appeared to increase their lean body mass, reduce excess fat, and thicken their skin. When the injections were stopped, these changes reversed, and the signs of aging returned. Researchers are continuing to explore whether or not the injections can also increase muscle strength in the elderly.

What the men were taking was recombinant human growth hormone (GH), a synthetic version of the hormone that is produced in the pituitary gland and plays a critical part in normal childhood growth and development. Now researchers are learning that GH, or the decline of GH, seems also to play a role in the aging process in at least some individuals.

The idea that hormones are linked to aging is not new. We have long known that some hormones decline with age. Human growth hormone levels decrease in about half of all adults with the passage of time. Production of the sex hormones estrogen and testosterone tends to fall off. Hormones with less familiar names, like thymosin, are also not as abundant in older as in younger adults.

16

Hormones and Research on Aging

Produced by glands, organs, and tissues, hormones are the body's chemical messengers, flowing through the blood stream and searching out cells fitted with special receptors. Each receptor, like a lock, can be opened by the specific hormone that fits it and also, to a lesser extent, by closely related hormones. Here are some of the hormones and other growth factors of special interest to gerontologists.

Estrogen. The female hormone estrogen is used in hormone replacement therapy to relieve discomforts of menopause. Produced mainly, by the ovaries, it slows the bone thinning that accompanies aging and may help prevent frailty and disability. After menopause, fat tissue is the major source of a weaker form of estrogen than that produced by the ovaries.

Growth Hormone. This product of the pituitary gland appears to play a role in body (composition and muscle and bone strength. It is released through the action of another trophic factor called growth hormone releasing hormone, which is produced in the brain. It works, in part, by stimulating the production of insulin-like growth factors which comes mainly from the liver. All three are being studied for their potential to strengthen muscle and bones and prevent frailty among older people.

Melatonin. This hormone from the pineal gland responds to light and seems to regulate sleep onset, timing of sleep-wake phases, and seasonal changes in the body. Researchers are examining how melatonin supplements affect sleep patterns in the elderly, among other topics.

Testosterone. The male hormone testosterone is produced in the testes and may decline with age, though less frequently or, significantly than estrogen in women. Researchers are investigating its ability to strengthen muscles and prevent frailty and disability in older men. They are also looking at its side effects, which may include an increased risk of certain cancers, particularly prostate cancer.

DHEA. Short for dehydroepiandrosterone, DHEA is produced in the adrenal glands. It is a weak male hormone and a precursor to some other hormones, including testosterone and estrogen. DHEA is being studied for its possible effects on selected aspects of aging.

Hormone Replacement

We also know that when some declining hormones are replaced, various signs of aging diminish. Most, like growth hormone, are still in the experimental stage, but one, estrogen, is used in medical practice to alleviate the discomforts of menopause. Estrogen replacement therapy also lessens the accelerated bone loss that comes with menopause and helps prevent cardiovascular disease. However, questions about cancer and other risks surround hormone therapy and have not yet been resolved.

Growth Factors

Hormones are aided and abetted by an arsenal of other substances that also stimulate or modulate cell activities. Known collectively as growth or trophic factors, these include substances such as insulin-like growth factor (IGF-1), which mediates many of the actions of GH. Another trophic factor of interest to gerontologists is growth hormone releasing hormone, which stimulates the release of GH.

The mechanisms—how hormones and growth factors produce their effects—are still a matter of intense speculation and study. Scientists know that these chemical messengers selectively stimulate cell activities which in turn affect critical events, such as the size and functioning of skeletal muscle. However, the pathway from hormone to muscle is complex and still unclear.

Consider growth hormone. It begins by stimulating production of insulin-like growth factor. IGF-1 enters and flows through the blood stream, seeking out special IGF-1 receptors on the surface of various cells, including muscle cells. Through these receptors it signals the muscle cells to increase in size and number, perhaps by stimulating their genes to produce more of special, muscle-specific proteins. Also involved at some point in this process are one or more of the six known proteins that bind with IGF-1; their regulatory roles are still a mystery.

As if the cellular complexities weren't enough, the action of growth hormone also may be intertwined with a cluster of other factors—exercise, for example, which stimulates a certain amount of GH secretion on its own, and obesity, which depresses production of GH. Even the way fat is distributed in the body may make a difference; lower levels of GH have been linked to excess abdominal fat but not to lower body fat.

Biochemistry and Aging: Selected Readings

Ames, B.N., "Endogenous DNA Damage as Related to Nutrition and Aging," in Ingram, D.K., Baker, G.T., Shock, N.W., eds., *The Potential for Nutritional Modulation of Aging Processes*, Trumbull, CT: Food and Nutrition Press, 1991.

Blake, M.J., Udelsman, R., Feulner, G.J., Norton, D.D., Holbrook, N.J., "Stress-Induced HSP70 Expression in Adrenal Cortexi A Glucocorticoid Sensitive, Age-Dependent Response," *Proceedings of the National Academy of Sciences* 87:846-850, 1991.

Cerami, A., "Hypothesis: Glucose as a Mediator of Aging," *Journal of the American Geriatric Society* 33:626-634, 1985.

Harman, D., "The Free Radical Theory of Aging," in Warner, H.R., et al., eds., *Modern Biological Theories of Aging*, New York: Raven, 1987.

Rudman, D., Feller A.G., Nagraj, H.S., et al., "Effects of Human Growth Hormone in Men Over 60 Years Old," *The New England Journal of Medicine* 323:1-6, 1990.

Stadtman, E.R., "Protein Oxidation and Aging," *Science* 257:1220-1224, 1992.

Wallace, D.C., "Mitochondrial Genetics: A Paradigm for Aging and Degenerative Diseases?" *Science* 256:628-632, 1992.

Glossary

antioxidants: Compounds that neutralize oxygen radicals. Some are enzymes like SOD while others are nutrients such as vitamin C, vitamin E, and beta-carotene.

anti-proliferative genes: Genes that inhibit cell division or proliferation; also known as tumor suppressor genes.

average life span: The average number of years that members of a population live.

biomarkers: Biological changes that characterize the aging process; because biomarkers are considered a better measure of aging than chronological time, studies are under way to identify biomarkers in cells, tissues, and organs.

caloric restriction: An experimental approach to studying longevity in which life spans of laboratory animals have been extended by reducing calories while the necessary level of nutrients is maintained.

cell senescence: The stage at which a cell has stopped dividing permanently.

chromosomes: Structures in the cell's nucleus, made up of protein and DNA, that contain the genes.

cytokines: Proteins that are secreted by cells and regulate the behavior of other nearby cells through signals. Cytokine signals trigger activity in some types of immune cells, and cause changes in many different types of cells throughout the body.

DNA (deoxyribonucleic acid): A large molecule that carries the genetic information necessary for all cellular functions, including the building of proteins. Damage to DNA and the rate at which this damage is repaired may help determine the rate of aging.

free radicals: Molecules with unpaired electrons that react readily with other molecules. Oxygen free radicals, produced during metabolism, damage cells and may be responsible for aging in tissues and organs.

gene: A segment of DNA that contains the "code" for a specific protein or other product.

gene expression: The process by which genes are transcribed and translated into proteins. Age-related changes in gene expression may account for some of the phenomena of aging.

glycation: The process by which glucose links with proteins and causes them to bind together, thus stiffening tissues and leading to the complications of diabetes and perhaps some of the physiologic problems associated with aging.

Hayflick limit: The finite number of divisions of which a cell is capable.

interleukins: A type of cytokine. The amount present in the body varies with age.

lymphocytes: Small white blood cells that are important to the immune system. A decline in lymphocyte function with advancing age is being studied for insights into aging and disease.

maximum life span: The greatest age reached by any member of a given species.

mitochondria: Cell organelles that metabolize sugars into energy. Mitochondria also contain DNA, which is damaged by the high level of free radicals produced in the mitochondria.

photoaging: The process initiated by sunlight through which the skin becomes drier and loses elasticity. Photoaging is being studied for clues to aging because it has the same effect as normal aging on certain skin cells.

proliferative genes: Genes that promote cell division or proliferation; also known as oncogenes.

proteins: Molecules made up of amino acids arranged in a specific order determined by the genetic code. Proteins are essential for all life processes. Certain ones, such as the enzymes that protect against free radicals and the lymphokines produced in the immune system, are being studied extensively by gerontologists.

telomeres: Repeated DNA sequences found at the ends of chromosomes; telomeres shorten each time a cell divides.

tumor suppressor genes: Genes that inhibit cell division or proliferation.

Chapter 2

With the Passage of Time: The Baltimore Longitudinal Study of Aging

A Treasury of Data

In 1991, 54 men took part in a study that discovered something new, and potentially very important, about one kind of cancer. Eighteen of the 54 had had prostate cancer. All were participants in the Baltimore Longitudinal Study of Aging (BLSA).

The researchers began with frozen blood samples provided by the men over a period of years, during their regular visits to the BLSA. Using a test already common in medical practice, this team of scientists from the National Institute on Aging (NIA) and The Johns Hopkins University analyzed each of the samples for an enzyme called prostate-specific antigen or PSA.

The medical community already knew that most men with prostate cancer have high levels of PSA in their blood. What these investigators wanted to explore was the rate of change in PSA levels over time and how that rate differed among the 54 men in the study. Did the men who had developed cancer have a rate of change different from the others?

The answer, reported by H. Ballentine Carter, Jay D. Pearson, and their colleagues in the *Journal of the American Medical Association*, was yes. In the 18 men who had cancer, PSA levels began to rise rapidly about 5 years before the disease had been diagnosed by traditional means. In the other men—including those with benign prostate

Excerpted from the booklet *With the Passage of Time: The Baltimore Longitudinal Study of Aging,* National Institute on Aging (NIA), NIH Pub. No. 93-3685, October 1993.

growth or hyperplasia (BPH) and those without prostate disease—no such dramatic rise occurred.

This medical discovery had its origin in the rich treasury of data that has been carefully collected for more than three decades at the Baltimore Longitudinal Study of Aging. Launched in 1958, the BLSA is America's longest running scientific examination of human aging. Its aims are to measure the usual or universal changes that occur as people age and to learn how these changes relate to the fundamental causes of aging and to the diseases that sometimes accompany aging.

With the Passage of Time tells the story of the BLSA—a study conceived as a partnership between volunteer participants and researchers. It is a story that revolves around these two groups: the men and women who travel to the NIA's Gerontology Research Center (GRC) in Baltimore every 2 years to take part in the study and the scores of investigators, from the GRC and other academic centers around the world, who conduct studies with BLSA participants and analyze the data, putting together a picture of how we age.

But the story told here is not complete. The prostate study, for example, has given hope and direction to other investigations. In Baltimore and elsewhere, researchers are testing a new hypothesis—that tracking PSA levels over time, or "serial testing," may be a better way of detecting prostate cancer than single, isolated tests. This is because the BLSA data showed that rate of change in PSA level may be a more reliable and earlier marker of prostate cancer than the actual PSA level.

In addition, BLSA and Johns Hopkins investigators are following up with a 10-year investigation involving all BLSA men over age 30. This study is looking at a multitude of factors related to prostate cancer and BPH. It will examine PSA levels, hormone levels, and urination patterns. It will use magnetic resonance imaging to detect changes associated with prostate cancer and BPH. It will look for the reasons that the incidence of prostate cancer rises so steeply with age. A particular focus will be African Americans who have the highest rate of prostate cancer in the world.

The prostate study is just one example of how BLSA volunteers and researchers are contributing to scientific knowledge of health and aging. Each year the study adds to its treasury of data, generating new findings and new questions. It is an unfolding story with many chapters still to come.

Every Two Years

Eyes intent on the computer screen in front of her, Louise Capone pulls up on the armrest of the Kin-Com chair. The armrest rises and a line ascends the screen. She pulls again, harder, and the line climbs a little higher.

"Pull, pull, pull, keep pulling, keep pulling," cheers Rosemary Lindle, the exercise physiologist who presides over strength tests at the Baltimore Longitudinal Study of Aging (BLSA), in which Ms. Capone is a participant. The Kin-Com, more officially known as a kinetic communications device, works in much the same way that weight resistance machines in gyms do. When someone applies force— pulling with the biceps muscle of the right arm, for instance—the apparatus resists. Inside the Kin-Com, intricate, state-of-the-art measuring devices register the degree of force and transmit this information to the computer.

"Pull, pull, pull, keep pulling." The third time the line peaks at 29 newton meters, its highest point so far. The computer, at a touch to the screen, commits the measurement to memory.

Louise Capone is one of more than a thousand BLSA participants who travel to Baltimore every 2 years to take part in this long-term study of human aging. Ranging in age from their twenties to their nineties, BLSA participants come from every part of the United States. Some have been with the study since it began. But every year new volunteers of all ages join the BLSA and make their first visit, drawn in, they say, by twin lures: the opportunity to learn more about themselves and the satisfaction of being part of a major scientific investigation.

On this Monday morning, five BLSA volunteers are here. Their schedules for the next two-and-a-half days are posted on a bulletin board outside the main office: a complete physical exam, tests of bone density, aerobic capacity, psychology, hearing, reaction time, glucose tolerance, lung function, and more. Each assessment will add detail and focus to the BLSA's slowly growing picture of how we age.

"This is really what keeps me coming back," says Ms. Capone, who is on her seventh visit. "We get the results of our own tests, which are nice to have, but also we learn what the study is learning, overall. There is a real sense of being a partner in the study, of working with the researchers toward a goal."

Themes

That goal, stated in its simplest form, is to describe systematically the process of aging. Often called a study of "normal aging," the BLSA is examining the usual and universal changes that affect all people as they age, changes that can be attributed to aging per se, rather than to a disease or to specific environments.

"There are two ways to study aging," explains James Fozard, the NIA's Associate Scientific Director for the BLSA. "You can study it cross-sectionally, by comparing people of different ages. Or you can study it longitudinally, which means studying changes in the same individuals over time, as they grow older." Much more can be learned from longitudinal studies. Cross-sectional studies cannot provide the same insight into the natural course of aging or the changes that lead to disease. But, longitudinal studies, by definition, are exhaustive, extended enterprises and therefore are relatively rare.

Because the BLSA is longitudinal, Louise Capone's muscle strength at 47, her current age, can be compared to her strength at, for example, ages 53 and 67 and 81. This profile of one individual's aging muscles goes into the BLSA's data bank, along with strength test results from all the other volunteers in the study. The result is a record of how muscle strength changes over an adult's life span.

One of the BLSA's objectives is to relate aging processes to one another. If Ms. Capone has a lower score on the Kin-Com when she reaches 53 or 67, that decline in strength may be associated with lower bone density and perhaps to declining glucose tolerance, the body's ability to use sugar. These possible interconnections intrigue Guest Scientists Ben Hurley and Rosemary Lindle, both from the University of Maryland and GRC/NIA researchers. They are using the Kin-Com data to explore such linkages. "We have smaller studies suggesting that when strength improves, bone density and glucose metabolism also improve," says Dr. Hurley. "The advantage of this study is the large number of participants and the wide range of ages. We're getting a big picture."

Theirs is one of many studies that is helping to map the territory that lies between health and disease. When and how do declines in glucose tolerance turn into diabetes? When does bone loss become osteoporosis? What difference do other factors—such as muscle strength—make?

"The BLSA is a study of transitions," points out Jeffrey Metter, the study's Medical Officer. "Not only the transitions of normal aging, but the transitions from the usual aging process to the disease processes that sometimes accompany aging."

If the strength study does find linkages between muscle strength and bone density or glucose tolerance, it could point the way to interventions, i.e., ways to keep bone loss from becoming osteoporosis.

Changes occur with aging not only in organs and tissues, but also in cells and molecules. "There are really three overall threads or themes to research with BLSA data," points out Dr. Fozard. "The longitudinal changes are one, and the relationships between health and disease are another. A third is the fundamental biology of aging. A number of studies here are looking at the mechanisms of aging in cells and molecules, using data from BLSA participants."

For example, while Louise Capone is recording her muscle strength on the Kin-Com, up one flight of stairs another BLSA participant could be having his muscle cell metabolism measured using nuclear magnetic resonance spectroscopy. "We'd like to find out whether the changes in metabolism—how the cell produces energy—are intrinsic to the cell or whether they are due to extrinsic factors, like changes in muscle mass," says Richard Spencer, who is conducting this study in the GRC's Laboratory of Cellular and Molecular Biology. "Do young and old people with the same muscle mass have the same muscle metabolism? Or are there some cellular mechanisms that change with age, independent of muscle mass?" The answers to these questions, he says, should help show what kinds of interventions might keep muscles strong.

Exploding Stereotypes

If Louise Capone fits the average, her glucose tolerance and bone density may decline as she ages. But this cannot be assumed. Many people do not conform to the average, according to BLSA data, which, in this and other areas, have overturned some once-common ideas about aging.

To date, two major conclusions have emerged from the Baltimore study: 1) aging cannot be linked to a general or universal decline in all physical and mental functions; and 2) there is no single, simple, pattern to human aging.

Consider heart function: It was once thought that resting cardiac output (the amount of blood pumped per minute) always declined with advancing age. However, studies with BLSA data have shown that when older persons' hearts are carefully screened and found free of disease, their cardiac output at rest is comparable to that of younger people.

Psychological stereotypes also are crumbling in the face of BLSA data. It was once believed that personality altered as people grew older. According to one popular image, age brought crankiness; according to another, people became mellower with age.

Neither view has held up under scientific scrutiny. The fact is that human personality remains remarkably stable. A person who is cheerful and optimistic when young usually stays that way throughout life.

Someone who is irritable and impatient in early life keeps those traits with advancing age.

BLSA data also show that aging is a highly variable, individualized process. To take glucose tolerance as an example, studies have shown that in some people it begins to decline in the mid-thirties. The rate of decline, however, differs markedly among individuals. In the GRC's Laboratory of Clinical Physiology, researchers have found that three factors—fatness, distribution of fat on the body, and level of physical inactivity—account for many of these individual differences.

Even within a single individual, organ systems can change at different rates. This suggests that several processes are at work in aging, says George Martin, Scientific Director of the NIA. These include genetic, lifestyle, and environmental factors, and because they differ so widely among individuals, no two people age in the same way. In fact, individual differences increase as we age, according to studies which show that older people differ from each other to a greater degree than do younger people. Yet accumulated, longitudinal data can be analyzed to yield knowledge about the many processes of aging.

Traditions

After the strength test, Louise Capone returns to the corridor that serves the volunteers as living quarters, a wide, quiet hallway that has the air of an informal hospital ward. A bulletin board displays news about participants and researchers, announcements, lists of Baltimore restaurants, and old cartoons. Across the hall there's a small kitchen and next to it the dayroom, where breakfasts are served at a wooden table that fills one end of the room.

Over in this corridor, with its well-used bulletin boards and lived-in dayroom, the remarkable continuity of the BLSA is striking. Dozens of small signs reflect the constancy, the year-by-year steadiness that lies near the heart of a longitudinal investigation.

Photograph albums, ranged along a shelf in the dayroom beneath the window, hold pictures of every volunteer in the study, past and present. They include Louise Capone's father, John Frederick Kirby, one of the first to sign up when the BLSA was launched in 1958. Her grandfather, husband, brothers, sisters, several in-laws, and two nephews,—fourth-generation volunteers—also have places in the albums. "My sons will probably join too," she says. "It borders on being a family tradition. "

Because of the word-of-mouth recruitment that has characterized the BLSA since its beginning, dozens of volunteers, like Louise, have relatives in the study. But the great majority do not. Why then do people join the BLSA? "Curiosity," says Lois Odell, who is here on her 9th visit. "I find it intriguing," agrees Charles Wolfe, on his 19th visit. "And I've gotten some excellent medical advice over the years that has been of benefit."

Many BLSA participants were recruited by friends and colleagues. Lenny Milner was persuaded to join in 1964 by two of his coworkers at the Federal government's Naval Ordnance Laboratory, and he later recruited two others from that office. "I've never missed a visit," says Mr. Milner. "It's something to look forward to, and there's a little challenge to some of it." The co-founder of two outdoor groups in Washington, D.C.—Black Ski, Inc. and Under-water Adventure Seekers—Mr. Milner savors challenges, and tests like the Kin-Com and the treadmill let him track his own fitness levels.

Dee Milner who joined the study in 1979, has been impressed by what people can learn about their own health. "There are no medicines, no treatments," she says. "It just allows you to monitor your own health. If there's a problem, they'll let you know. And if you don't want a test, you can say no."

Cathy Dent, one of several long-time staff members, schedules and guides the volunteers through their biennial round of tests.

One BLSA custom is celebrating anniversaries. Outside the dayroom, a small ceremony is being prepared for Alice Brands, who will receive a certificate on this, her 10th visit to the study. Mrs. Brands and Dr. Fozard are standing in front of the Founder's Bulletin Board, where a photographer, Edward Billips, is trying out various distances and light settings. The Founder's Bulletin Board is where many official BLSA photographs are taken, because the founders have come to stand as a symbol of the study itself. Nathan W. Shock, William W. Peter, and Arthur H. Norris were integral to the BLSA's beginnings, not only providing a strong original impetus but also, each in a different way, stamping the study with a character it still bears.

Their story goes like this: In 1958, Nathan Shock was the chief of the Gerontology Branch, now the GRC, of the National Institutes of Health. A pioneer in the relatively young science of gerontology, he had developed the Branch into the largest institution in the western hemisphere devoted entirely to studies of aging.

Dr. Shock was approached by William Peter, a retired medical missionary and officer of the U.S. Public Health Service. Then in his seventies, Dr. Peter wanted to make arrangements to bequeath his body to science when he died.

"We need live people," said Dr. Shock, who had for some time been convinced of the need to study healthy community-living volunteers. Up until then, most aging research had been carried out in hospitals or institutions where illness could mask normal age changes.

Convinced, Dr. Peter became the BLSA's first volunteer. As Dr. Shock began building the scientific framework, Dr. Peter embarked on a personal quest to find others. He organized an intensive word-of-mouth campaign, starting with his own family, friends, and neighbors. Each of the early recruits was asked to find friends and acquaintances, and by 1967, more than 500 people had signed up.

The Founder's Bulletin Board also tells the story of Arthur Norris, coordinator of the BLSA for 22 years, who implemented many of the original research designs. Renowned for his efforts to stay in close touch with volunteers, staff, and researchers, he knit together a cohesive and ongoing venture. One volunteer recalled that "he made me feel not like a guinea pig, but like a human being who is part of a great scientific enterprise."

One of Dr. Peter's early recruits was Andrew N. Thompson, the first husband of Mrs. Brands who has just received her certificate. When the study expanded to include women in 1978, Mrs. Brands recalls, the administrators called the long-timers, like her husband, and asked them to recruit their wives. Mrs. Brands herself was one of the first women to enter the study. But not, she recalls, before Eleanor Peter, who was William Peter's widow.

"She was wheeled in the door in a wheelchair at the age of 94, about a month before her 95th birthday," says the Peter's daughter, Jane Coffin, also a volunteer. "She had always wanted to be part of the study, and she was determined to live until they opened it to women."

As the study passed its 35th anniversary in 1993, it included about 500 women and nearly 700 men. Its goal is to expand, with new recruitment efforts focusing on women and minorities.

At the Cutting Edge

The next test on Louise's schedule is labeled "bones." It is in fact a measurement of both bone density and body composition using a state-of-the-art scanning device called the Dual Energy Xray Absorptiometer or DEXA.

Bones lose some of their density with age, an example of an aging process that is linked, through a transition not yet completely understood, to a medical condition. Bone loss can lead to brittle bones or osteoporosis. Osteoporosis is especially common among older women, although it also occurs in men, according to Jordan Tobin, who studies osteoporosis and osteoarthritis in a section of the GRC's Laboratory of Clinical Physiology. Data from BLSA bone scans help show when and how fast bone loss occurs at various ages.

The DEXA has an unassuming look. There is a long, narrow cushioned surface, like a doctor's examining table, and a small scanning arm. The arm is attached so that it rests about a foot above the head of the person reclining on the table. Beneath the cushioned surface, however, is an array of computer hardware that constitutes some of the most sophisticated scanning equipment now available.

The scanning arm moves from head to foot, taking its multiple measurements very quickly and at very low doses of radiation—"less than natural background radiation," points out researcher Tracey Roy. On a nearby computer screen, a slowly evolving image of Louise's bone structure marks the progress of the scanning arm. Two more times the scanning arm makes a sweep, measuring bone density in the lower part of the spine and the hip.

The DEXA tests are playing an important role in the BLSA's Perimenopausal Initiative, a special study-within-the-study, which is examining three major factors—hormones, bone density, and body composition—and how they are affected by menopause. This study will take an intensive look at what precisely happens before, during, and after menopause in 100 white and 100 African-American women.

"We think that even before menopause there are things happening in bone, maybe in body composition, certainly in hormones," explains Dr. Tobin. "This study will let us find out more about the rates of change and, most important, the interrelationships among these factors." It will show, for example, how obesity is related to estrogen levels and how hormone levels interact with bone turnover (the process of bone loss and replacement), which speeds up during menopause. Because the BLSA participants in this particular study come to Baltimore every 3 months (for one morning), the Perimenopausal Initiative will be able to track closely the changes that occur during menopause and provide more insight than has been available up to now.

"I really feel like sort of a pioneer," says Rosalie Carr, a BLSA volunteer who is on her first visit and has signed up for this initiative. "Menopause used to be something you couldn't talk about. I'm determined to talk about it. At least the next generation of women will know more than we do."

Data from the Perimenopausal Initiative will also be used to measure changes in cholesterol and other fats in the blood, since women, as they pass through menopause, develop a higher risk for heart and blood vessel diseases. Another GRC research group will carry out these tests. "That's the strength of this building," says Dr. Tobin, "this potential for studying interrelationships that you can't do anywhere else and the different kinds of expertise and laboratories in one place."

The last test on Louise Capone's schedule is hearing. At a desk in the hearing room, she first fills out a questionnaire on which she reports any difficulties in hearing that she herself has noticed. Then, in a small booth that blocks outside noises, she listens to a series of sounds of varying intensity, signaling with a push-button device whenever she hears one.

As part of this test, researcher James Wood plays a tape that sounds like people talking at a party. This is the babble threshold test, he explains. One sentence is made to stand out above the background babble, and the participant must repeat the last word of the sentence. Sometimes it's a word that makes sense in the context of the sentence, sometimes it is not. The percentage of word recognitions is used to determine babble threshold.

Sandra Gordon-Salant, a BLSA Guest Investigator from the University of Maryland, is working with the data from these tests to learn whether self-reported difficulties in hearing are predictable from the results of the babble threshold test. Because this study is just getting underway, no longitudinal findings will be available for several years—not until participants have gone through at least two cycles of testing. Eventually, though, the results will provide a clearer picture than is now available of the kinds of hearing loss that occur over time.

BLSA data on hearing have already surprised researchers on one front. In another study, Dr. Gordon-Salant and her BLSA colleagues have looked for links between hearing loss and three other factors— smoking, alcohol use, or high blood pressure. So far there is a suggestion—only a suggestion, she emphasizes—that high blood pressure in women may be linked in some way to a loss of hearing. More research will follow up on this possibility.

This sequence of events—data collection, analysis, findings, surprises, new questions—is a familiar one at the BLSA. "Many more surprises concerning the aging process are likely to be forthcoming," notes Reubin Andres, Clinical Director of the NIA and chief of the GRC's Laboratory of Clinical Physiology. "We did not think up all the important questions in the beginning .... The questions never end, they just get more complex."

The BLSA at a Glance

Objectives:

- to measure changes in biological and behavioral processes as people age;
- to relate these measures to one another; and
- to distinguish universal aging processes from those associated with disease and particular environmental effects.

Founded: 1958. Women entered the study in 1978.

Location: Gerontology Research Center (National Institute on Aging), Frances Scott Key Medical Center, Baltimore, Maryland.

Participants: Over the life of the study, the BLSA has had 2,227 participants. In 1993, active participants included 675 men and 503 women from their 20s to their 90s.

Researchers: NIA/GRC scientists in six laboratories and guest investigators and collaborators.

Training: Pre-and post-doctoral students.

To Volunteer: Baltimore Longitudinal Study of Aging, NIA Gerontology Research Center, 4940 Eastern Avenue, Baltimore, MD 21224; 800-225-2572 or 410-558-8139.

To Inquire About Collaboration and Training: Associate Scientific Director, BLSA, NIA Gerontology Research Center, 4940 Eastern Avenue, Baltimore, MD 21224; 800-225-2572 or 410-558-8139.

Chapter 3

Profile of Older Americans

The Older Population

The older population—persons 65 years or older—numbered 34.1 million in 1997. They represented 12.7% of the U.S. population, about one in every eight Americans. The number of older Americans increased by 2.8 million or 9.1% since 1990, compared to an increase of 7.0% for the under-65 population.

In 1997, there were 20.1 million older women and 14.0 million older men, or a sex ratio of 143 women for every 100 men. The sex ratio increased with age, ranging from 119 for the 65-69 group to a high of 248 for persons 85 and over.

Since 1900, the percentage of Americans 65+ has more than tripled (4.1% in 1900 to 12.7% in 1997), and the number has increased eleven times (from 3.1 million to 34.1 million).

The older population itself is getting older. In 1997 the 65-74 age group (18.5 million) was eight times larger than in 1900, but the 75-84 group (11.7 million) was 16 times larger and the 85+ group (3.9 million) was 31 times larger.

In 1997, persons reaching age 65 had an average life expectancy of an additional 17.6 years (19.0 years for females and 15.8 years for males).

A child born in 1997 could expect to live 76.5 years, about 29 years longer than a child born in 1900. The major part of this increase occurred

U.S. Department of Health and Human Services, Administration on Aging, November 1998.

because of reduced death rates for children and young adults. Life expectancy at age 65 increased by only 2.4 years between 1900 and 1960, but has increased by 3.3 years since 1960.

Almost 2 million persons celebrated their 65th birthday in 1997 (5,335 per day). In the same year, over 1.7 million persons 65 or older died, resulting in a net increase of 214,000 (587 per day). (Data for this section were compiled primarily from Internet releases of the U.S. Bureau of the Census and the National Center for Health Statistics).

Future Growth

The older population will continue to grow significantly in the future (see Figure 3.1.). This growth slowed somewhat during the 1990's because of the relatively small number of babies born during the Great Depression of the 1930's. But the older population will burgeon between the years 2010 and 2030 when the "'baby boom" generation reaches age 65.

NUMBER OF PERSONS 65 +: 1900 to 2030

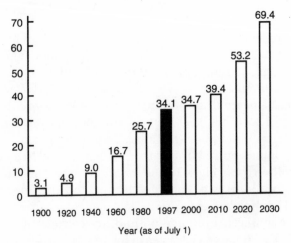

Note: Increments in years on horizontal scale are uneven.

Based on data from U.S.Bureau of the Census

Figure 3.1.

By 2030, there will be about 70 million older persons, more than twice their number in 1997. People 65+ are projected to represent 13% of population in the year 2000 but will be 20% by 2030.

Minority populations are projected to represent 25% of the elderly population in 2030, up from 15% in 1997. Between 1997and 2030, the white nonhispanic population 65+ is projected to increase by 79% compared with 238% for older minorities, including Hispanics (368%) and nonhispanic blacks (134%), nonhispanic American Indians, Eskimos, and Aleuts (159%), and nonhispanic Asians and Pacific Islanders (354%).

*(See "Population Projections of the United States by Age, Sex, Race and Hispanic Origin: 1995-2050," *Current Population Reports*, P25-1130).

Marital Status

In 1997, older men were much more likely to be married as older women—74% of men, 42% of women (figure 3.2.).

Almost half of all older women in 1997 were widows (46%). There were four times as many widows (8.5 million) as widowers (2.1 million).

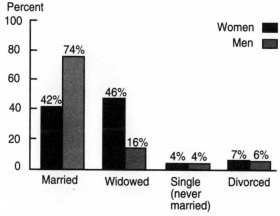

MARITAL STATUS OF PERSONS 65 +: 1997

Based on data from U.S.Bureau of the Census

Figure 3.2.

Although divorced older persons represented only 7% of all older persons in 1997, their numbers (2.2 million) had increased five times as fast as the older population as a whole since 1990 (2.8 times for men, 7.4 times for women).

Living Arrangements

The majority (66%) of older noninstitutionalized persons lived in a family setting in 1997. Approximately 10.7 million or 80% of older men, and 10.5 million or 57% of older women, lived in families (Figure 3.3.). The proportion living in a family setting decreased with age. Only 47% of those 85+ years old lived in family setting. About 13% of older persons (8% of men, 17% of women) were not living with a spouse but were living with children, siblings, or other relatives. An additional 3% of men and 2% of women, or 776,000 older persons, lived with nonrelatives.

About 31% (9.9 million) of all noninstitutionalized older persons in 1997 lived alone (7.6 million women, 2.3 million men). They represented 41% of older women and 17% of older men. Living alone correlates with advanced age. Among women aged 85 and over, for example, three of every five lived outside a family setting.

**LIVING ARRANGEMENTS OF PERSONS
65+:1997**

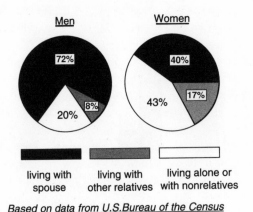

Based on data from U.S.Bureau of the Census

Figure 3.3.

(See "An Overview of Nursing Homes and their Current Residents: Data from the 1995 National Nursing Home Survey," published by the National Center for Health Statistics, January 23, 1997)

While a small number (1.4 million) and percentage (4%) of the 65+ population lived in nursing homes in 1995, the percentage increased dramatically with age, ranging from 1% for persons 65-74 years to 5% for persons 75-84 years and 15% for persons 85+.

Racial and Ethnic Composition

In 1997 about 15.3% of persons 65+ were minorities—8.0% were Black,** 2.0% were Asian or Pacific Islander,** and less than 1% were American Indian or Native Alaskan.** Persons of Hispanic origin (who may be of any race) represented 4.9% of the older population.

Only 7.1% of minority race and Hispanic populations were 65+ in 1997 (8.4% of nonhispanic blacks, 7.2% of Asians and Pacific Islanders, 7.0% of American Indians and native Alaskans, 5.7% of Hispanics), compared with 14.8% of nonhispanic whites.

(Data for this section were compiled from Internet releases of the U.S. Bureau of the Census).

Geographic Distribution

In 1997, about half (52%) of persons 65+ lived in nine states. California had over 3.5 million, Florida (2.7) and New York (2.4) million, Texas and Pennsylvania had almost 2 million, and Ohio, Illinois, Michigan, and New Jersey each had over 1 million (Figure 3.4.).

Person 65+ constituted 14.0% or more of the total population in 10 states in 1997 (Figure 4): Florida (18.5%); Pennsylvania and Rhode Island (15.8%); West Virginia (15.1%); Iowa (15.0%); North Dakota and Connecticut (14.4%); Arkansas and South Dakota (14.3%); and Massachusetts (14.1).

In thirteen states, the 65+ population increased by 14.0% or more between 1990 and 1997(Figure 5): Nevada (49%); Alaska (43%); Hawaii and Arizona (25% each); Utah and Colorado (19% each); Delaware (17%); North Carolina and Wyoming (15 % each); South Carolina, Florida, and Texas (14% each).

The ten states with the highest poverty rates for elderly over the period 1994-1996 were: the District of Columbia (20%); South Carolina (17.9%); Louisiana (17.8%); Tennessee (17.7%); Mississippi (17.4%); Arkansas (17.0%); New Mexico (15.9%); Georgia (15.1%); Texas (14.6%); and Alabama (14.0%).

Table 3.1.

THE 65+ POPULATION BY STATE: 1997

State Number of Persons	Number (000's) 1997	Percent of all ages 1997	Percent increase 1990-97	Percent below poverty level*** 1994-96
U.S., total	34,075,611	12.7	9.1	11.0
Alabama	560,974	13.0	7.5	14.0
Alaska	32,041	5.3	42.7	5.4
Arizona	602,409	13.2	25.3	10.7
Arkansas	359,909	14.3	3.0	17.0
California	3,571,964	11.1	13.9	9.2
Colorado	393,602	10.1	18.9	6.7
Connecticut	469,600	14.4	5.4	6.8
Delaware	94,371	12.9	16.7	9.8
District of Columbia	73,375	13.9	-4.8	20.2
Florida	2,708,804	18.5	14.1	10.1
Georgia	738,154	9.9	12.8	15.1
Hawaii	156,701	13.2	25.3	8.6
Idaho	136,867	11.3	12.6	7.4
Illinois	1,481,303	12.5	3.3	8.6
Indiana	733,847	12.5	5.3	8.2
Iowa	429,264	15.0	0.6	9.6
Kansas	351,595	13.5	2.6	11.1
Kentucky	488,893	12.5	4.8	11.4
Louisiana	496,789	11.4	6.0	17.8
Maine	173,264	13.9	6.0	11.0
Maryland	583,854	11.5	12.7	9.2
Massachusetts	862,493	14.1	5.5	9.0
Michigan	1,214,010	12.4	9.4	9.1
Minnesota	577,744	12.3	5.5	10.9
Mississippi	332,982	12.2	4.1	17.4
Missouri	740,595	13.7	3.2	9.4
Montana	116,143	13.2	9.0	10.1
Nebraska	227,538	13.7	2.0	10.3
Nevada	192,645	11.5	49.2	7.1
New Hampshire	141,454	12.1	13.0	8.4
New Jersey	1,105,688	13.7	7.3	9.1
New Mexico	192,941	11.2	18.2	15.9
New York	2,427,365	13.4	3.5	12.3
North Carolina	927,739	12.5	15.1	13.6
North Dakota	92,545	14.4	1.6	11.4
Ohio	1,494,482	13.4	6.1	10.6
Oklahoma	444,453	13.4	4.7	12.6
Oregon	430,276	13.3	9.7	6.2
Pennsylvania	1,904,822	15.8	4.1	10.4
Rhode Island	156,103	15.8	3.9	12.5
South Carolina	453,825	12.1	14.4	17.9
South Dakota	105,198	14.3	2.8	11.5
Tennessee	670,142	12.5	8.3	17.7
Texas	1,959,722	10.1	14.0	14.6
Utah	180,029	8.7	19.4	5.1
Vermont	72,213	12.3	9.2	10.6
Virginia	755,546	11.2	13.5	13.7
Washington	647,348	11.5	12.3	6.9
West Virginia	274,333	15.1	2.1	13.4
Wisconsin	683,357	13.2	4.8	7.9
Wyoming	54,300	11.3	14.8	10.5

Based on data from U.S. Bureau of the Census.
See:http://www.census.gov/population/www/estimates/97ageby5.txt

Persons 65+ were slightly less likely to live in metropolitan areas in 1997 than younger persons (77% of the elderly, 81% of persons under 65). About 29% of older persons lived in central cities and 48% lived in the suburbs.

The elderly are less likely to change residence than other age groups. In 1997 only 5% of persons 65+ had moved since 1996 (compared to 18% of persons under 65). A large majority of those elderly (81%) had moved to another home in the same state.

(Data for this section and for Table 3.1. were compiled primarily from Internet releases of the U.S. Bureau of the Census).

PERCENT DISTRIBUTION BY INCOME:1997

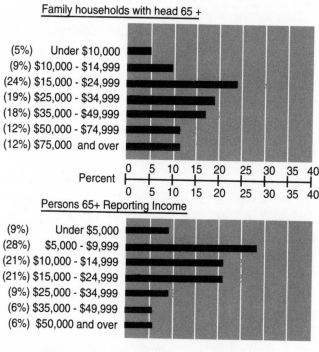

Family households with head 65 +

(5%)	Under $10,000
(9%)	$10,000 - $14,999
(24%)	$15,000 - $24,999
(19%)	$25,000 - $34,999
(18%)	$35,000 - $49,999
(12%)	$50,000 - $74,999
(12%)	$75,000 and over

Percent   0 5 10 15 20 25 30 35 40

Persons 65+ Reporting Income

(9%)	Under $5,000
(28%)	$5,000 - $9,999
(21%)	$10,000 - $14,999
(21%)	$15,000 - $24,999
(9%)	$25,000 - $34,999
(6%)	$35,000 - $49,999
(6%)	$50,000 and over

$30,660 median for 11.3 million family households 65 +
$13,049 median for 31.4 million persons 65 + reporting income

Based on data from *Current Population Reports,*
"Consumer Income," P60-200 Issued September 1998
by the U.S. Bureau of the Census

Figure 3.4.

Income

The median income of older persons in 1996 was $17,768 for males and $10,062 for females. In terms of real median income (after adjusting for inflation), these figures represent a increase in real income from 1996 for men (+4.2%) and women (+2.2%)

Households containing families headed by persons 65+ reported a median income in 1997 of $30,660 ($31,167 for Whites, $23,420 for Blacks, and $22,677 for Hispanics). Approximately one of every seven (14.2%) family households with an elderly head had incomes less than $15,000 and 42.3% had incomes of $35,000 or more (figure 3.4.).

For all older persons reporting income in 1997(31.4 million), 37% reported less than $10,000. Only 21% reported $25,000 or more. The median income reported was $13,049.

The major sources of income as reported by the Social Security Administration for older persons in 1996 were Social Security (reported by 91% of older persons), income from assets (reported by 63%), public and private pensions (reported by 41%), earnings (reported by 21%), and public assistance (reported by 6%).

Older households were less likely than younger households in 1994 to have received public assistance income (8% vs. 9%), food stamps (6% vs. 10%), or to have members covered by Medicaid (12% vs. 14%). About one-third (31%) of older renter households lived in publicly owned or subsidized housing in 1994 (14% for younger renters).

The median net worth (assets minus liabilities) of older households ($86,300), including those 75+ years ($77,700), was well above the U.S. average ($37,600) in 1993. Net worth was below $10,000 for 16% of older households but was above $250,000 for 17%.

Poverty

About 3.4 million elderly persons were below the poverty*** level in 1997. The poverty rate for persons 65+ was 10.5%, slightly less than the rate for persons 18-64 (10.9%). Another 2.1 million or 6.4% of the elderly were classified as "near-poor" (income between the poverty level and 125% of this level). In total, one of every six (17.0%) older persons was poor or near-poor in 1997

One of every eleven (9.0%) elderly Whites was poor in 1997, compared to (26.0%) of elderly Blacks and (23.8%) of elderly Hispanics.

Older women had a higher poverty rate (13.1%) than older men (7.0%) in 1997. Older persons living alone or with nonrelatives were much more likely to be poor (21.0%) than were older persons living with families (6.0%).

Two-fifths (40.0%) of older black women who lived alone were poor in 1997. The poverty rate in 1997 for people 65+ was also high for those who lived in the South (13.1%).

(Based on data from *Current Population Reports*, "Poverty in the United States: 1997," P60-201, Issued September, 1998 by the U.S. Bureau of the Census).

Housing

Of the 20.8 million households headed by older persons in 1995, 78% were owners and 22% were renters. The median family income of older homeowners was $21,627. The median family income of older renters was $10,151.

About 53% of homes owned by older persons in 1995 were built prior to 1960 (35% for younger owners) and 6% had physical problems.

The percentage of income spent on housing (including maintenance and repair) in 1995 was higher for older persons than for the younger consumer population (34% vs. 27%).

In 1995, the median value of homes owned by older persons was $81,956 ($56,15 for Blacks and $85,521 for Hispanics). About 80% of older homeowners in 1995 owned their homes free and clear.

(Based on data from the "American Housing Survey for the United States in 1995," H150/95 RU.)

Employment

About 3.9 million older Americans (12%) were in the labor force (working or actively seeking work) in 1997, including 2.3 million men (17%) and 1.6 million women (9%). They constituted 2.9% of the U.S. labor force. About 3.3% of them were unemployed.

Labor force participation of older men decreased steadily from 2 of 3 in 1900 to 15.8% in 1985, and has stayed at 16%-17% since then. The participation rate for older females rose slightly from 1 of 12 in 1900 to 10.8% in 1956, fell to 7.3% in 1985, and has been around 8%-9% since 1988.

Approximately half (53%) of the workers over 65 in 1997 were employed part-time: 46% of men and 63% of women.

About 680,000 or 18% of older workers in 1997 were self-employed, compared to 6% for younger workers. Two-thirds of them (67%) were men.

(Data compiled from unpublished data provided by the Bureau of Labor Statistics).

Education

The educational level of the older population is increasing. Between 1970 and 1997, the percentage who had completed high school rose from 28% to 66%. About 15% in 1997 had a bachelor's degree or more.

The percentage who had completed high school varied considerably by race and ethnic origin among older persons in 1997: 68% of Whites, 44% of Blacks, and 30% of Hispanics.

(See *Current Population Reports*, "Educational Attainment in the United States: March 1997," P20-505).

Health and Health Care

In 1995, 28.3% of older persons assessed their heath as fair or poor (compared to 9.4% for all persons). There was little difference between the sexes on this measure, but older Blacks were much more likely to rate their health as fair or poor (43%) than were older Whites (28%).

Limitations on activities because of chronic conditions increase with age. In 1995, over one-third (37.2%) of older persons reported they were limited by chronic conditions. Among all elderly, (10.5%) were unable to carry on a major activity. In contrast, only (13.9%) of the total population were limited in their activities, and only (4.3%) had a major restriction.

In 1994-95 more than half of the older population (52.5%) reported having at least one disability. One-third had a severe disability (ies). The percentages with disabilities increase sharply with age (Figure 3.5.). Over 4.4 million (14%) had difficulty in carrying out activities of daily living (ADLs) and 6.5 million (21%) reported difficulties with instrumental activities of daily living (IADLs). IADLs include bathing, dressing, eating, and getting around the house. IADLs include preparing meals, shopping, managing money, using the telephone, doing housework, and taking medication].

Most older persons have at least one chronic condition and many have multiple conditions. The most frequently occurring conditions per 100 elderly in 1994 were: arthritis (50), hypertension (36), heart disease (32), hearing impairments (29), cataracts (17), orthopedic impairments (16), sinusitis (15), and diabetes (10).

Older people accounted for 40% of all hospital stays and 49% of all days of care in hospitals in 1995. The average length of a hospital stay was 7.1 days for older people, compared to only 5.4 days for people under 65. The average length of stay for older people has decreased 5.0 days since 1964. Older persons averaged more contacts with doctors in 1995 than did persons under 65 (11.1 contacts vs. 5 contacts).

In 1995, 33.1 million persons aged 65 and over were enrolled in Medicare. Four out of every five (82.6%) received health and medical services covered by Medicare at an average annual payment of $15,074. (Data excludes HMO enrollees).

Over 11 million older persons received services under the Medicaid Program in 1995. While the average vendor payment for all Medicaid recipients was $3,311, that for persons aged 65 and over was $8,868.

Footnotes:

*Principal sources of data for the Profile are the U.S. Bureau of the Census, the National Center of Health Statistics, and the Bureau of Labor Statistics.

**Excludes persons of Hispanic origin.

***Calculated on the basis of the official poverty definitions for the years 1994-1997

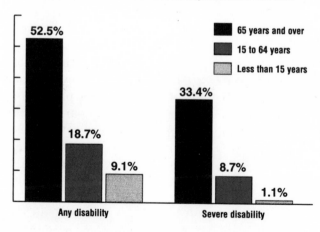

PERCENT WITH DISABILITIES, BY AGE: 1994-95

Source for Figure 8 and for the accompanying data on disabilities, including the definition of disability, is Current Population Reports, "Americans with Disabilities: 1994-95," P70-61, August 1997

Figure 3.5.

Chapter 4

Aging among Minority Populations

Aging among Minority Populations: An Overview

Information Summary

Introduction

The U.S. population is aging dramatically. Already the number of persons over the age of 65 living in the U.S. is greater than the entire population of Canada. According to the 1990 U.S. Census, an estimated 31.6 million persons were age 65 or older, representing one in eight Americans. By the year 2030, the number of persons 65 or older is expected to more than double to 66 million, or one in five Americans.

Minority persons constitute the fastest growing segment of the elderly population. The number of minority group elderly is expected to increase more than 500% by the middle of the next century, from 4.3 million persons in 1990 to 22.5 million by the year 2050. Whereas minority elders currently represent only 10% of all older adults, they will account for more than 15% of older persons by 2020 and more than 21% of older persons by 2050. Although Whites will continue to represent the majority of the aged population, minority elderly will become "an even larger and more important component of the aging of America" (Angel and Hogan, 1991:1).

Reprinted with permission from the Resource Center for Aging, University of California at Berkeley.

This Overview provides a summary of key issues in minority aging. Topics covered include diversity among minority elders, demographic trends, life expectancy, economic status, health conditions, and family relationships. The Overview is followed by separate sections summarizing existing information regarding older adults in four general minority groups: African-Americans, Hispanics, Asian/Pacific Islanders, and American Indians.

The Overview and each of the following sections is accompanied by an in-depth interview with a selected expert regarding a particular minority elderly population. The five interviews converge on a number of key points:

1. Existing theories of the aging process do not adequately address cultural factors;

2. There is great diversity within as well as between ethnic groups;

3. There is a tremendous need for additional research;

4. We need to acknowledge how little we actually know about each other;

5   Minority aging presents a wide field of opportunities both for scholarship and for career development in the social and health sciences.

Who are the Minority Elderly?

Minority elderly persons are generally identified as members of four non-European populations: African-American, Hispanic, Native American, and Asian/Pacific Islander. Amendments to the Older Americans Act in 1987 focused national attention on the needs of these groups by mandating that services be targeted to those in greatest social and economic need, particularly minority elderly. These minority categories represent diverse, heterogeneous populations. The category of Asian/Pacific Islander, for example, embraces numerous distinct cultural groups, including native and foreign-born Americans from diverse backgrounds such as Korean, Japanese, Chinese, Filipino, Samoan, and refugee Hmong and Mien peoples. The category of Native American includes the extremely heterogeneous population of American Indians, Aleuts, and Inuits from approximately 278 federally recognized reservations, 500 tribes, bands or Native Villages, and 100 non-recognized tribes.

Definitions of the four ethnic minority categories are generally accepted across disciplines but are not absolute. Native Hawaiians, for example, are considered an Asian/Pacific Islander population by demographers; however, since 1987, policy makers have included Native Hawaiians under the category of Native Americans/ Alaskan Natives with regard to the funding provisions of Title VI of the Older Americans Act.

The Hispanic category is unified by linguistic and some cultural traditions, although it includes significant differences between Puerto Rican, Cuban, Latin American, Mexican and Central American populations. While the other three minority groups may also represent broad racial groups, persons of Hispanic origin may be of any race.

While the heterogeneity of Native American, Asian/Pacific, and Hispanic populations may seem obvious, the heterogeneity in the African-American population should not be overlooked (Jackson, 1988). Differences among elderly African-Americans, based largely on life experience, are reflective of the great variation in the American experience among rural and urban lifestyles, geographic regions and socio-economic conditions.

Dramatic Growth in the Numbers of Minority Elders

The population of minority elderly is expected to increase 500% in the next 55 years. While fewer than one in ten minority persons are now elderly, by the year 2050 the proportion will increase to one in five. Already, the fastest growing segment of the African-American population is composed of those persons over the age of 65, and the number of Afro-American elderly increased 21% between 1980 and 1990. The number of Hispanic elderly grew 64% between 1980 and 1990. The biggest growth is expected to occur among the "oldest old," those who are 85 years of age and older.

The projected changes in the number of minority elders from 1990 to 2050 are shown in Table 4.1. (taken from Taeuber, 1990):

Table 4.1. Projected Growth of Minority Populations, Age 65+

	1990	2050
Blacks	2.6 million	9.6 million
Other Races (Not White or Black)	600,000	5.0 million
Hispanic (any race)	1.1 million	7.9 million

Perspectives on Minority Aging

Two hypotheses which describe minority aging have received considerable attention. The "double jeopardy" hypothesis argues that minority elderly are at a double disadvantage in American society, particularly with regard to economic status and health (Dowd & Bengston, 1978; Jackson, 1968). Minority elders are discriminated against by virtue of being a member of a minority group and by being identified as aged in an ageist society. However, a review of various studies of the double jeopardy concept (Jackson, 1985a) found the hypothesis to have limited theoretical or empirical validity, despite its usefulness as an advocacy concept.

A competing perspective, the "age as leveler" hypothesis, maintains that differences in status between minority and Anglo populations are reduced over the course of a lifetime, particularly as both groups experience similar problems and societal barriers in old age (Kent, 1971). Analyses of inter-group differences in later life are generally consistent with the predictions of the "age as leveler" hypothesis (Markides, 1983). Differences between African-Americans and Anglos with regard to income and health, for example, tend to decline from middle age to old age.

As noted in the accompanying interviews with leading experts in the field of minority aging, many contemporary researchers find these and other theoretical formulations unsatisfactory because they tend to ignore the experience and effect of cultural factors. "Diversity in aging" is now being considered in a new light (Bass, Kutza & Torres-Gil, 1990; Stanford & Torres-Gil, 1991). The use of a Euro-American standard model from which other populations deviate is now rejected. Diversity is taken to include not only a multi-ethnic perspective, but also the many individual and social differences that are related to the aging process.

Ethnic and cultural diversity are woven into American society. Within any minority group there are differences in individual status with regard to health, housing, marital status, social network, income, etc. These differences cut across all social categories.

America can acknowledge its diversity and accept the challenge to develop a new language that validates and affirms differences as an essential part of the economic and social fabric of one's society. America's diversity is not a melting pot, and it may but be a "mosaic" or a "tossed salad." How our diversity will be characterized, named, and tolerated is as much a challenge in gerontology as in other disciplines. (Stanford & Yee, 1991:22)

Life Expectancy and Racial Mortality Cross-over

Minorities tend to have shorter life expectancies than do Anglos. In 1986 the average U.S. life expectancy at birth was 74.8 years. The average life expectancy of a minority individual was 69.2 years, more than five years less (Harper, 1991). However, those African-Americans and Hispanic persons who do survive to old age tend to live longer than their Anglo counterparts (Wing et al., 1985). This "mortality cross-over" phenomenon has not been found among Japanese, Chinese, or Native American populations (Harper, 1991).

Although there are no definitive answers explaining this crossover phenomenon, one suggestion is that early mortality selects the least hardy individuals, leaving among the older cohort a disproportionate population of more hardy persons who have been successful in coping with stress throughout their lifetime (Greene & Siegler, 1984). In any case, this phenomenon is an indication that chronological age may not be an adequate measure in developing policies to meet the needs of older adults (Jackson, 1985b; Markides & Machalek, 1984).

Economic Status

Despite substantial decreases in the poverty rate of America's senior citizens over the last twenty years, the incidence of poverty among minority elders remains high. Whereas the 1990 Census found 10.1% of older Anglos living in poverty, 33.8% of elderly African-Americans lived in poverty as did 22.5% of older persons of Hispanic origin (Chen, 1991). Data from the 1990 Census also indicated that the percentage of older American Indians living in poverty ranged from 21.3% in urban areas to 37.5% in rural and/or reservation areas.

Higher poverty rates among minority elders result from a combination of factors over the life course: inadequate education, discrimination in hiring and rates of pay, work histories of low wage jobs, high unemployment, and intermittent employment. Frequent and/or extended periods of unemployment or underemployment create immediate financial hardship and reduce the possibility of adequate pension benefits. Because Social Security payments are based on a person's average yearly income including incomeless years, periods of unemployment reduce monthly benefits eligibility.

Many minority elders worked at manual labor, domestic service, and/or temporary or part-time jobs that offered neither pensions nor social security benefits. Moreover, low paid workers had little opportunity to accumulate assets on which to live in their later years. Savings provide a major source of income for 72% of all households of elderly Anglos, in contrast to only 27% of elderly African-American households and 37% of elderly Hispanic households (Chen, 1991).

Health

Minority elders experience higher rates of morbidity and mortality than do Anglo elders. Seventeen percent of African-American elders and 11% of Hispanic elders rate their health as poor, as compared with 7% of Anglo elders. Even when controlling for income, minority elders in 1976 had an average of 58 days on which their activity was restricted due to health reasons as opposed to an average of 45 days for Anglos (Manuel, 1982).

Risk factors contributing to greater morbidity and mortality among minority elders include higher rates of smoking, poor nutrition, inadequate housing, and reduced access to or use of health care services. These differences are largely attributable to a number of social, economic and political realities: increased poverty among minority elders, lack of adequate health care throughout life, and a greater likelihood of working at manual jobs that are potentially physically debilitating. Moreover, despite more problematic health conditions on average, older minority members are less likely than Anglo elders to have health insurance or to visit a doctor.

The rates of mortality and morbidity for specific diseases vary among the various racial or ethnic groups. The current level of research does not readily allow comparisons across groups, however the following are some important variations:

- American Indian elders tend to experience aging-related physical, psychological and social changes at much younger ages than do non-Indians (NICOA, 1981). The characteristics associated with Anglos of age 65 often are found among urban elders at age 55 and among reservation elders at age 45. Heart disease recently has become the leading cause of death among Indian elders, perhaps as a result of the increasing incidence of diabetes and non-traditional behaviors such as habitual and excessive use of tobacco, poor dietary practices, and increased levels of life stressors (Rhoades, 1991).

- Gillum and Liu (1984) note that American Blacks have the highest rate of mortality due to coronary heart disease of any population in the world. Since many of the risk factors for heart disease can be modified, there is hope that its incidence can be reduced for this population (Harper & Alexander, 1991:203).

- The first national assessment of the health of older Hispanics, conducted under the auspices of the Asociacion Nacional por Personas Mayores, found that 73% of Hispanic elderly reported impaired activities as a result of their health conditions (LaCayo, 1980). Data on specific diseases awaits the completion of the national Hispanic Health and Nutrition Examination Survey (HHANES).

- Chinese and Japanese Americans have lower mortality rates and longer life expectancies than do Anglos (Markides & Mindel, 1987). Data remain scarce on health issues affecting Asian Americans and Pacific Islanders (Harper, 1991). However, adoption of majority U.S. lifestyles appears to be having a negative impact on health. The higher sodium diet in the U.S., for example, has been associated with increased rates of hypertension and arteriosclerotic disease (Liu, 1985).

It is noteworthy that the higher proportion of health problems among minority elders do not lead to higher institutionalization rates for this population. In fact, a much smaller percentage of non-white (3%) than Anglo (5.8%) elderly live in nursing homes. Reasons for this difference include discrimination in referrals to long term care services, geographical separation from support networks, potential linguistic isolation, shorter life spans for most minority individuals, and greater involvement of families and other unpaid sources of assistance (Manuel, 1982). In addition, some ethnic groups place high value on caring for elderly members within the family context and/or attach a social stigma to institutionalization.

Communal and Religious Participation

Religion and peer support are important resources for many minority elders. Strong communal support systems have developed for many minority groups as a reaction to discrimination and to facilitate support, interaction and functioning among group members. These economic, emotional and social support systems often are particularly important for elderly persons, especially those who are foreign born and have limited English language skills. The church often occupies a central role in the provision of support within minority communities. It provides a political structure for helping minority group members, particularly Hispanics and Afro-Americans, to deal with "social, economic, and political inequities" (George, 1988); it provides a mutual aid system to provide economic, emotional and spiritual assistance to a disenfranchised population; and, it provides an opportunity for minority elders to perform meaningful roles that are valued by their community.

Family

Research on all four minority populations documents the traditional and cultural importance of the family in providing informal support to elderly members. Minority families often have developed and retain distinctive models of interaction that combine traditional patterns of roles and responsibilities with adaptations called forth by the American experience.

Among African American families, intergenerational relationships have been found to be extremely significant (Mutran, 1985); the American Indian elder is considered the "heart and soul" of family and tradition (Lyons, 1978; Red Horse, 1980); Confucian ideals of filial piety influence many Asian families (Koh and Bell, 1987); and, an intergenerational compact underlies relationships in Hispanic families (Markides and Krause, 1985).

Afro-American, Hispanic and Native American families have traditionally been structured to involve at least three generations. The grandparents frequently see their role as passing on the traditions and heritage of the culture, including the teaching of Spanish language skills in Hispanic families. In addition, grandparents may act as surrogate parents when parents work outside the home, are disabled, or are otherwise unavailable (Barresi, 1987).

Generalizations about family support among minority groups must be tempered with the knowledge that the family's resources often are scarce and inconsistent (Manson, 1990). The realities of family diversity and of the barriers to accessing formal support systems belie the simple belief that minority families "take care of their own" (Lockery, 1991). Immigrant families may have particular difficulty dealing with the potential "generation gap" between grandparents and grandchildren who may speak different languages and have different beliefs and expectations regarding filial piety.

Cultural values regarding the provision of care to older family members also are being challenged by demographic forces which affect the entire society. Declining birth rates, increasing female labor force participation, decreasing rates of marriage, increasing rates of divorce, wide-spread unemployment, and abuse of drugs and alcohol all limit the number of persons available to provide care and assistance to increasing numbers of older family members (Antonucci and Cantor, 1991). As the number of adults living longer lives continues to increase, this will be a challenge throughout the entire society.

Approaches to the Study of Minority Aging

To date, most research regarding the elderly has focused on the majority Euro-American population. However, as current demographic trends have become more widely recognized, there has been increasing attention to the special needs of minority elders in the United States.

The available data, while limited, are sufficient to convince even a critical observer that race and ethnicity affect the health and welfare of elderly minority group members. Unfortunately, the existing data can tell us neither why nor what interventions might improve the status of older minority people. (Gerontological Society of America, 1991:vii)

Many studies of minority aging compare minority elders to an Anglo standard, largely ignoring intragroup heterogeneity. In so doing, they gloss over the dimensions of culture which distinguish the various ethnic groups that comprise the minority elderly. This approach ignores the positive experience of participating in an ethnic minority community in which shared cultural values facilitate individual adjustment to aging (see for instance studies on the anthropology of aging in Sokolovsky, 1990, or Myerhoff and Simic, 1978). In addition, focusing on minorities as social classes within a stratified society can contribute to a deficit model that views minority status only in terms of discrimination and exclusion (Holtzberg, 1982).

Conclusion

The cohort of minority persons who are now elderly has experienced a unique history, typically including substantial family and social involvement, problems associated with immigrant status, as well as great perseverance in the face of racism and institutionalized prejudice. The unique assets and problems of minority elders have, to a large extent, been ignored by mainstream social scientists, policy makers and service providers. There is a need for accurate, relevant knowledge regarding minority elders in order to assure that the needs of all older persons are adequately met and understood.

References

Angel, J. L., & Hogan, D. P. (1991). "The Demography of Minority Populations." *In Minority Elders: Longevity, Economics and Health, Building a Public Policy Base* (pp. 1-13). Washington, DC: Gerontological Society of America.

Antonucci, A. C., & Cantor, M. H. (1991). "Strengthening the Family Support System of Older Minority Persons." *In Minority Elders: Longevity, Economics and Health, Building a Public Policy Base* (pp. 32-37). Washington, DC: Gerontological Society of America.

Bass, S. A., Kutza, E. A., & Torres-Gil, F. M. (Eds.). (1990). *Diversity in Aging.* Glencoe, IL: Scott, Foresman.

Chen, Y-P. (1991). "Improving Economic Security of Minority Persons As They Enter Old Age." *In Minority Elders: Longevity, Economics and Health, Building a Public Policy Base* (pp. 14-23). Washington, DC: Gerontological Society of America.

Dowd, J. J., & Bengston, V. L. (1978). "Aging in Minority Populations: An Examination of the Double Jeopardy Hypothesis." *Journal of Gerontology*, 33, 427-436.

Gillum, R., & Liu, K. C. (1984). "Coronary Heart Disease Mortality Among United States Blacks, 1940-1978: Trends and Unanswered Questions." *American Heart Journal*, 108, 728-732.

Harper, M. S. (1991). Introduction. In M. S. Harper (Ed.), *Minority Aging: Essential Curricula Content for Selected Health and Allied Professions.* Health Resources and Services Administration, Department of Health and Human Services. DHHS Publication No. HRS (P-DV-90-4). Washington, DC: U.S. Government Printing Office.

Harper, M. S., & Alexander, C. E. (1991). "Profile of the Black Elderly." In M. S. Harper (Ed.), *Minority Aging: Essential Curricula Content for Selected Health and Allied Professions.* Health Resources and Services Administration, Department of Health and Human Services. DHHS Publication No. HRS (P- DV-90-4). Washington, DC: U.S. Government Printing Office.

Holtzberg, C. S. (1982). "Ethnicity and Aging: Anthropological Perspectives On More Than Just the Minority Elderly." *The Gerontologist*, 22, 249-257.

Jackson, J. J. (1985a). "Double Jeopardy Re-examined." *Journal of Minority Aging*, 10, 25-61.

Jackson, J. J. (1985b). "Race, National Origin, Ethnicity and Aging." In R. H. Binstock and E. Shanas (Eds.), *Handbook of Aging and Social Sciences* (2nd ed., pp. 78-84). New York: Van Nostrand Reinhold.

Jackson, J. J. (1970). "Aged Negroes: Their Cultural Departures From Statistical Stereotypes and Rural-Urban Differences." *The Gerontologist*, 10, 140-145.

Jackson, J. S. (1988). *Black American Elderly*. New York: Springer.

Kent, D. P. (1971). "The Elderly in Minority Groups: Variant Patterns of Aging," *The Gerontologist*, 11, 26-29.

Koh, J. Y., & Bell, W. G. (1987). "Korean Elders in the United States: Intergenerational Relations and Living Arrangements." *The Gerontologist*, 27, 66-71.

LaCayo, C. G. (1980). *A National Study to Assess the Service Needs of the Hispanic Elderly*. Los Angeles: Asociacion Nacional por Personas Mayores.

Liu, W. T. (1985). "Asian Pacific Elderly: Mortality Differentials, Health Status and Use of Health Services." *Journal of Applied Gerontology*, 4, 35-64.

Lockery S. A. (1991). "Caregiving Among Racial and Ethnic Minority Elders." *Generations*, 15(4), 58-62.

Lyons, J. P. (1978). *The Indian Elders: The Forgotten American. Final Report of the First National Indian Council on Aging Conference*, 1976. Washington, DC: National Tribal Chairmen Association.

Manson, S. M. (1990). "Older American Indians: Status and Issues in Income, Housing and Health." *In Aging and Old Age in Diverse Populations* (pp. 17-40). Washington, DC: American Association of Retired Persons.

Markides, K. S. (1982). "Ethnicity and Aging: A Comment." *The Gerontologist*, 22, 467-472.

Markides, K. S., & Krause, N. (1985). "Intergenerational Solidarity and Psychological Well-Being Among Older Mexican Americans: A Three Generations Study." *Journal of Gerontology*, 40, 390-392.

Markides, K. S., & Machalek, R. (1984). "Selective Survival, Aging and Society." *Archives of Gerontology and Geriatrics*, 32, 207-222.

Markides, K. S., & Mindel, C. H. (1987). *Aging and Ethnicity*. Beverly Hills: Sage.

Morrison, B. J., & Gresson III, A. D. (1991). "Curriculum Content Pertaining to Black Elderly for Selected Health Care Professions." In M. S. Harper (Ed.), *Minority Aging: Essential Curricula Content for Selected Health and Allied Professions*. Health Resources and Services Administration, Department of Health and Human Services. DHHS Publication No. HRS (P-DV-90-4). Washington, DC: U.S. Government Printing Office.

Mutran, E. (1985). "Intergenerational Family Support Among Blacks and Whites: Response to Culture or to Socioeconomic Differences." *Journal of Gerontology*, 40, 383-389.

Myerhoff, B. G., & Simic, A. (Eds.). (1978). *Life's Career -Aging: Cultural Variations on Growing Old*. Beverly Hills: Sage.

National Indian Council On Aging. (1981). *American Indian Elderly: A National Profile*. Albuquerque, NM: National Indian Council on Aging.

RedHorse, J. G. (1980). "American Indian Elders: Unifiers of Indian Families." *Social Casework*, 61, 491-493.

Rhoades, E. R. (1991). "Profile of American Indians and Alaskan Natives." In M. S. Harper (Ed.), *Minority Aging: Essential Curricula Content for Selected Health and Allied Professions*. Health Resources and Services Administration, Department of Health and Human Services. DHHS Publication No. HRS (P-DV-90-4). Washington, DC: U.S. Government Printing Office.

Sokolovsky, J. (1990). *The Cultural Context of Aging: Worldwide Perspectives*. New York: Bergin & Garvey.

Stanford, E. P., & Torres-Gil, F. M. (Eds.). (1991). "Diversity: New Approaches to Ethnic Minority Aging." *Generations*, 15(4).

Taeuber, C. (1990). "Diversity: The Dramatic Reality." In S. A. Bass, E. A. Kutza, & F. M. Torres-Gil (Eds.), *Diversity in Aging*. Glencoe, IL: Scott, Foresman.

Wing, S., Manton, K. G., Stallard, E., Haines, C. G., & Tyroles, H. A. (1985). "The Black/White Mortality Cross-Over: Investigation in a Community Based Study." *Journal of Gerontology*, 40, 78-84.

Minority Elderly

Based on an interview with Percil Stanford, Director, National Resource Center on Minority Aging, University Center on Aging, San Diego State University.

Who Are the "Minority Elderly"?

Minority older persons are those persons who are underserved and in many instances economically deprived. Some years ago, we had to narrow down the definition to be consistent with the civil rights definition: African American or Black, the Hispanic or Chicano or Latino, the American Indian and the Asian/Pacific Islanders. About six or seven years ago it became clear that these particular groups were still the target groups. But, we've gotten more individuals from some of the Eastern European countries who are also showing some of the same needs in terms of services, language needs, and diet. So we've had to pay more attention to a broader kind of concern than color and race and deal with cultural tradition and value systems, or ethnicity. So more and more we talk about ethnic as well as minority older persons.

Most of the time ethnic minority persons are not effective or politically powerful enough to make a difference in the political agenda. So I think that's very definitely a defining factor. Another aspect that we just don't deal with, and I don't see any signs of dealing with, is racism. Historical racism underlies much of the inattention to older minorities, not only from those who are in a position to make a difference, but also from the reactions of older people. The real tragedy is that we expect minority older people to somehow become involved in doing things that will empower their own plight, when in most instances they have been denied the pathway to do anything to enhance their own plight, over and over for years. So it's very difficult for them to automatically, or to just suddenly, take the position to step forward and say "I'm going to be a spokesperson. I'm going to speak out. I'm going to make a difference." I think those are some of the underlying things that make a difference in terms of who those individuals are that might be labeled as minority.

What Is the Popular Image of Minority Elders?

Outside of AARP's image of a rainbow collection of older people, I don't see much being done to foster any kind of public image of the underserved ethnic minority older people. It's still kind of a hidden group of individuals. When people talk about the minority aged quite often the image is an older black person. And when you question them further they will say, "oh, yeah, that's who I'm talking about," or "Oh no, I'm really talking about two groups: Hispanic, and black or African American." Very seldom is there the notion that the category minority collectively includes the groups that I've mentioned.

I think, with the language in the Older Americans Act which dealt with targeting services to low income and minority aged, there was a resurgence of attention to minority concerns. But I see a backing away from putting money into programs. I wouldn't say that there was any kind of drive on the part of politicians and legislators and others to include the minority older person under "the umbrella." I think part of what has happened is that older people themselves have indicated the need to pay more attention to their basic needs in their particular communities. So I think recent interest in minority aging is more from the ground up, rather than from any kind of real political agenda. Even from a research standpoint, there has been very little effort, except maybe in the last two years, to really address an agenda that would take aggressive action toward highlighting minority research. The major effort recently has come through the National Institute on Aging looking at some specific issues related to long-term care and Alzheimer's Disease.

What Public Policies Particularly Impact Minority Elders?

Basic policies affecting older minorities include the Older Americans Act: Title III (the social support services) or Title VII (the nutrition program). There have been situations where programs were not accepted by the Feds because they didn't meet all the criteria for appropriate nutrition programs. In fact, given the conditions and the circumstances, the equipment and training of individuals in those minority communities were adequate in terms of their needs. There were no adjustments for the particular cultural values and expectations even for nutrition programs. In some of the American Indian communities, for example, the expectation was that if there was food available, then according to their particular cultures it was not to be reserved just for the old. It was to be used for the children as well. When you look at a broader issue of targeting, up until the last couple of years, there has been very little attention given to the distribution of funds for programs and projects. So now that's being addressed a little bit better.

What Are the Greatest Service Needs of Minority Elders?

I think one of the major things that needs to happen now is to look at some of the issues around employment. There are a lot of older people who are in need of some kind of supplementary income. Many of the individuals in this group have not had jobs that would even provide social security. Another issue is how well-prepared are they to be involved in job situations that would require a certain level of literacy. We talk about the growing number of older persons in minority ranks and the fact that older people are going to be increasingly more visible in the workforce, but we don't stop and assess very carefully who those people are going to be and what their preparation is. Training for effective participation in the job market is very critical. Another area that has a tremendous impact on this group is being victims of crime in their own neighborhoods. We know for a fact that the crime rates are quite often higher in some of the areas where minority elder people reside, so it is somewhat prohibitive for them to get out and participate without fear.

Retirement is basically a misnomer for minority older people. The majority in fact never retire. Most of the individuals that we look at are people who have gone from job to job and haven't had the benefit of any kind of systematic retirement or pension plan. So most, I would say probably 60% or more, may use the word "retirement" but are saying that they have reached an age, but do not necessarily have the benefits or the wherewithal to assume the retired role. So I would say that the situation in a nutshell is that we have terminology that doesn't meet with fact.

What Special Challenges Are Faced by Today's Minority Elders?

The current generation of minority elders probably is not going to be tremendously different from the next cohort. We would like to think that they would; but, if you stop and think about the next cohort, those will be people who are probably right now in their early sixties. These are individuals who were born in the early 1930's or when the country was coming out of the Depression. These are still people who have been subject to a lot of laws and reprisals because of their race and ethnicity. I don't think you are going to see much difference between cohorts until you get to the baby boom generation. These individuals, not the majority but a substantial number, will exhibit more of the traits of the mainstream society elders. That will include better economic opportunities and perhaps better retirement lifestyles in a true sense. But that's another generation down the road. And then after that group, I think we're going to be back to where this current cohort is to a great extent, because the kinds of economic and social supports that the baby boom generation has received, would have been and have been withdrawn to a great extent. So you are going back to another deprived cohort where there is a struggle to have full participation in our various societal systems.

What Do People Most Need to Understand about Minority Elders?

I think one of the first things that instructors and teachers have to do, is to compare themselves to the minority older persons that they are teaching about to understand their similarities and their differences. Understand that there are some cultural differences that they won't understand immediately and not be afraid to explore those differences. Then once that exploration has taken place, it's important to work with people to highlight the fact that there are some basic differences. Contrary to what we've thought over the years, we're not going to automatically have a melting pot in this society. There may be some assimilation and acculturation; but, for the foreseeable future, we're going to have multiple cultures which need to co-exist.

Having said that, I think the focus needs to be on understanding the true history of the minority groups. I think the celebration of Columbus Day is a good example. We say that Columbus discovered America when in fact American Indians were here for years. Well, when you stop to look at the ridiculous nature of that, it's a powerful statement as to the disregard for human beings that occupied a territory. We need to understand, and to make people understand, how the African-American population was integrated into this land. And look at that for what it is, and what it was, and how that has unfolded. The succeeding groups, Hispanics and Asian/Pacific Islanders, had their roles in building this country. So all of that, then, would serve to put some reality into the existence of different groups in our society.

Deal with the stereotypes and understand what the stereotypes are. Have people ask themselves very carefully how they have come about the stereotypes that they have. Whether it's first hand, second hand, or tertiary. Get people to acknowledge that they, in fact, quite often don't know very much about the reality of other groups, only the stereotype.

Older people are a tremendous resource that we don't use enough. The minority older person is a very good resource that we need to take more advantage of in a positive way. We need to set up situations where interested parties can interface with minority older persons, learn from them, and have a chance to see them as real people. We need to get people to a point where they can appreciate the beauty of the differences which many older people bring to a situation rather than saying, "it's not like me," or "not like what I know," and therefore it's not good.

I think the other thing that is very important to stress is that intragroup variations are very important, yet they often get ignored in the emphasis on inter-group affairs. Too often, we use mainstream EuroAmerican vs. all other non-EuroAmerican groups as our primary context for examining issues. In doing so, we may ignore some very real concerns from an intra-ethnic and minority standpoint.

Suggested Readings

American Association of Retired Persons (AARP). (1987). *A Portrait of Older Minorities*. Washington, DC: AARP.

This is a comprehensive, concise overview of sociodemographic characteristics of minority elders in the United States. Included is information on demography, marital status, living arrangements, education, employment, income and health.

American Society on Aging (ASA). (1992). *Serving Elders of Color: Challenges to Providers and the Aging Networks*. San Francisco, CA: ASA.

This report provides a concise overview of the demographic and social trends affecting elders of color, their role as a resource in their communities and the country, and the problems and barriers they face. The report discusses an approach to change based on a commitment to empowerment of elders of color, and concludes with suggestions for future directions for improving the status of elderly persons of color.

Angel, Jacqueline L., & Hogan, Dennis P. (1992). "The demography of minority aging populations." *Journal of Family History*, 17, 95-115.

This article examines historical and demographic trends in the ethnic and racial composition of older cohorts in the United States.

It projects future trends in the relative size of different racial and ethnic populations, considers their likely impact on family structure, and discusses implications for social policy and for the welfare of the minority elderly in the 21st century.

Gelfand, Donald, & Barresi, Charles. (1987). *Ethnic Dimensions of Aging.* **New York: Springer.**

This edited volume examines the interrelationships between ethnicity and aging from the perspective of leading researchers and practitioners. The volume includes chapters on theoretical issues related to ethnicity and aging, examples of conceptually grounded research on various ethnic groups, and practice and policy implications. This is an important book, which does an excellent job of summarizing many key issues regarding the ways in which aging and ethnicity interact in the lives of individuals and society.

Gerontological Society of America (1991*). Minority Elders: Longevity, Economics and Health, Building a Public Policy Base.* **Washington, DC: GSA.**

Background papers on demography, income, social support and health status review current state-of-the art knowledge and include findings on the 1990 U.S. Census. A fifth paper provides excellent background on American Indian Aging.

Harper, Mary S. (1990). *Minority Aging: Essential Curricula Content for Selected Health and Allied Professions.* **Health Resources and Services Administration, Department of Health and Human Services. DHHS Publication No. HRS (P-DV-90-4). Washington, DC: U.S. Government Printing Office.**

This volume provides an excellent overview on each of the four minority populations in terms of demography, health status and cultural background. Focusing on health care, the collection has applied research to recommendations for improving health status and health car within each group.

Kramer, B. Josea, & Barker, Judith C. (1991). "Ethnic Diversity in Aging and Aging Services in the U.S." *Journal of Cross Cultural Gerontology,* **6(2).**

This special issue is devoted to research on smaller ethnic populations located mainly in California.

Markides, Kyriakos S. (1983). "Minority Aging." In Mathilda W. Riley, Beth B. Hess, and Kathleen Bond (Eds.), *Aging in Society* (pp. 115-138). Hillsdale, NJ: Lawrence Erlbaum Associates.

This article provides an excellent review of research regarding the "double jeopardy" versus "age as leveler" perspectives on minority status and aging. Markides compares the two perspectives in terms of their ability to explain existing knowledge about Afro-American, Hispanic and Anglo elders with regard to income, health, primary group relations, and psychological well-being. This chapter will undoubtedly promote class discussion.

Sokolovsky, Jay. (1990). "Bring Culture Back Home: Aging, Ethnicity, and Family Support." In Jay Sokolovsky (Ed.), *The Cultural Context of Aging* (pp. 201-212). New York: Bergin & Garvey Publishers.

This chapter provides a concise overview of family and community involvement of minority elders. It argues that public policy has relied too heavily on family-based "informal support systems" for service provision to the minority elderly, and that family support must be coupled with publicly funded non-familial systems of care to avoid inadequacies in service delivery and excessive demands on minority families.

Stanford, E. Percil, & Torres-Gil, Fernando. (Eds.). (1991, Fall). "Diversity: New Approaches to Ethnic Minority Aging." *Generations*, 15(4)

This entire issue of Generations, the journal of the American Society on Aging, is devoted to a variety of new approaches to policy and planning to meet the needs of a culturally diverse and heterogeneous aging society. Of special interest to Californians will by Hayes-Bautista's article on young Latinos, older Anglos, and public policy.

Stoller, Eleanor P., & Gibson, Rose C. (Eds.). (1994). *Worlds of Difference: Inequality in the Aging Experience*. Thousand Oaks, CA: Pine Forge Press.

This anthology includes a rich mosaic of selections—some scholarly, some fictional, some autobiographical—representing diverse experiences of the aging process. Major sections of the book address race, class, and gender differences among older adults with regard to (1) life course and cohort influences, (2) cultural images about old age, (3) productive activity in late life, (4) family diversity, and (5) health and mortality. Whether read selectively or as a whole, this anthology provides a stimulating and provocative introduction to the topic of aging and diversity.

Yeo, Gwen, & Hikoyeda, Nancy. (1992). *Cohort Analysis as a Clinical and Educational Tool in Ethnogeriatrics: Historical Profiles of Chinese, Filipino, Mexican and African American Elders.* **Stanford, CA: Stanford Geriatric Education Center.**

This monograph provides historical profiles of American elders from four racial/ethnic groups. Each profile traces some of the major periods and events in each group's history since coming to the United States. Major historical periods also are examined in terms of the approximate age at which today's elders may have experienced them, making this an extremely useful resource for gaining an overview of how ethnicity-related historical events have influenced the lives of older individuals.

Periodicals

Journal of Cross-Cultural Gerontology (published quarterly by Kluwer AcadeMic Publishers). Anthropology Library (UC Berkeley) (HQ1060.J68).

Journal of Minority Aging (published semi-annually by the National Council on Black Aging).Social Welfare Library (UC Berkeley) (HQ1064.U5.B4).

Audiovisual Resources

Alzheimer's: A Multicultural Perspective
Running time: 34 minutes/video
ATTN: Andrew Scharlach
School of Social Welfare
329 Haviland
University of California at Berkeley
Berkeley, CA 94720
(510) 642-0126

This tape examines the experience of caring for an elderly relative through the eyes of four families: Chinese, Japanese, Latino, and Vietnamese. The stories portray some of the difficulties families can experience when traditional cultural values conflict with majority societal norms and the pressures of daily life. Included is a discussion of services available to assist families caring for someone with Alzheimer's Disease, as well as potential barriers to service utilization. Produced by the School of Social Work at San Jose State University.

Geriatric Assessment: A Functionally Oriented, Ethnically Sensitive Approach to the Older Patient **Running time: 20 minutes/ video**
(1990) Stanford Geriatric Education Center
703 Welch Rd., Suite H-1
Stanford, CA 94305
(415) 723-7063

An introductory video designed to acquaint the learner with the concepts underlying assessment of the geriatric patient using formal instruments in different domains of function. The tape demonstrates four patients of differing ethnic/racial groups in four separate health care settings.

Responsive Health Care for Minority Elderly
Running time: 38 minutes/video
University of Maryland—Video Services Dept. of Physical Therapy
32 S. Greene Street
Baltimore, MD 21201
(301) 528-7720

A series of actual patient interviews demonstrates the need for health professionals working with elderly minority patients to expand the traditional concept of assessment to include psychosocial, cultural, educational, economic, and environmental factors. Emphasized is the importance of integrating the patient into the health care system, patient education and preventive medicine.

—by Andrew E. Scharlach, Ph.D.,
Esme Fuller-Thomson, MSW, Ph.D.,
B. Josea Kramer, Ph.D.

Chapter 5

African American Elderly

Demographic Overview

There are approximately two million African Americans age 65 or older in the U.S., representing about 8% of the African American population. The African American elderly population has been increasing at a rate almost twice that of the African American population as a whole. This rate of growth also exceeds that of the general elderly population. It is estimated that, by the year 2050, the number of elderly African Americans could nearly quadruple to more than nine million persons, representing 15% of all African Americans. Increasing percentages of elderly persons are primarily a result of declining death and birth rates, which act together to bring about an increase in the number and proportion of elderly. The percentage of elderly remains lower in the African American population than in the white population because death and birth rates, though declining, still are higher than in the white population (Cowgill, 1988).

Life Expectancy and the Crossover Phenomenon

African Americans continue to have shorter life expectations than does the white majority. The estimated life expectancy for African American men is 67.7 and for African American women is 75, considerably lower than the 72.7 and 79.6 years estimated for their white

Reprinted with permission from the Resource Center for Aging, University of California at Berkeley.

counterparts (AARP, 1987). Possible reasons for this shorter lifespan include poverty, dramatic health status differences, and reduced access to health care services.

Despite lower life expectancies for African Americans from birth, a mortality crossover phenomenon occurs at age 73 for black males and age 85 for black females, whereby African American elders that reach these ages tend to live longer than their white contemporaries. Although there are no definitive answers explaining this crossover, one suggestion is that high early mortality selects the least hardy African American individuals, producing among the older cohort a disproportionate population of more hardy persons. Another possible explanation is that many African American elders have had to cope with stress and few economic resources throughout their lifetime; therefore, negative outcomes in old age may appear less serious or the elder may simply have developed a more reliable set of coping strategies to deal with the stresses of old age (Greene & Siegler, 1984).

Socioeconomic Situation

African American elders tend to have significantly lower socioeconomic status than do white elders. In 1990 the median income for urban African American elderly men was $7078 versus $13,745 for urban white elderly men. Urban African American older women earned an average of only $5,555 while white elderly women's earnings averaged $9,827. In 1990, the poverty rate for older African Americans was 30.7%, and only 9.6% for older white Americans.

There are many possible reasons for the high poverty rate among African American elders, including inadequate education, discrimination in hiring and rates of pay, work histories of low wage jobs, and high unemployment resulting in lower Social Security and private pension plan coverage.

With regard to educational background, the proportion of high school graduates is substantially less among African Americans (17%) than among white elders (41%). Perhaps even more significantly, many African American elderly never received any formal education. Six percent of older African Americans never attended school compared to only 2% of white elderly (AARP, 1987).

Discrimination is another important contributor to the high rates of poverty experienced by African American elders who often were denied access to jobs commensurate with their experience and capabilities. Moreover, minority elders often were (and are) paid lower salaries than their white counterparts for the same job responsibilities

(Manuel, 1982). Low wage jobs not only provide less of an income from which to save for one's retirement, they are also much less likely to be covered by a private pension. In addition, low paying jobs form the least stable part of the labor market, leaving workers in these jobs more vulnerable to unemployment.

Frequent and extended periods of unemployment and underemployment do not just provide immediate financial hardship, they also can disqualify a worker from receiving pension benefits. To be fully insured by Social Security, workers must be in jobs covered by Social Security for ten years. The elderly cohort of African Americans tended to work in manual labor, domestic service, temporary and/or part time jobs, the majority of which were not covered by Social Security. Social Security also computes incomeless years into an average yearly income; thus, scattered periods of unemployment can cause a significant reduction in monthly benefits. Moreover, only 20% of African American workers compared to 43% of white workers were covered at some point in their work career by a private pension. Of those workers who were covered by private pensions, only a little more than half (52%) of the African American workers actually collected pension benefits, as compared to 77% of white workers.

Health

African American elders tend to perceive their health as more problematic than do white elders. Seventeen percent of African American elders rate their health as poor, as compared with 7% of white elders. Much of this differential in health status can be attributed to increased rates of poverty among African American elders, lack of adequate health care throughout life, and a greater likelihood of working at manual, physically debilitating jobs. Moreover, older African Americans are less likely than white elders to have health insurance or to have seen a doctor in the previous year.

A higher proportion of health problems among minority elders does not lead to higher institutionalization rates for this population. In fact, a much smaller percentage of African American (3%) than white elderly (5.8%) live in nursing homes. Among the oldest population of elderly, 12% of African Americans and 23% of whites are institutionalized. Reasons for these differences include discrimination in referrals to long term care services, potential social isolation, geographical discrimination in nursing homes and shorter life expectancies (Manuel, 1982), as well as a culturally-based ethic that elderly should be cared for by "blood" (Carter, 1988). A strong, supportive family orientation may have its roots in the necessity to provide care unavailable from other sources due to the "racial discrimination and the social historical exclusion of African Americans from public and private social welfare and health services" (Watson, 1982, p. 145).

Family Roles

African American families have developed and retain distinctive models of family interaction that combine traditional patterns of roles and responsibilities with adaptations called forth by the American experience. Some of the African American family's strengths include: strong parent, child and sibling ties; greater likelihood of providing economic and social support to extended family members; large proportions of family members residing within the same neighborhood or area; care for ill and dependent family members; strong work orientation; adaptable family roles; strong religious orientation; and emphasis on respect for elders (Aschenbrenner, 1978, and Hill, 1972, as cited in Brown, 1990).

The black kinship system tends to be more extensive and cohesive than the family system of whites. The family is a mutual aid society where favors and obligations are taken when needed from other family members and paid back sometime in the future. Most studies comparing older African Americans and whites suggest older African Americans more frequently interact with their families and receive more social support from them. In addition, African American elders are more likely to provide help and money to their adult children (George, 1988).

African American elders are less likely than white elders to be married and living with a spouse, however. In 1983, 27% of older African American women compared to 40% of white women were living with their spouses, as were 63% of African American men versus 78% of white men. This difference is largely due to higher rates of widowhood and divorce among African American men and women.

African American families have traditionally been structured to involve at least three generations. It is estimated that 20% to 30% of African American older women head a multigenerational household. Older African American women are four times more likely than their white peers to live with young dependent relatives under 18 years of age (Tate, 1983). The grandparents frequently see their role as passing on the traditions and heritage of their culture and religion. In addition, grandparents may act as surrogate parents when parents work outside the home or are unavailable (Barresi, 1987). The African

American grandmother has held and typically retains a central role in the family kinship system, often attempting to allocate limited family resources to ensure that all members are adequately provided for (LesnoffCaravaglia, 1982).

There is much historical precedence for the respect of elders within the African American family. In preslavery days, the elders were the oral historians and the guardians of communal wisdom, customs and legends (Watson, 1982). Traditional organization was structured around kinship groups, in which elders had a great deal of authority and respect. Although the experience of slavery changed the structure of the family, families still retained their traditional importance and served to support the individual in the hostile American environment.

Even in post-Civil War America, African American families had to adapt cultural practices in order to deal with prejudices and inequalities associated with widespread racism. Extended families pooled economic resources to ensure survival and improve living standards. Grandparents were important to provide childcare and also to contribute to the economic viability of the extended family. In this context, older family members maintained the position of respect and authority they historically had held within the family. The extended matriarchal coresident family, which describes a significant minority of African American families today, can be perceived as a continuation of this tradition.

Social, Community And Religious Involvement

Communal support and responsibility is a central feature of the African American community. It is not uncommon for nonrelated individuals to address each other as kin through endearments such as "granny" or "uncle", illustrating the closeness and importance of the bond. African Americans tend to utilize support from friends and neighbors to a greater degree than do whites. Even greater importance is put upon friendships for those elders without children or spouses (Taylor, 1988).

African Americans developed distinct ethnic enclaves in reaction to racial discrimination and segregation from the dominant society and to facilitate support, interaction and functioning among group members. Faced with impoverished circumstances, vulnerable to the stresses of frequent racial slurs and humiliations from the racist majority, economic and social support systems developed among African Americans to help community members in times of need. Historically, the church has fulfilled numerous functions within African American communities. It provided a political structure for helping African Americans to deal with "social, economic, and political inequities" (George, 1988); it instituted a mutual aid system to provide economic, emotional and spiritual assistance to a disenfranchised population; and, it provided an opportunity for minority elders to perform meaningful roles that were valued by their community. In recent decades, the church has retained its prestige in the community through the leadership position it adopted in the fight for equal rights.

The present cohort of elderly, in both the AngloAmerican and African American population, tends to be more religious than younger cohorts. Consequently, elders are both the mainstay of the church and significant recipients of its services and help. Individual members and church groups support each other with material, emotional and spiritual assistance. Many churches have programs to provide food and clothing and to visit the sick as well as elderly shut-ins. In addition, the church plays a significant role in promoting self worth and self esteem through the validation of "shared beliefs and attitudes held by the congregation" (Taylor, 1988).

References

American Association of Retired Persons Minority Affairs Initiative (1987). *A Portrait of Older Minorities.* Washington, DC: AARP.

Aschenbrenner, J. (1978). "Continuities and Variations in Black Family Structures." In D. B. Shimkin, E. N. Shimkin and D. A. Frate (Eds.), *The Extended Family in Black Societies.* Paris: Mouton Publishers.

Barresi, C. (1987). "Ethnic Aging and the Life Course." In D. Gelfand and C. Barresi (Eds.), *Ethic Dimensions of Aging* (pp. 18-34). New York: Springer.

Carter, J. J. (1988). "Health Attitudes/Promotions/Preventions: The Black Elderly." In J. S. Jackson (Ed.), *The Black American Elderly.* New York: Springer.

Cowgill, D. O. (1988). "Aging in CrossCultural Perspective: Africa and the Americas." In E. Gort (Ed.), *Aging in CrossCultural Perspective.* New York: Phelps Stokes Fund.

Davis, L. G. (1989). *The Black Aged in the United States: A Selectively Annotated Bibliography.* Westport, CT: Greenwood Press.

George, L. K. (1988). "Social Participation in Later Life: Black-White Differences." In J. S. Jackson (Ed.), *The Black Elderly: Research on Physical and Psychosocial Health*. New York: Springer Publishing Co.

Greene, R. L., & Siegler, I. C. (1984). "Blacks." In E. Palmore (Ed.), *Handbook on the Aged in the United States*. Westport, CT: Greenwood Press.

Harel, Z., McKinney, E., & Williams, M. (Eds.). (1990). *Black Aged: Understanding Diversity and Service Needs*. Newbury Park, CA: Sage Publications.

Harper, M. S., & Alexander, C. (1990). "Profile of the Black Elderly." In M. S. Harper (Ed.), *Minority Aging: Essential Curricula Content for Selected Health and Allied Health Professions*. Health Resources and Services Administration, Department of Health and Human Services. DHHS Publication No. HRS (PDV904). Washington, DC: U.S. Government Printing Office.

Hill, R. B. (1972). *The Strengths of Black Families*. New York: National Urban League.

Jackson, J. J. (1985). "Race, National Origin and Ethnicity." In R. H. Binstock and E. Shanas (Eds.), *Handbook of Aging and the Social Sciences* (2nd Ed.). New York: Van Nostrand Reinhold.

Lesnoff Caravaglia, G. (1982). "The Black 'Granny' and the Soviet 'Babushka': Commonalities and Contrasts." In R. Manuel (Ed.), *Minority Aging: Sociological and Psychological Issues*. Westport, CT: Greenwood Press.

Manuel, R., & Reid, J. (1982). "A Comparative Demographic Profile of the Minority and Nonminority Aged." In R. Manuel (Ed.), *Minority Aging: Sociological and Psychological Issues*. Westport, CT: Greenwood Press.

Markides, K. S. (1983). "Minority Aging." In M. White Riley, B. B. Hess and K. Bond (Eds.), *Aging in Society*. Hillsdale, NJ: Lawrence Erlbaum Associates.

Peterson, J. (1990). "Age of Wisdom: Elderly Black Women in Family and Church." In J. Sokolovsky (Ed.), *The Cultural Context of Aging*. New York: Bergin & Garvey Publishers.

Robinson Brown, D. (1990). "The Black Elderly: Implications for the Family." In M. S. Harper (Ed.), *Minority Aging: Essential*

Curricula Content for Selected Health and Allied Health Professions. Health Resources and Services Administration, Department of Health and Human Services. DHHS Publication No. HRS (PDV904). Washington, DC: U.S. Government Printing Office.

Staples, R. (1976). "The Black American Family." In C. H. Mindel and R. W. Habenstein (Eds.), *Ethnic Families in America*. New York: Elsevier Scientific.

Tate, N. (1983). "The Black Aging Experience." In R. McNeely and J. Colen (Eds.), *Aging in Minority Groups*. Beverly Hills: Sage.

Taylor, R. J. (1988). "Aging and Supportive Relationships Among Black Americans." In J. S. Jackson (Ed.), *The Black Elderly: Research on Physical and Psychosocial Health*. New York: Springer.

Watson, W. H. (1982). *Aging and Social Behavior: An Introduction to Social Gerontology*. Monterey, CA: Wadsworth Health Sciences Division.

African American Elderly

Based on an interview with Charlotte Perry, Medical Anthropology Department, UC San Francisco.

What Term Do African American Elders Use to Identify Themselves?

Many folks in the African American community at this time use the term "African-American." They also use "Black" and, at times, they use "Colored."

What Is the Popular Image of African American Elders?

If there would be a popular image of the African-American elder, I suppose it would be one of a grandparent surrounded by great-grandchildren, perhaps cooking, or enjoying television shows. What is close to reality is that a good many of them are female.

In the cohort of the oldest old, it is surprising that a good number of them are childless. They were in the childbearing age during the depression and some of them chose not to become parents because of the economic picture at the time. And then others have outlived their children and so they are also childless.

What Theories Best Describe How African Americans Respond to the Aging Process?

In terms of theories that describe African American aging the best model that I have seen thus far entails the aging process but it goes beyond that. I like to use Kahn and Antonucci's "Convoy of Social Support" approach in looking at older African Americans because it takes into consideration the lifespan approach, looking at their roles over their lifespan, personal characteristics, situational characteristics, support structure, and support functions. It incorporates role theory, continuity theory and interaction theory.

How Do African American Elders Differ from Elders of Other Ethnic Groups?

One of the differences between African Americans and older white Americans has been the whole notion of social support. African Americans tend to take on friends and see them as part of the family network. In that network, friends may become the providers of expressive or instrumental support, which I find to be very different from older white Americans. For the latter, if it's not family and it's not spouse, then it may not be anyone. The literature says that Hispanics are more family-based, tend to keep connected over the years, and may even live in extended family situations. Whereas, older African Americans have moved away from that model. They are now in what we, as researchers, term the "modified extended model," and many families have incorporated either friends or fictive kin.

What Are the Greatest Service Needs of African American Elders?

The major health and support service needs of older African Americans are something better than Medicare and the Medicare gap insurance, such as the senior HMOs with a cap on out-of-pocket expenses. As far as social support, I think the United States social policy should move to compensating those families that provide long-term care in a community setting, as opposed to institutionalization. There should be some monetary compensation to shore up the efforts of family and friends. I did a study in the Southeastern part of the United States of a large group of widows living in subsidized housing. The widows who were "weller" (for lack of a better term) were in fact taking care of those in the housing complex that weren't as well. The housing complex management took no responsibility for making assessments on health status beyond the initial application that showed that applicants were able to manage their daily lives. People didn't come forth and say, "Well, now I'm unable to do this," because if they did, they would no longer be able to live there. What we found was that younger widows were taking care of those who were frail.

What Do People Most Need to Understand about African American Elders?

The major message I would send to new people in the area, would be to learn as much as they can about the culture. Then they would best understand the ways of some of the older African American adults. If we're thinking about health in this large group, some practice folk medicine. They also take over-the-counter drugs with prescription medications. There is also a strong spiritual belief. A good many of them leave everything up to God. I ask them whom they trust in and they say, "it's God." And I ask who is their confidante and they will say, "He is the one." We really need more African American researchers to conduct research with older African Americans. Research is needed in all areas, across the board. If I were to pick any particular area, I would say we need more research in family support and health care delivery. We need more individuals to serve this community in social work and public administration, for housing developments, senior centers, adult day care centers, and other community services.

Suggested Readings: African-American Elderly

Gibson, Rose C. (1986). *Blacks in an Aging Society.* **Daedalus, 115, 349-371.**

This chapter addresses the social problems facing African American teenagers, middle-aged and elderly, as our population ages, as well as the implications they pose for society as a whole. The author uses census data to identify and summarize such critical issues as health care, shrinking federal funds, education, poverty and retirement among African Americans.

Greene, Ruth L., & Siegler, Ilene C. (1984). "Blacks." In Erdman Palmore (Ed.), *Handbook on the Aged in the United States* **(pp. 219-233). Westport, CT: Greenwood Press.**

This chapter provides a concise introductory overview on Afro-American elders in the United States. A cohort historical analysis is done contextualizing the experience of the elderly through the Segregation era and Civil Rights era. Social and economic characteristics are discussed including population, education, labor force participation, income, and poverty. Coping, adaptation and mental health are also discussed and several research issues are presented.

Harel, Zev, McKinney, Edward, & Williams, Michael. (Eds.). (1990). *Black Aged: Understanding Diversity and Service Needs.* **Newbury Park, CA: Sage.**

This book is of particular use for health care and social welfare service providers to Afro-American elderly. Federal social welfare policies, health issues and diversity amongst the aged Afro-American population are discussed. A chapter by Stewart, Gerace and Noelke provide case studies to illustrate clinical social work practice with Afro-American elderly and their family caregivers.

Harper, Mary S., & Alexander, Camille. (1990). "Profile of the Black Elderly." In Mary S. Harper (Ed.), *Minority Aging: Essential Curricula Content for Selected Health and Allied Health Professions* **(pp. 193-222). Health Resources and Services Administration, Department of Health and Human Services. DHHS Publication No. HRS (P-DV-90-4). Washington, DC: U.S. Government Printing Office.**

This chapter provides a comprehensive overview of aged Afro-American's demography, marital status, living arrangements, education, employment history, poverty levels, and family life. A one page scenario is presented of a life history of a 74 year old Afro-American elder.

Jackson, James S. (Ed.). (1988). *The Black American Elderly: Research on Physical and Psychological Health.* **New York: Springer.**

This collection provides a comprehensive overview of recent research. Of particular interest are Taylor's article on aging and supportive relationships, George's article on social participation in later life, and Carter's article on health issues.

Peterson, Jane. (1990). "Age of Wisdom: Elderly Black Women in Family and Church." In Jay Sokolovsky (Ed.), *The Cultural Context of Aging* **(pp. 213-228). New York: Bergin & Garvey Publishers.**

This readable chapter is an anthropological study of an Afro-American great-grandmother. Through this woman's life-story, the importance of family and religion for many older Afro-American women is richly portrayed. The roles of elderly women discussed by the author include creating relationships, teaching values, helping raise children, being religious role models, and supporting fellow church members. This article will generate class discussion on the role of Afro-American Elders in the Afro-American community.

Richarson, Julee. (1990). *Aging and Health: Black American Elders.* **Stanford, CA: Stanford Geriatric Education Center.**

This monograph provides a concise but comprehensive overview of existing knowledge regarding the physical health and well-being of older African Americans, including information regarding morbidity, mortality, service barriers, and health practices and beliefs. While intended for health care providers and trainees, this review is an excellent resource for all people interested in understanding health-related issues affecting this population.

Robinson Brown, Diane. (1990). "The Black Elderly: Implications for the Family." In Mary S. Harper (Ed.), *Minority Aging: Essential Curricula Content for Selected Health and Allied Health Professions* **(pp. 275-295). Health Resources and Services Administration, Department of Health and Human Services. DHHS Publication No. HRS (P-DV-90-4). Washington, DC: U.S. Government Printing Office.**

The author discusses the structure, organization and importance of the family for Afro-American elders. Relationships within Afro-American families and the family impact on the elder's interaction in the community are also discussed.

Audiovisual Resources

Family Counseling with an Older Black Family
Running time: 15 minutes/video
ATTN: Professor Andrew Scharlach
School of Social Welfare
329 Haviland Hall
University of California
Berkeley, CA 94720
(510) 642-0126

Created to demonstrate family counseling skills appropriate to work with older Black families and to serve as a trigger for discussion, the tape portrays work with an older parent and their adult children where health-related issues have resulted in tensions and misunderstandings. The major issue presented is the conflict between a daughter and her recently disabled mother over the mother's desire to live among her friends, and the daughter's insistence that she move far away to live with her. The theme is the importance of understanding the value of the Black church and extended kin networks to the life of many Black elderly people. Produced by the School of Social Work at San Jose State University.

Old, Black, and Alive!
Running time: 28 minutes/film (1974)
University of California at Berkeley
Extension Media Center
2176 Shattuck Avenue Berkeley, CA 94704
(510) 642-0618 or 642-0460

Seven elderly blacks share their insight, faith and strength in a compelling documentary on aging. Aging touches everyone. Its universality is reflected in this film with candidness and humor. Filmed in a rural area of the south, this film shows people who have something to say about aging. "A beautiful, thoughtful film ... full of humor and love." (*Film Library Quarterly*) "A vibrant film done with feeling and respect. An excellent addition to programs on aging, death, black social problems, and religion." (*Religious Film Newsletter*).

Older, Stronger, Wiser
Running time: 28 minutes/video or film (1990)
Indiana University Audio Visual Center
Bloomington, IN 47405
(812) 335-2103

Importance of black women as foundations of community through life-long dedications to church, education, and family. Profiles 5 remarkable women who have struggled to rise above the indignities of racism that have characterized the black experience for years.

On My Own: The Traditions of Daisy Turner
Running time: 28 minutes/video
(call # Video/C2163) Media Center,
Moffitt Library University of California at Berkeley

Presents the life of a daughter of a former slave, 102-year old Daisy Turner. She recalls childhood incidents and her father's Civil War experiences and talks about life in her homestead in Vermont. Folklorist Jane Beck fills in details about traditions preserved in the Turner family.

— by Andrew E. Scharlach, Ph.D.,
Esme Fuller-Thomson, MSW, Ph.D.,
B. Josea Kramer, Ph.D.

Chapter 6

Hispanic Elderly

Demographic Overview

The U.S. Census Bureau defines the Hispanic population as consisting of Mexicans, Puerto Ricans, Central Americans and others of Hispanic origin. Hispanic groups have different histories and cultures but share the Spanish language and some cultural features. Among older Hispanics in the United States, the majority (54%) are of Mexican descent, 14% are Cuban, 9% are Puerto Rican, and 24% are from other Spanish-speaking countries.

In 1990 there were one million Hispanic Americans age 65 or older, comprising 5% of all Hispanic Americans and less than 3% of all elderly Americans. The population of Hispanic elderly has increased by 150% since 1970, a rate three times that of the increase in the older Anglo population. Moreover, it is estimated that, by the year 2050, the number of Hispanic elderly could reach twelve million persons, representing 15% of all Hispanic Americans.

The proportion of elderly in the Hispanic population is considerably smaller than the Anglo population for a variety of reasons. The Hispanic population has a lower life expectancy and higher fertility than the Anglo population, so a large proportion of the population is quite young. In addition, ongoing immigration of young families contributes to a youthful age structure (Markides & Martin, 1983). It also is likely that some older Hispanic immigrants

Reprinted with permission from the Resource Center for Aging, University of California at Berkeley.

return to their homeland, further decreasing the proportion of elderly in the community.

Patterns of immigration and repatriation vary markedly among the various Hispanic groups, contributing to substantial differences in the proportion of older persons. Cuban Americans, for example, have a much higher proportion of elderly (13.3%) than do Puerto Rican Americans (2.2%) and Mexican Americans (3.7%); they also have a larger proportion of elders than the Anglo population (12%). Many Cubans immigrated in the 1960's as well established professionals fleeing communism. A significant proportion of these Cubans are now seniors, and political and economic factors make it unlikely that they would return to Cuba. Also, there has been very little ongoing large scale immigration of younger persons from Cuba. It also is possible that Cuban Americans' better socioeconomic conditions may result in longer life expectancies than for persons from Puerto Rico and Mexico.

Socieoeconomic Situation

Median incomes for Hispanic-American elders are significantly lower than for White elders, for both men and women. More than 20% of older Hispanics have incomes below the poverty level, compared to less than 10% of older Anglos. There are many possible reasons for the high poverty rate among Hispanic-American elders, including inadequate education, discrimination in hiring and rates of pay, work histories of low wage jobs, and high unemployment resulting in lower Social Security and private pension plan coverage.

Elderly Hispanics are the most educationally deprived of all elderly groups. The proportion of Hispanic elderly with no formal schooling is eight times the rate for Anglo elderly. For Hispanic-American elders born in the United States, inadequate education can be attributed to the segregation practices common during this cohort's youth. Immigrants often experienced inadequate and/or prohibitively expensive schooling opportunities in their country of origin. Also, it was often an economic necessity for all family members to be generating income to support the family, thereby curtailing the number of years of schooling possible.

Discrimination is another important contributor to the high rates of poverty experienced by Hispanic-American elders, who often were denied access to jobs commensurate with their experience and capabilities. Moreover, Hispanic elders often were (and are) paid lower salaries than their white counterparts for the same job responsibilities

(Manuel, 1982). In addition, linguistic difficulties significantly decrease access to higher paying jobs. Older Hispanics often are much more comfortable speaking Spanish than English, with over 80% reporting that they speak Spanish most of the time.

Poverty among elderly Hispanics is also due to a work history of high levels of unemployment and low wage jobs. Frequent and extended periods of unemployment not only provide immediate financial hardship, they also can disqualify a worker from receiving pension benefits due to vesting problems. To be fully insured by Social Security, workers must be in jobs covered by Social Security for ten years. This elderly cohort of Hispanics tended to work as agricultural laborers or domestic workers, in temporary and in part-time jobs, most of which were not covered by Social Security. Social Security also computes incomeless years into an average yearly income, so that scattered periods of unemployment cause a significant reduction in monthly benefits (Becerra, 1984).

Hispanic elders are much less likely than Anglo elders to have income from private pension sources. Two cross-cultural studies in the late 1970's indicated that three times as many Anglos as Hispanics received private pensions. This discrepancy can be attributed to a variety of causes. In addition to many of the reasons mentioned in the discussion on Social Security, Hispanics are less likely than Anglos to work in manufacturing, professional or technical jobs offering pension plan coverage. Furthermore, until the government relaxed vesting restrictions governing private pensions in 1974, it was not unusual for a worker to have to remain with a company for twenty years before his/her private pension would be guaranteed. Undoubtedly, the vesting requirements have proved detrimental to older Hispanic Americans who were often in unstable, temporary jobs (Becerra, 1984).

Health

Hispanic elders tend to perceive their health as more problematic than do Anglo elders. A study by the Asociation National pro Personas Mayores (Lacayo, 1984), for example, found that 28% of Hispanic elders rated their health as poor or very poor, as compared with 4% of older Anglo respondents. Other studies indicate that 85% of elderly Hispanics report at least one chronic health problem and 45% experience some functional limitations (Cuellar, 1990). Moreover, older Hispanics are twice as likely as Anglos to have impairments that prevent them from shopping or attending social functions.

Health problems often begin at an earlier age for Hispanics. A study of Los Angeles Mexican Americans found that between the ages of 45 and 50 one third of Hispanic respondents versus 5% of Anglos had health problems impairing their ability to work (Becerra, 1984). Hispanic life expectancy, between 55 and 59 years, is considerably shorter than the life expectancy of Anglos (Lacayo, 1984). Despite more problematic health conditions on average, older minority members are less likely than Anglo elders to have health insurance or to have seen a doctor in the last year.

Among the oldest population of elderly, 10% of Hispanic Americans and 23% of Whites are institutionalized. Reasons for these differences include discrimination in referrals to long term care services, potential social and linguistic isolation, geographical discrimination in nursing homes and shorter life spans (Manuel, 1982). Probably the major reason for low institutionalization rates is the widespread ethic in the Hispanic-American population that the elderly should be cared for by family. Failure to care for one's own elderly is often seen as deviant behavior in Mexican-American communities (Becerra, 1984). Culture and kinship patterns that historically have promoted home-based care for impaired elders may also be a response to the difficulty obtaining public and private health services, due to inadequate funds and racial discrimination (Watson, 1982).

Family

Hispanic-American families have developed and retain distinctive models of family interaction that combine traditional patterns of roles and responsibilities with adaptations called forth by experiences in the United States. Some typical features of Hispanic families include: strong family ties; greater likelihood of providing economic and social support to extended family members; large proportions of family members residing within the same neighborhood or area; care for ill and dependent family members; strong work orientation; and emphasis on respect for elders (Cuellar, 1991).

Hispanic families traditionally have been structured to involve at least three generations. The grandparents frequently see their role as passing on the traditions and heritage of the culture, including the teaching of Spanish language skills. In addition, the grandparents often provide child care services for their working children as well as exerting their influence in family decisions. There is evidence, however, that elderly Hispanics' role in religious training and transmission of culture to younger members of the family is lessening (Barresi,

1987). In general, however, the transition to the grandparent role seems to be a more significant life change for Hispanic elders than it does for members of the dominant Anglo majority.

Hispanic Americans generally interact more frequently with family members and are more satisfied with the frequency of the family interaction than are Anglos. Close residential proximity among members of Hispanic families is due in part to poverty and low wage jobs, which tend to discourage social and geographic mobility. High fertility ensures that elders have, on average, many children and therefore there is more likelihood of at least one child living in the neighborhood. Language barriers and housing discrimination also often serve to restrict residential choice. In addition, because the proportion of Hispanic women having children in their late 40's and early 50's is twice the Anglo rate, many elders have dependent teenagers or young adult children living with them. Finally, many older Hispanics, particularly widows, must live with family because they are impoverished and cannot support themselves independently (Markides & Martin, 1983).

Intergenerational relationships frequently can be problematic for HispanicAmerican immigrant families. It is not uncommon for a grandchild to be monolingual in English, while the grandparent is monolingual in Spanish. Also, many immigrant elders grew up with a strong belief in filial piety and reverence for the elderly, which may not be supported by their Americanized grandchildren. Consequently, immigrant families may be more vulnerable to the problems of the "generation gap" than minority families who have resided in the United States for many generations.

References

American Association of Retired Persons Minority Affairs Initiative (1987). *A Portrait of Older Minorities*. Washington, DC: AARP.

Barresi, C. (1987). "Ethnic Aging and the Life Course." In D. Gelfand and C. Barresi (Eds.), *Ethnic Dimensions of Aging* (pp. 18-34). New York: Springer.

Becerra, R. (1983). "The MexicanAmerican: Aging in a Changing Culture." In R. L. McNeely and J. N. Colen, *Aging in Minority Groups*. Beverly Hills: Sage.

Becerra, R. M. (1984). *The Hispanic Elderly*. Lanham, MD: University Press of America.

Cuellar, J. (1990*). Aging and Health: Hispanic American Elders.* Stanford, CA: Stanford Geriatric Education Center.

Cuellar, J. (1990). "Hispanic American Aging: Geriatric Education Curriculum Development for Selected Health Professionals." In M. S. Harper (Ed.), *Minority Aging: Essential Curricula Content for Selected Health and Allied Health Professions* (pp. 365-414). Health Resources and Services Administration, Department of Health and Human Services. DHHS Publication No. HRS (P-DV-90-4). Washington, DC: U.S. Government Printing Office.

Hendricks, J., & Hendricks, C. D. (1986). *Aging in Mass Society: Myths and Realities.* Boston: Little, Brown and Co.

Lacayo, C. G. (1984). Hispanics. In E. B. Palmore (Ed.), *Handbook on the Aged in the United States.* Westport, CT: Greenwood Press.

Manuel, R., & Reid, J. (1982). "A Comparative Demographic Profile of the Minority and Nonminority Aged." In R. Manuel (Ed.), *Minority Aging: Sociological and Psychological Issues.* Westport, CT: Greenwood Press.

Markides, K. S. (1983). "Minority Aging." In M. White Riley, B. B. Hess and K. Bond (Eds.), *Aging in Society.* Hillsdale, NJ: Lawrence Erlbaum Associates.

Markides, K. S., & Martin, H. W. (1983). *Older Mexican Americans: A Study in an Urban Barrio.* Austin, TX: University of Texas Press.

Queralt, M. (1983). "The Elderly of Cuban Origin: Characteristics and Problems." In R. L. McNeely and J. N. Colen, *Aging in Minority Groups.* Beverly Hills: Sage.

SanchezAyendez, M. (1991). "Puerto Rican Elderly Women: Shared Meanings and Informal Supportive Networks." In M. Hutter (Ed.), *The Family Experience: A Reader in Cultural Diversity.* New York: MacMillan.

Watson, W. H. (1982). *Aging and Social Behavior: An Introduction to Social Gerontology.* Monterey, CA: Wadsworth Health Sciences Division.

Hispanic Elderly

Based on an Interview with Ramon Valle, Professor, School of Social Work, College of Health & Human Services, San Diego State University.

What Term Do Hispanic Elders Use to Identify Themselves?

One term, "Hispanic," is generally accepted as a research term but Latino is more popular actually. Many of the people will say, "Soy Latino" or they will actually tell you, "I am Mexican" (or Chilean or Cuban). They identify with a specific Latin American nation. There isn't just one term used by this population.

What Divisions Exist among Hispanic Elderly?

The heterogeneity of this population reflects not only the different cultural backgrounds and countries of origin, but also the reasons for immigration. For instance, in Miami about 88% of the Cuban population came in the 1960s; another 8% percent were here a long time before that; then, in late 1979 and 1980 came another influx of Cubans, the Marielitos. Those who immigrated in 1960 are ultraconservative. They fled Cuba for political reasons when their property was seized. The other groups came because of opportunity. They really wanted to migrate, and they have very different political and even economic profiles. Another contrasting set would be Puerto Ricans who belong to a commonwealth and are U.S. citizens. They don't have the same group experiences as Mexican, Salvadoran or Guatemalan people.

Looking at the elderly, the social history would be quite varied because some of the elderly would have been here many years, while some came following their adult children. Elders who followed their children to the U.S. may or may not be able to be linked to services, whereas those who can demonstrate that they have been here for some time can get services.

It's a very heterogeneous group. A lot of Latinos have had positions that permit retirement. If they worked for private corporations, The Feds, or State and local governments, the retirement concept applies. Then there is the other group that is constantly in flux, coming to the U.S. basically to flee from poverty or political situations. For them, retirement is somehow being able to maybe get on MediCal or Medicaid. Each day brings literally thousands of immigrants to all over the United States for whom retirement is a very unclear picture.

What Is the Popular Image of Hispanic Elders?

I don't know whether the general public has a concept of Latino elderly. They probably identify the youth gangs or law and order problems with Latinos, but no elderly cohort comes up on their "radar screen." Probably the most profoundly telling image of the Latino would be the 1941 movie with Tyrone Power, "Zorro." During the afternoon siesta, Zorro comes into the village to display his defiance against the Alcalde. In the village are all these hats, these hats listing very slowly. People all ultimately run out from under the hats. That's the image of Latinos. They sleep in the big hats and pop up somewhere. But the reality is most of the people we know work pretty hard and for long hours. They scraped and scrounged all their lives and they are very ambitious.

How Do Hispanic Elders Feel about Aging?

The concept of aging as the "golden years" isn't necessarily true. I would say that aging is seen as an inevitable outcome of life but not necessarily anything positive. The population suffers from a higher level of morbidity so it's a lot harder to enjoy, or look forward to enjoying, those years. Even though the traditional value system supports the role of an old person, the reality is that elders have less of a role, or no role, in a complex society such as ours. Like other older adults immigrating from traditional societies, they don't understand why their kids don't come to them more for advice.

What Are the Greatest Service Needs of Hispanic Elders?

One problem is the lack of attention within the communities themselves to the phenomenon of aging. We're not ready for the vast numbers of Hispanic elderly that will be present in the environment in the upcoming century. It would seem to me that we need to do a great deal of public health education, very similar to what has taken place in the Anglo community about life after age 60 or 65, but pitched to the Hispanic elderly. We need to have an extensive campaign to attract non-Hispanics as well as Hispanics to the Hispanic community, because we are not going to have enough professional resources to handle the issue. I would also to very strongly target the age 40-60 group to prepare for lifestyle changes, diet changes, and things that need to be done to handle the later years. The public health campaign done for the general population should be tailored to this group. Fourth, there still is a residual value on the family (even though it doesn't always mean all positive experiences), and I would work with that value to develop approaches to health care.

What Is the Role of the Family in Providing Support to Hispanic Elders?

There is no question that language and communication are very important and that creates a different style than other minorities or than Anglos. There is a value on family. (I either get along with them or I don't get along with them but they are my family). When these older people lived in a smaller community, they were embedded in social networks with their family members. There was an expectation that younger family members would pass by grandfather's house and check on the household. Today, younger people, their children who could be in the forties or fifties or their grandchildren, are busy with their urban active life. They don't touch base. There is not enough touching contact and a lot of older people complain about that. They won't ask for help but there is the expectation that their children should come by and say hello. This is the way it should be done but isn't being done.

The importance of family is separate from whether the family is supportive or not. Counter to stereotype, the Hispanic family does not necessarily pull together more in response to illnesses like Alzheimer's Disease. These kinds of illnesses put a very heavy strain on families and are considered a private family matter. You don't tell strangers. So, instead of getting help you then are more secretive.

When a catastrophic illness like Alzheimer's Disease strikes we find that the larger and more extended the family, the more confusion and depression and other problems prevail because the issues are not really understood. While there is a desire to act on behalf of "my" family, it doesn't always get acted out in the sense of a cohesive concerted plan for either care or attention. However, once you can mobilize the whole family, there are a lot of positive outcomes because then you've got sort of a natural setting, a bond of family trying to work together.

In working with Alzheimer's families, what we do, in essence, is become like their family. We touch base with them and then provide something of a surrogate family. In turn, we are almost seen by them as a member of their family. Some of them will say "oh, you are just like my daughter. You are like a daughter to me or a granddaughter to me." They are pleased by this style of contact and that's part of what is expected. Those are certainly at least two of the areas of difference that are subtle, and have not been clearly identified in the literature.

What Do People Most Need to Understand about Hispanic Elders?

As people approach this community, it's easier to focus on socio-economic differences and more difficult to approach this group from a cultural understanding. There need to be frameworks for specific values, interactions, meaning and importance of language and symbols. Yes, there is inequality and it's a form of racism that affects the oldest Hispanics. But there also is much in understanding the background of older persons at this time in their lives.

Understand the cultural values because we can't resolve the problems presented without that. We spend a great deal of time upfront establishing rapport, and if that isn't done first, forget all the work. There needs to be an appropriate interactional style before any work is done for an older Hispanic client. Even economic aid is rejected when it's presented by an alien style of communication.

Three-quarters of the world is built on the family system. The Western world has developed an organizational system and sees organizations as solutions. Hispanics tend to see them as impediments. The way to reach the Hispanic community is to develop surrogate familistic approaches for health and social services. You certainly can't be family, but you can act like a family member.

Suggested Readings: Hispanic Elderly

Becerra, Rosina. (1983). "The Mexican-American: Aging in a Changing Culture." In Robert L. McNeely and John N. Colen (Eds.),*Aging in Minority Groups* (pp. 108-118). Beverly Hills: Sage.

Becerra reviews the literature on aging Mexican-American's roles and family interactions. She upholds that immigration, urbanization and acculturation are resulting in changes in family structure, social support systems and social roles of elders. Ethnically similar communities provide support and new coping models for elders and families who are experiencing this transition.

Becerra, Rosina. (1984).*The Hispanic Elderly*. Lanham, MD: University Press of America.

This book summarizes research findings regarding elderly Hispanic Americans. Notable is the inclusion of Spanish language research instruments which are designed for use with the Hispanic elderly.

Brink, Terry L. (Ed.). (1992). *Hispanic Aged Mental Health.* **Binghamton, NY: The Haworth Press.**

This edited volume describes the influence of cultural factors on the aging process of elderly Hispanic persons in the United States. Emphasizing a clinically relevant presentation of mental health issues in this population, it focuses on incidence and assessment of dementia and depression and describes various forms of intervention with Hispanic elders.

Cuellar, Jose. (1990). *Aging and Health: Hispanic American Elders.* **Stanford, CA: Stanford Geriatric Education Center.**

This monograph provides a concise but comprehensive overview of existing knowledge regarding the physical and mental health of older Hispanic Americans, including information regarding demographic characteristics, morbidity and mortality, cultural traditions and values, and health practices. While intended for health care providers and trainees, this review is an excellent resource for all people interested in understanding health-related issues affecting this population.

Lacayo, Carmela G. (1984). "Hispanics." In Erdman B. Palmore (Ed.), *Handbook on the Aged in the United States.* **Westport, CT: Greenwood Press.**

This chapter is an excellent summary of data regarding elderly Hispanic Americans. Information is presented on demography, immigration history, and Hispanic family relations. In addition, the chapter covers issues related to community supports, social service utilization, health care, and emerging trends regarding Hispanic elderly.

Markides, Kyriakos S. (1983). "Minority Aging." In Mathilda White Riley, Beth B. Hess and Kathleen Bond (Eds.), *Aging in Society* **(pp. 115-138). Hillsdale, NJ: Lawrence Erlbaum Associates.**

This article provides the definitive overview of the research literature in the context of the double jeopardy versus "age as leveler" theories. Markides used the two theories to analyze the available literature on the Afro-American, Hispanic and Anglo-American elderly population in the areas of income, health, primary group relations, and psychological well-being. It will undoubtedly promote debate.

Queralt, Magaly. (1983). "The Elderly of Cuban Origin: Characteristics and Problems." In Robert L. McNeely and John N. Colen (Eds.), *Aging in Minority Groups* (pp. 50-65). Beverly Hills: Sage.

Cuban-American's have the highest proportion of elderly of any Hispanic-American group. This article briefly outlines Cuban-American immigration history and demography and discusses problems of the elderly including income inadequacy, physical health, life satisfaction, English language difficulties and housing. Queralt recommends various actions to minimize or overcome these problems.

Sanchez-Ayendez, Melba. (1991). "Puerto Rican Elderly Women: Shared Meanings and Informal Supportive Networks." In Mark Hutter (Ed.), *The Family Experience: A Reader in Cultural Diversity.* New York: MacMillan.

The author analyzes the meaning of motherhood, family unity and family interdependence in the Puerto Rican community in the United States. Quotes from interviewed older women are used to illustrate their interpretation of the social supports they receive from adult children, spouses, neighbors and friends.

Torres-Gil, Fernando. (1986). "The Latinization of a Multigenerational Population: Hispanics in an Aging Society." *Daedalus*, 115, 325-348.

This chapter assesses the impact of an aging society on the Hispanic population, and poses problems, challenges and implications for policy and cultural change. The author challenges both the Hispanic population and society at large to share in an opportunity to redefine the American character for the next century.

Audiovisual Resources

Family Counseling with an Older Hispanic Family
Running time: 15 minutes/video
ATTN: Andrew Scharlach
School of Social Welfare
329 Haviland
University of California at Berkeley
(510) 642-0126

Created to demonstrate family counseling skills appropriate to work with older Hispanic families and to serve as a trigger for discussion, the tape portrays work with an older parent and their adult children where health-related issues have resulted in tensions and misunderstandings. The major issue presented is the conflict between a brother and sister over whether to use community services for care of their father. The theme is the cultural clash of values between traditional expectations of "familia" as sole caretaker, and the limitations of providing this care by contemporary Mexican-American women. Produced by the School of Social Work at San Jose State University.

Luisa Torres
Running time: 29 minutes/video or film
Centre Productions, Inc. (Barr Films)
12801 Schabarum Avenue
Irwindale, CA 91706

Weaves Spanish and English as it beautifully follows one day in the life of a 79 year old woman who follows the traditions of her ancestors in the mountains of northern New Mexico. Her life is a simple one, filled with work, but out of her relationship to the work has come peace and contentment, and in old age, grace, and wisdom.

Nosotros Los Viejos; Your Challenge, Your Reward
Running time: 22 minutes/video (1987)
National Hispanic Council on Aging, Inc.
2713 Ontario Rd. N.W., Washington, DC 20009
(202) 745-2521

Produced by the National Hispanic Council on Aging, this video highlights the views of aging Hispanics in America and addresses the need for more Hispanic professionals in the field of Gerontology. Leading Hispanic scholars, professionals, advocates, and politicians present their views on the growing Hispanic aging population and its unmet needs. César Chávez, Dr. John Santos, and Congressman Edward R. Roybal are among those featured.

Siempre Viva: Latino Family's Struggle With Alzheimer's
Running time: 49 minutes/video (Spanish)
Maria Aranda
P.O. Box 23401
Los Angeles, CA 90023
(213) 806-4921

A story of a Latino family living in the United States and the family's struggle with the devastating experience of Alzheimer's Disease. The story is based on real-life accounts of Spanish-speaking caregivers of Alzheimer's Disease victims and their desire to unite people of color to understand this chronic, degenerative disease in their own communities.

Triple Jeopardy
Running time: 18 minutes/video or film (1983)
Center on Aging
590D University Hall
University of California at Berkeley
(510) 643-6427

This tape is based on A National Study to Assess the Service Needs of the Hispanic Elderly, published by the Asociacion Nacional Pro Personas Mayores. It illustrates the three major problems reported by the Hispanic elderly: health, income, and morale (life-satisfaction). As many as 30% of elderly Hispanic people live alone. Older Hispanics are more than two times as apt to live in poverty as other aged members of our population. They struggle to survive under triple jeopardy: they are old, they are poor, and they are members of a minority group.

—by Andrew E. Scharlach, Ph.D.,
Esme Fuller-Thomson, MSW, Ph.D.,
B. Josea Kramer, Ph.D.

Chapter 7

Asian American and Pacific Islander Elderly

Demographic Overview

Asian Americans and Pacific Islanders encompass a large number of ethnic and cultural groups, including Asian Indian, Cambodian, mainland Chinese, Filipino, Guamanian, Hawaiian, Hmong, Japanese, Korean, Laotian, Samoan, Taiwanese, Vietnamese, and others. These groups are diverse with regard to language, culture, immigration history, and treatment by United States laws.

There currently are almost 500,000 Asian American and Pacific Islander elders in the United States, representing 6% of the Asian American and Pacific Islander population (by comparison, older adults represent 12% of the overall United States population). Since 1970, the number of Asian American and Pacific Islander elderly has increased 500%, in part because of liberalization of immigration laws since 1965. The end of immigration quotas also has led to large numbers of predominantly young Asian and Pacific Islander immigrants in the recent decades, so that the composition of these groups is considerably younger than it would have been without the recent surge of immigrants (Kii, 1984). As these younger members age in the second quarter of the next century, the number of elderly Asian American and Pacific Islanders could swell to more than seven million persons by the year 2050, representing 16% of all Asian Americans and Pacific Islanders.

Reprinted with permission from the Resource Center for Aging, University of California at Berkeley.

Age distributions vary greatly among the different Asian American and Pacific Islander groups, reflecting each group's unique immigration history. Among Southeast Asian Americans, only 2% of the population are elderly. The refugee experience limited the number of elders who could immigrate, and as relative newcomers to America, few of the immigrants have reached age 65 since their arrival in this country (Sakauye, 1990). In contrast, the proportion of elderly is much higher among the Japanese, at 7.1%. In this population, current immigration is limited and therefore there is not a wave of younger people coming into the country. In addition, both the surviving original immigrants from the turn of the century and most of their children are now elderly (Kim, 1990). These diverse backgrounds directly and indirectly impact these elders' past and present adjustment to life in the United States (Kii, 1984).

Immigration History

Chinese American Elderly

The first major wave of Asian or Pacific Islander immigration began in the mid-1800's when Chinese men were imported to work on railways, farms, and in mines in California, Hawaii, and other Western states. Many immigrants left their wives and children behind in China, motivated by the opportunity to earn adequate income abroad. The majority of these early Chinese immigrants expected their stay in the United States to be temporary; however, many never returned home.

Chinese immigrants were restricted primarily to menial jobs and were forced to live in ethnic ghettos that developed into Chinatowns in the big Western cities. As the numbers of Chinese immigrants increased, hostility from the Anglo-American majority grew, leading to anti-miscegenation laws, taxes applicable only to Chinese workers, and culminating in the Chinese Exclusion Act of 1882, which limited entry of Chinese women into the United States. These laws effectively prevented many of the Chinese immigrants from establishing families, leaving them to grow old alone in urban Chinatowns. In the 1930's, the sex ratio was 4 males for every female (Kim, 1990). The Japanese occupation of mainland China during World War II and the subsequent communist take-over of the country prohibited many Chinese American immigrants from ever returning home.

Since the repeal of quota restrictions in 1965, large numbers of Chinese have immigrated to this country. These individuals have much higher educational levels and are more likely to be employed in professional jobs than were the Chinese immigrants of the last century. Some members of this recent wave of immigrants brought their elderly parents, and some of these immigrants themselves are entering their retirement years after two decades in this country.

Consequently, the Chinese American elderly are predominantly composed of three groups: (1) primarily male immigrants who have lived in the United States the majority of their lives; (2) children of immigrants who have lived here all their lives; and (3) those who entered this country in the last twenty years, usually in the company of family. In total, there currently are over 50,000 Chinese American elderly, representing 6% of the Chinese American population (Kim, 1990).

Japanese American Elderly

After the Chinese Exclusion Act essentially ended the influx of Chinese workers in the late 1880's, Japanese indentured laborers began to fill the need for cheap agricultural workers. Unfortunately, as the numbers of immigrants increased, the Japanese also became subject to widespread discrimination by the Anglo-American majority. In 1905, the *San Francisco Chronicle* supported an anti-Japanese movement, and numerous incidents of individual harassment occurred. In 1908, the Japanese government signed a "Gentleman's Agreement" which substantially restricted the entry of Japanese men into the United States, primarily limiting immigration to the parents, wives and children of Japanese already in the U.S. In an attempt to avoid this prohibition, some unmarried male immigrants married "picture brides," who were then able to join husbands they had never met in the United States.

Discrimination continued after the 1908 agreement. In 1913, the Alien Land Law was passed, which restricted the ability of Japanese to purchase land. In 1924, the Asiatic Immigration Exclusion Act effectively ended all immigration of both Chinese and Japanese. However, as most Japanese had families, the population continued to grow, unlike the predominantly male Chinese community.

A distinctive event in Japanese-American history was the incarceration of 110,000 Japanese-Americans living in the Western states after the Japanese attack on Pearl Harbor in 1942. These Japanese, two-thirds of whom were American citizens, were interned in concentration camps by the United States government. Often their property was lost or damaged when they returned after the war. Moreover, fearful of further discrimination, many of these now-elderly Japanese Americans tried to suppress their Japanese ancestry and "fit in" with Euro-American values, often teaching their children to do the same. In many cases, this experience negatively impacted attitudes of subsequent generations regarding their Japanese heritage and disrupted traditional intergenerational roles.

Filipino American Elderly

Filipino immigration began in the early part of the century and increased dramatically after 1924 when the Asian Exclusion Act restricted Chinese and Japanese immigration. Since the Philippines was made a United States territory after the Spanish-American war, Filipinos were exempted from the restrictions imposed upon Asian immigration. The immigrants predominantly were men seeking work in agriculture and in the canning factories; consequently, there were 10 Filipino men to every one woman by 1930 (Kim, 1990). However, with the onset of the Depression, anti-Filipino sentiment became widespread, resulting in the Tydings-McDuffie Act of 1934, which restricted Filipino immigration to 50 people per year. Many of the young men who immigrated prior to 1934 are still single, often living alone in hotels and rooming houses in urban centers. These elders' education level and English skills tend to be low and they are predominantly poor.

The abolition of the quota system in 1965 promoted a second surge of immigration from the Philippines, composed largely of highly educated professionals. Some elderly came with their families in this wave of immigration, but they represent a much different profile than those who came in their youth. This population tends predominantly to be female, middle class and to live with adult children in suburban areas. By the mid-1980's there were 50,000 to 60,000 older Filipinos living in the United States, comprising a little over 6% of the Filipino-American population, with elderly Filipino men continuing to outnumber women by more than four to one (Hendricks and Hendricks, 1986).

Southeast Asian American Elderly

Immigration of Southeast Asians to the United States began primarily after the fall of Saigon in 1975. These Indochinese refugees were driven from their homeland by regional strife, often having to leave family members behind in their home country or in refugee camps. The first wave of refugees, arriving prior to 1978, had contact with American servicemen during the Vietnam War and often brought with them substantial educational and economic resources. Those who came later were more likely to have fled Communist regimes; they were from rural areas and tended to be less Westernized, less educated, and less well-equipped for adapting to a highly technological society such as the United States. Southeast Asian American elders, most of whom accompanied their children to the United States, have in many cases become dependent upon their children and grandchildren for negotiating with their new American environment, in some cases contributing to a dramatic role reversal in the family.

As this brief overview of immigration history illustrates, there are dramatic differences in the life experiences and present situation of elders between and within the various Asian American and Pacific Islander ethnic groups. However, there have been few group-specific studies of these various ethnic groups. The following discussion will primarily consider Asian American and Pacific Islander elderly in general, although as many specific group examples will be included as possible.

Economic Situation

The median income of urban Asian American and Pacific Islander elderly men in 1990 was $9,269, almost $4,500 less than that of urban Anglo-American elderly men. Urban Asian American and Pacific Islander women made an average of $7,742, while urban white American women made an average of $9.827. Reasons for generally lower incomes include limited English ability among a significant portion of the Asian American and Pacific Islander elderly, inadequate education, discrimination in hiring and rates of pay, work histories of low wage jobs, and high unemployment resulting in lower Social Security and private pension plan coverage (Manuel, 1982). Even independent farmers were affected by land-owning restrictions in the early part of this century, which restricted upward economic mobility for farming immigrants.

With regard to educational background, the proportion of high school graduates among Asian American and Pacific Islander elderly is substantially lower (26%) than among Anglo elders (41%). Thirteen percent of Asian American and Pacific Islander elders lack any formal education whatsoever, as compared to only 1.6% of-Anglo-American elderly.

Health

The mean life expectancy of Asian Americans and Pacific Islanders is higher than for the Anglo-American population. In 1980, the mean for Japanese-Americans was 79.7 years; for Chinese-Americans, 80.2; for Filipino-Americans, 78.8; and for Anglo-Americans, 76.4 years (Kitano & Daniels, 1988). However, despite their greater longevity, Asian American and Pacific Islander elders are more likely to have debilitating health problems than are their Anglo-American peers. Tuberculosis rates among Asian-Americans and Pacific Islanders, for example, are 12 times the national average (Hendricks and Hendricks, 1986). Hawaiians and certain other Pacific Islander groups are particularly likely to experience serious health conditions such as heart disease, cancer, and diabetes. Chinese American elders have a suicide rate three times higher than the general elderly population and a greater prevalence of mental illness, possibly due to social and emotional isolation (Kii, 1984).

Much of this differential in health status can be attributed to lower income levels among Asian American and Pacific Islander elders, lack of adequate health care throughout life, and a greater likelihood of working at manual, physically debilitating jobs. Moreover, health care service utilization by Asian American and Pacific Islander elders is restricted because of language difficulties, a preference for traditional folk medicine, distrust of services from the dominant culture which has historically discriminated against them, reduced eligibility for Medicare because of work histories, and an unwillingness to use Medicaid because it is perceived as a sign of inability to take care of oneself.

A much smaller percentage of Asian-American (3%) than Anglo elderly (5.8%) live in nursing homes. Among the oldest of the elderly population, only 10% of Asian American and Pacific Islanders are institutionalized, as compared with 23% of Anglo-Americans. Reasons for this difference include discrimination in referrals to long term care services, potential linguistic isolation, geographical discrimination in nursing homes, and greater involvement of families and other unpaid sources of assistance (Manuel, 1982). In addition, Asian American and Pacific Islander groups place a high value on caring for elderly members within the family context, attaching a social stigma to institutionalization.

Family

Asian American and Pacific Islander families typically have developed distinctive models of family interaction that combine traditional patterns of roles and responsibilities with adaptations called forth by the American experience. Thus, although Asian cultures traditionally emphasize the primacy of family bonds and unquestioned respect for elderly family members, the extent to which individual families subscribe to these traditional values and beliefs varies widely. For most Asian American and Pacific Islanders, however, the family performed a crucial function in the immigrants' new surroundings, providing a haven from a racist society and an environment where self-esteem could be developed and creative coping tactics could be promoted.

Many traditional Asian practices and beliefs regarding family interaction are based on Confucian philosophy, which asserts the importance of social order within families and society. Roles, responsibilities, and status in the family are clearly prescribed, and transcend personal desires or affectional bonds. Loyalty to the family is a long-term commitment and is maintained through a system of obligations that must be repaid by family members. For example, filial piety must be paid to older family members because they gave life to younger members and also because they provide a special connection to the spirits of previous generations. In addition, elders in traditional Asian families were the authority figures, who controlled the family's finances and had the final say over decisions affecting the lives of younger family members.

Asian American and Pacific Islander families are faced with conflict between these traditional Asian values and the popular culture of the United States, which tends to value independence, autonomy, and youth. To the extent that Americanized family members no longer abide by prescribed roles, duties, and responsibilities, elderly members are apt to have less control over family financial resources and decision-making, sometimes experiencing the shame of becoming dependent upon children and grandchildren for support and for negotiations with an unfamiliar environment.

Immigration also has impacted the structure and roles of the Asian American family. The skewed sex ratio in the Chinese and Filipino population disrupted traditional family life as many men did not marry, and therefore have no offspring to aid them in their old age. Change occurred even among those who had families. Many Asian immigrants left their home countries in their youth and came to the U.S., often sending money to support their parents; but, as their parents were not present, they could not model traditional filial behavior for their American-born children. In addition, Americanized children had the example of the dominant society and with their upward mobility were often required to relocate for employment, altering traditional patterns of family support and involvement (Kii,

1984). Despite the ongoing pressures of assimilation and acculturation, Asian American and Pacific Islander families continue to place
greater importance on family bonds and filial responsibility than do
many other American ethnic groups.

Social Relationships and Communal Involvement

Strong peer and communal support systems are important resources that Asian American and Pacific Islander elders rely on as
they adapt to their later years. As a result of impoverished circumstances and racial discrimination, immigrants were forced to rely
heavily upon peer, family and informal communal support systems
in times of difficulty. Assistance from majority culture institutions
typically was not available or was not considered a viable option, and
therefore economic, emotional and social support was sought primarily within ethnic enclaves. These enclaves often were the only environment where the monolingual immigrant could function
independently. There, most social relationships developed and cultural
institutions such as community-specific churches flourished. In addition, ethnic-specific service centers such as On Lok in San Francisco
developed to serve the needs of the elderly who were concentrated in
these enclaves.

Social relationships and social networks among Asian Americans
and Pacific Islanders continue to evidence an ethic of mutual support,
although relationships among members of particular ethnic groups
vary greatly. For Japanese, Chinese, and Filipino families who have
been in the United States for generations, the pattern of social relationships more closely approximates the dominant Anglo pattern, although their elderly members continue to be more likely to live with
their adult children than are middle-class Anglo elders.

Many Korean American elders have immigrated recently with
their well-educated, professional adult children and have embraced
many aspects of the dominant culture. Although a relatively high
proportion of these elders live with their children in suburbs that
have no Korean enclaves, they prefer to live independently. However, as recent immigrants, they have not had the opportunity to
develop an adequate support network; nor do they typically have
English skills to interact outside their ethnic community. They
generally cannot drive and therefore may be isolated from regular
contact with the friends that they have made. The Korean church
is the predominant structure for socializing with other Koreans,
but there is not usually a formal structure for ongoing informal

socializing for the elders, leaving the Korean elderly vulnerable to loneliness and isolation.

Southeast Asian refugees and other recent immigrant groups tend to have more traditional expectations regarding living arrangements and filial behavior. More than 85% of Southeast Asian American elders live with their families, with family members providing almost all of their economic and social support. Such extensive dependence on younger family members, reversing the traditional family roles, can exacerbate the difficulties of adapting to a new environment already experienced by both generations.

References

American Association of Retired Persons Minority Affairs Initiative. (1987). *A Portrait of Older Minorities*. Washington, DC: AARP.

Hendricks, J., & Hendricks, C. D. (1986*). Aging in Mass Society: Myths and Realities*. Boston: Little, Brown and Co.

Kii, T. (1984). Asians. In E. B. Palmore (Ed.), *Handbook on the Aged in the United States*. Westport, CT: Greenwood Press.

Kim, P. (1990). "Asian-American Families and the Elderly." In M. S. Harper (Ed.), *Minority Aging: Essential Curricula Content for Selected Health and Allied Health Professions*. Health Resources and Services Administration, Department of Health and Human Services. DHHS Publication No. HRS-(P-DV-90-4). Washington, DC: U.S. Government Printing Office.

Kitano, H., & Daniels, R. (1988). *Asian Americans*. Englewood Cliffs, NJ: Prentice-Hall.

Manuel, R., & Reid, J. (1982). "A Comparative Demographic Profile of the Minority and Nonminority Aged." In R. Manuel (Ed.),*Minority Aging*. Westport, CT: Greenwood Press.

Sakauye, K. (1990). "Differential Diagnosis, Medication, Treatment and Outcomes: Asian American Elderly. " In M. S. Harper (Ed.), *Minority Aging: Essential Curricula Content for Selected Health and Allied Health Professions* (pp.-331-340). Health Resources and Services Administration, Department of Health and Human Services. DHHS Publication No. HRS (P-DV-90-4). Washington, DC: U.S. Government Printing Office.

Asian and Pacific Islander Elderly

Based on an interview with Barbara W. K. Yee, Associate Professor, University of Texas, Medical Branch at Galveston.

What Term Do Asian American Elders Use to Identify Themselves?

Many of the elderly do not use the term "Asian American," but instead will identify themselves by their primary ethnic group. For instance they will say, "Well, I'm Japanese," and drop off the term American because they may or may not be citizens. Some of the younger cohorts of Asian elderly may use the term Asian-American if they are American born or more Westernized.

What Is the Popular Image of Asian American Elders?

There are very few media presentations of Asian elderly. But, the ones that I've seen tend show people who are middle aged. Older adults portrayed tend to be like the sansei, or teacher, in Karate Kid, who is teaching the young Italian boy about how to fight.

This image reflects a resurgence in the 1970s of older adults teaching the younger generation about their culture. That is true in families where there are younger grandchildren who are in their late high school and early college years. The older person often times will be called upon to help them in the process of rediscovering the family history and the cultural roots. When grandchildren are born there is a resurgence of interest and appreciation of the family, and along with that come more traditional ideas of what it means to be Chinese, Japanese, Vietnamese, Korean, etc.

What Divisions Exist among Asian American Elderly?

There are more than 16 groups in the category we call Asian/ Pacific Islanders. They range from the Asian groups who have been coming over since the 1800s, to the current groups immigrating right now in large numbers, such as Cambodians and Vietnamese. The major Asian groups include Japanese, Chinese, Filipinos, Korean, Vietnamese, Cambodian, Laotian, Hmong, Asian-Indian, Thai, Pakistani, Indonesian. Pacific Islanders also have a number of different ethnic groups. The largest populations are, in descending order: Hawaiians, Samoans, Guamanians, Tongans and Fijians. There are many other smaller islands that could be included as well. The Asians have common cultural similarities among them because many of them have Confucian roots. But the extent to which an individual older person abides by some of those cultural roots depends on how acculturated they are.

Asian elderly today are very diverse. Some of them are very Americanized, especially the younger ones aged 65-74 years. Many of them are American born and many of them had grandparents who were born in the United States. Many Chinese elderly had grandparents who were born in the United States. But we also have many Chinese elderly immigrants who just came over from Hong Kong last year.

What Special Challenges Are Faced by Today's Asian American Elders?

The challenges for Asian Americans have changed. In the past, more people focused on survival issues. Many elders who have recently come to the United States are in a much more privileged position because of changes in the immigration laws. Immigration laws in the past restricted Asian immigration, so family members who were supposed to come were never able to. In the late 1800s and early 1900s, for example, the flow of Chinese and Filipino immigrants was stopped suddenly. Many single Chinese elderly men were forced to stay in the United States, single and alone. They always expected to go back to their home countries to rejoin their families. They were restricted from intermarrying American women by law, so they were also prevented from starting new families in the United States.

Recent immigrants, on the other hand, often come to the United States as a result of family reunification, which is encouraged by current immigration law. So, the new immigrants have an established family in the United States, and they usually migrate to areas of the country where there are also other Asians. However, they still have to deal with the rapid acculturation to American lifestyles. Not only do they have language barriers but they have had less time to become familiar with how to survive in this culture. They also suffer from much more depression (there is a linear relationship between years in this country and depression). In addition, if the family is very Americanized and does not abide by many traditional beliefs (e.g. living together and providing care), there can be a breakdown of inter-generational relationships.

How Do Asian American Elders Feel about Aging?

Older Asian-Americans expect to be taken care of in old age. The extent of care varies across families, by social class and whether they are more traditional or not. My research indicates that after a number of years in the United States, the elders no longer hold very traditional beliefs of what behavior constitutes taking care of an older person; they modify some beliefs to be much more consistent with perhaps American ideas. One example is that we are now seeing elderly Vietnamese being put in nursing homes, something that was not condoned 15 years ago.

While they accept disabilities, in many traditional Chinese and Asian cultures they don't accept it passively. They do a lot of health promotional kinds of activities, like Tai Chi, that will either forestall disabilities or maintain their health. But once the disability occurs they don't have any resistance to engage in rehabilitative types of therapy. The problem is access to services that are appropriate such as facilities that provide bilingual services.

What Theories Best Describe How Asian Americans Respond To the Aging Process?

Theoretical formulations of aging often do not capture the important elements of culture, and how people cope with aging once transplanted from one culture to the other. That's why most theories fail. We need to develop better theories about aging and acculturation because it applies across the minority groups, as well as to other immigrants coming to this culture.

How Do Asian American Elders Differ from Elders of Other Ethnic Groups?

I see major differences between minority elderly and non-minority elderly in terms of the cultural differences. But, I also see, and find intriguing, major differences in terms of some genetic components for being at risk for certain kinds of diseases (for example diabetes, cardiovascular problems, or certain kinds of cancer). Lifestyle factors, acculturation, nutrition habits, and stress also affect health risk. We see some interesting kinds of comparisons for health in Asians. Japanese living in Japan have a very low risk of cardiovascular disease. Japanese living in Hawaii have a lifestyle which is between the traditional Japanese of Japan and the American lifestyle of the west coast Japanese. Japanese living in Hawaii are moderately at risk for cardiovascular problems. The highest risk group is Japanese living on the west coast.

Asian elderly may be much healthier than the Caucasian elderly today. But in a generation that difference may be totally wiped out because of the selective migration factor. In terms of health we should look at the protective factors and ask why they are healthier. What protects Asians from some of these dread diseases that other minorities have to deal with? What are the protective factors? Is it merely genetics or is it lifestyle habits like nutrition and exercise and stress levels? I think we can learn from what happens in the Asian American communities and perhaps help other groups as well.

What Are the Greatest Service Needs of Asian American Elders?

We really need to improve access to health services for Asians. There are a lot of factors that form barriers, including language and culture. The elderly often times will not seek services if they can't communicate. Language is a critical issue to providing good care and services.

Access to services depends on where the Asian elderly live. If the Asian elderly live in an urban community where there is an ethnic enclave, there usually will be some targeted services or some bilingual services at least. Asians in rural areas, on the other hand, typically have very little access to services, especially if they are only monolingual in their own language.

One cost efficient way to offer services to Asian elderly is to have a "one stop shopping" concept where some services for Asian elders can be integrated with services for other generations within the family. For instance, the grandparent might bring the grandchild to have a health checkup, while the grandparent uses the center for him or herself. That seems to work best in the urban areas where there is a high density of people in a specific Asian group.

Utilization of mental health services among Asian elderly is very limited. They don't accept it; they find it to be threatening. One way to enhance utilization is to provide that service within a one stop service center, so that users of mental health services aren't stigmatized. Service providers need to show concrete examples of how the service can be used in the initial stages, or they won't see the client again. This is true regardless of age, but it is most true with the elderly.

What Is the Role of the Family in Providing Support to Asian American Elders?

Asians heavily rely on their families for many of the resources they need. This can be a Catch-22 situation. Many service providers believe

that Asian families always take care of their own; but, in many circumstances, that is no longer true. The elders have changed their
expectations about what the family should provide and what government should provide.

Family relationships continue to be the most important social issue for Asian elders. The elders are worried about relationships within
their families and often are concerned with the decline they see in
many of the family's cultural traditions and rituals. Asian elders traditionally feel responsible for maintaining family harmony and family relationships; when something goes wrong they often times will
take the blame for it, even though they may not be at fault.

In many Asian American families, there are wide gaps between the
generations in terms of acculturation level. So, there may be family
conflicts because of differing views of each generation about what is
appropriate behavior between the old, middle aged, and younger
people. Asian elderly also are worried about the success of their children and grandchildren in the United States. Survival is important
for many of the newly arrived groups; but, once survival is taken care
of, they often may not meet their own goals for what they would like
to do in their lives or what they are capable of doing. Instead, their
goals will be transferred to the younger generation, which is expected
to succeed. This can create all kinds of family problems, as well.

In a traditional Asian family, elders are the liaison between the family and the community. What you often times will see in the rural areas,
or other areas where the family elders cannot speak English, is the
younger generations in the family will often have to translate. You see
role reversal in terms of the status of the older generation in the family:
now a kid in elementary school is looked upon as the family spokesperson. This role reversal is very demeaning to the elders in the household.
The elder's status has been lowered and the child's status has been raised
in the eyes of the American community as well as within the family.

What Do People Most Need to Understand about Asian American Elders?

I think that one thing that people should understand is that there
is really a lot of diversity among Asian American elders. For example,
each Asian group has a distinct language. Although Japanese and
Chinese can communicate through a pictorial language, they cannot
communicate verbally. The health status among the groups of Asian
and Pacific Islanders is startling different, also. Some of the best
health status in the world comes from the Japanese, Chinese and

Filipinos living in Hawaii. They are some of the longest lived people in the world. But native Hawaiians suffer from cardiovascular disease, diabetes, and high mortality and morbidity rates equal to some American Indian and black groups. So, even among Asian and Pacific Islanders groups health status varies.

The level of education also varies dramatically. We see doctorally trained people at the highest levels in some of the Asian and Pacific Island elderly, and we also see those who don't have a written language and currently are illiterate. Another example is immigration history and how groups came to the United States, whether they voluntarily immigrated or were forced from their country, like some of their Vietnamese. Income status is another area. People talk about Asian American elderly as doing much better than other groups. Yet, often times family status is taken as total family income, even though there are more individuals within the Asian elder's family pooling their income than other groups. So this great diversity is one thing that I want people to understand.

Secondly, we need to pay attention to cultural norms. We should not assume that because a person has an Asian face that they are very traditional or that they can't understand English. That is a very common mistake. You will find many Asian elderly today who are quite articulate in English, because they were born in this country. Acculturation has a significant impact, and the extent of acculturation varies depending on a family's history and the individual's history as well. It is important to treat Asians as individuals.

And the third thing that people should know is that this is a wide area for research. We need to know much more about this population than we do currently. It's an area where it's pretty exciting because, if you believe the data, there are some lifestyle habits in the Asian population that truly provide protective factors for certain kinds of health risks. We need to know whether there are protective factors and what they are. Exactly what is it that improves their health or makes them live longer? It's an interesting empirical question that needs to be answered.

Finally, it is important to remember that Asians are quite heterogeneous. Moreover, there is apt to be increasing diversity among the groups with age, and growing diversity even within the population of Asian elders. Rather than emphasizing commonalities and generalizations, we need to pay attention to diversity and how that may impact such areas as providing services to the elderly, understanding how he or she will grow older, and how a service professional can handle diverse cultural expectations.

Suggested Readings: Asian/Pacific Islander Elderly

Overview

Barker, Judith C. (1991). "Pacific Migrants in the US: Some Implications for Aging Services." *Journal of Cross-Cultural Gerontology*, **6, 173-192.**

This article discusses ethnic identity as both a strength and a stressor for Samoan, Tongan and Fijian migrants to the U.S. Development and delivery of aging services to older Pacific Islanders is discussed.

Hayes, Christopher. (1987). "Two Worlds in Conflict: The Elderly Hmong in the United States." In Donald E. Gelfand and Charles M. Barresi (Eds.), *Ethnic Dimensions of Aging* **(pp. 75-95). New York: Springer.**

This anthropological study clearly illustrates the dramatic role transitions elderly caused by the migration experience. The article discusses the ramifications for Hmong elders of changes in family structure, authority, customs and religious role. This article will provoke class discussion on migration's effects upon the elderly's status within the family.

Kii, Toshi. (1984). "Asians." In Erdman B. Palmore (Ed.), *Handbook on the Aged in the United States* **(pp. 201-218). Westport, CT: Greenwood Press.**

This chapter provides the best single summary of information on Asian-American elderly as a whole, with illustrations from specific groups. Information is presented on demography, immigration history, and Asian-American family relations and their development. In addition, the chapter covers issues related to ethnic communities, social service utilization and delivery, and health. Kii consistently attempts to explain possible causes of trends in the Asian-American community.

Morioka-Douglas, Nancy, & Yeo, Gwen. (1990). *Aging and Health: Asian/Pacific Island American Elders.* **Stanford, CA: Stanford Geriatric Education Center.**

This monograph provides a concise but comprehensive overview of existing knowledge regarding the physical health and well-being of older Asian Americans, including information regarding morbidity, mortality, service barriers, and health practices and beliefs. While intended for health care providers and trainees, this review is an excellent resource for all people interested in understanding health-related issues affecting this population.

Family Issues

Kim, Paul. (1990). "Asian-American Families and the Elderly." In Mary S. Harper (Ed.), *Minority Aging: Essential Curricula Content for Selected Health and Allied Health Professions* (pp. 349-364). Health Resources and Services Administration, Department of Health and Human Services. DHHS Publication No. HRS (P-DV-90-4). Washington, DC: U.S. Government Printing Office.

This chapter provides a brief overview of immigration history for the Chinese, Japanese, Korean, Filipino and Southeast Asian groups. Recent surveys of the groups are presented. The chapter identifies three problems most elderly Asians face: the erosion of the law of primogeniture; the myth that Asian-American families care completely for their elderly; and overt and covert prejudice against Asian-Americans resulting in societal injustice, inconsistency and individual powerlessness.

Kim, Paul. (1983). "Demography of the Asian-Pacific Elderly: Selected Problems and Implications." In Robert L. McNeely and John N. Colen (Eds.), *Aging in Minority Groups* (pp. 29-41). Beverly Hills: Sage.

Kim presents many of the needs of the Asian-Pacific elderly including health care, income, social services, nutrition and housing. Policy implications discussed include a need for an Asian-American elderly data base, and for unified national policy and service programs for Asian-American elderly with the flexibility to adapt to the needs and desires of the ethnic group served.

Audiovisual Resources

A Tale of Nisei Retirement
Running Time: 29 minutes/video
Japanese American Citizens League
1765 Sutter Avenue
San Francisco, CA 94115

In an effort to stimulate the Nisei (2nd generation Japanese Americans) to think about and plan for retirement, and to confront those cultural and historical factors which impact satisfaction with retirement, this video presents a Nisei family's struggle to cope with passage to retirement.

All Rivers Flow Home to the Sea: Caring Cultural Communities
Running Time: 28 minutes/video (1982)
Health Education Media, Inc.
1207 De Haro St.
San Francisco, CA 94107
(415) 282-9318

The objective of this videocassette is to provide the knowledge and the incentive to all communities to build a network of support for their citizens which will permit them to remain at home and as independent as possible. Two very dissimilar communities, in San Francisco, the Japanese through Kimochi, their community service center, and the Russian using the Russian American Service Center, show the tremendous impact of their cultural and nutritional programs in promoting the health of their elderly.

— by Andrew E. Scharlach, Ph.D.,
Esme Fuller-Thomson, MSW, Ph.D.,
B. Josea Kramer, Ph.D.

Chapter 8

American Indian and Native Alaskan Elderly

Demographic Overview

The Bureau of the Census defines Native Americans as Indians, Eskimos and Aleuts. Within this population there is enormous diversity. There are approximately 278 federally recognized reservations, 500 tribes, and an estimated 100 nonrecognized tribes in the U.S. Although Native American elders share a number of characteristics in common with other minority group elders, including poor health, lower life expectancy, general economic deprivation, disproportional levels of poverty and large family structures. However, Native Americans are the only indigenous minority group in the U.S. and maintain a special legal relationship with state and federal governments.

The number of elderly Native Americans has been estimated at more than 100,000, comprising about 6% of the Native American population (older persons comprise 12% of the entire U.S. population). Native Americans have higher birth rates and higher mortality rates than the white population, so that there is a disproportionate number of Native Americans who are young or in their early childbearing years compared with the population at large. However, life expectancy at birth for Native Americans, while still considerably less than the average for the Anglo-American population, has been increasing rapidly in recent years, and the number of Native American elders has increased more than 150% since 1970. It is estimated that, by the

Reprinted with permission from the Resource Center for Aging, University of California at Berkeley.

year 2050, the number of elderly Native Americans could exceed 500,000 persons, representing 12% of all Native Americans.

Both elderly Native American and white women outnumber their male peers. However, significantly smaller percentages of elderly Native Americans than whites are married. In 1980, 31% of older Native American women compared to 36% of white women were married, as were 60% of Native American men versus 74% of white men.

The migration of Native Americans to urban areas during and after World War II has created two distinct worlds of Native American elderly. Half of all Native American elders live in rural areas, including 25% who live on reservations (AARP, 1987). The other half live in urban environments, where they have little tribal community or tribal government concerned with their welfare.

Health

Health problems are a significant element affecting Native Americans' life expectancy, their work history, and quality of life. Native American elders have been found to have a poorer perception of their physical health than do other elderly persons, and they are twice as likely to exhibit mental health symptoms. Furthermore, reservation Indians aged 55 and above have levels of physical and social impairment comparable to those of non-Indians who are 65 and older (National Indian Council on Aging, 1984). Seventy-three percent of middle-aged and older Native Americans are impaired to some degree in their ability to perform basic activities of daily living (Hendricks & Hendricks, 1986).

Because of their unique relationship with the federal government, Native Americans who are members of federally recognized tribes and who live in rural or reservation environments are entitled to health care services provided directly by or through contracts with the Indian Health Service (IHS). However, these services are not widely available to urban Native American elders nor to the 14% of Native American elderly who are not registered in a tribe. Moreover, on reservations, barriers to suitable health care include lack of a national strategy for the delivery of preventive care; lack of information about health care; insufficient transportation to medical facilities; and lack of culturally sensitive care (National Indian Council on Aging, 1984). In cities Native American elders are vulnerable to the lack of health care services for individuals who have no health care insurance and do not have sufficient funds to pay for care.

Recent improvements in life expectancy are largely due to the efforts of the IHS to eliminate infectious disease and to meet the acute care needs of Native Americans. Although tuberculosis continues to be a health threat, these health problems have now been superseded by injuries, violence, cardiovascular disease, alcoholism, diabetes, cancer, and mental illness (most notably, depression). Because the IHS still interprets its mission in terms of providing acute care, however, it has concentrated its resources on child and adolescent care at the expense of programs for the elderly.

Socioeconomic Situation

Median incomes for Native American elders are significantly lower than for white elderly. In 1980, the median income for Native American elderly men was $4,257 versus $7,408 for white elderly men. Native American older women earned an average of $3,033 while white elderly women earned $3,894 (AARP, 1987). The poverty rate was 21.3% for urban Native American elders and more than 37.5% for rural elders, as compared to an overall white poverty rate of 9.5%.

Widespread poverty among Native Americans contributes directly to the high rates of morbidity and mortality mentioned earlier. In 1984, 25% of all Native Americans lived in households without plumbing. Overcrowding is also an issue, as one quarter of the elders reported that their bedroom was occupied by three or more people (National Indian Council on Aging, 1984). Malnutrition has been and continues to be a serious problem. In 1980, 45% of Native American elderly living in rural or reservation environments did not have a telephone, and only 50% lived within 30 minutes of the nearest health care facility. This lack of access limits the ability of the Native American elderly to seek medical care, and contributes to mortality in emergency situations.

There are many possible reasons for the high poverty rate among Native American elders, including inadequate education, discrimination in hiring and rates of pay, work histories of low wage jobs, and high unemployment. The Native American elderly have been educated in the U.S. school system, but the quality of education often has been poor. Only about 22% graduate from high school, and approximately 12% have no formal education at all as compared with only 2% of white elderly (AARP, 1987). This has many implications for occupational success during adult years.

Many elderly Native Americans also have a work history of high levels of unemployment and low wage jobs. Sixty five percent of elder

Native Americans worked as semi-skilled, unskilled, or farm workers (Stuart & Rathbone, McCuan, 1988). Low wage jobs not only provide less income from which to save for one's retirement, they are also much less likely to be covered by private pensions. They form the least stable part of the labor market and therefore workers in these jobs are very vulnerable to unemployment. High levels of involuntary retirement at early ages, often due to ill health or ageist hiring policies, contribute to a lower proportion of Social Security beneficiaries among Native Americans. Lastly, Social Security includes incomeless years in computing average yearly income, so that scattered periods of unemployment cause a significant reduction in monthly benefits even for those who do achieve eligibility for benefits. The vesting requirements of private pension funds have also proved detrimental to those Native American elders who were in unstable, temporary jobs.

Family Roles

Family involvement remains very important among Native American elders. Over half (58%) of all Native American elders live in households with two or more persons. About 20-25% of the elders' households have one or more foster children, often their grandchildren or children of other relatives. This percentage is many times higher than is found in the majority community (National Indian Council on Aging, 1984).

Native American families on reservations have traditionally involved three generations. The grandmother role is particularly important because of the family responsibilities that a woman assumes for the rearing of grandchildren. The grandparents often see their role as passing on the traditions and heritage of the culture. Models of grandparenting in Native American families are discussed in greater detail in the suggested reading by Weibel-Orlando (1990).

Sixty five percent of Native American elders live within five miles of relatives. In a primarily urban California study, 11% of unmarried older Native Americans lived in an adult child's household. Extended family is relied upon for assistance, support and companionship. Elder Native Americans tend to socialize less outside of the family than is common among their white peers, probably due to the frequency and importance of interaction within the family. Because Native American elders living in multigenerational households are more likely to have significant disabilities, they may be vulnerable to a sense of isolation, particularly when they lack transportation and have no telephone.

Social Relationships and Social Resources

There is a distinct division in the Native American population between urban and rural areas. While there is great diversity within this group, the urban Native American population is largely assimilated, predominantly sharing the values of the majority culture. Rural populations adhere more closely to traditional Native American patterns. The social structure of Native American tribes is characterized by the importance of the family or clan. Relationships among individuals who are part of the clan are considered to be extremely important, and the needs of the clan typically come before individual needs. Sharing what one has with clan members is expected. Hospitality is taken for granted, and family and friends have an open invitation to the home. However, more and more young adult Native Americans are choosing to leave the reservations in favor of better employment opportunities in urban settings, thereby diminishing the help available to Native American elders. Nor can these adult children and grandchildren be depended upon to provide financial support, since they also are vulnerable to economic deprivation.

References

American Association of Retired Persons (AARP). (1987). *A Portrait of Older Minorities*. Washington, DC: AARP.

Block, M. R. (1979). "Exile Americans: The Plight of the Indian Aged in the United States." In D. E. Gelfand and A. J. Kutzik (Eds.), *Ethnicity and Aging: Theory, Research, and Policy*. New York: Springer.

Cuellar, J. (1990). *Aging and Health: American Indian/Alaska Native*. Stanford, CA: Stanford Geriatric Education Center.

Hendricks, J., & Hendricks, C. D. (1986). *Aging in Mass Society: Myths and Realities* (3rd Edition). Boston: Little, Brown and Co.

National Indian Council on Aging (1984). "Indians and Alaskan Natives." In E. B. Palmore (Ed.), *Handbook on the Aged in the United States*. Westport, CT: Greenwood Press.

Schweitzer, M. M. (1983). "The Elders: Cultural Dimensions of Aging in Two American Indian Communities." In J. Sokolovsky (Ed.), *Growing Old in Different Societies*. Belmont, CA.

Wadsworth. Stuart, P., & Rathbone McCuan, E. (1988). "Indian Elderly in the United States." In E. Rathbone McCuan and B. Havens (Eds.), *North American Elders: United States and Canadian Perspectives.* New York: Greenwood Press.

Weibel-Orlando, J. (1990). "Grandparenting Styles: Native American Perspectives." In J. Sokolovsky, *The Cultural Context of Aging.* New York: Bergin & Garvey Publishers.

American Indian Elderly

Based on an interview with Robert John, Associate Scientist, Gerontology Center, University of Kansas.

What Is the Preferred Term for Identifying This Population?

American Indian elders, and people who work on behalf of elders, have disputed whether "Native American" is an appropriate term. Many Indians feel that the inclusion of native Hawaiians in the Native American title of the Older Americans Act meant that native Hawaiians would be using resources that should properly go to American Indians. Therefore, elders themselves said that they want to be known as "American Indian elders" to make the distinction between native Hawaiians and other native people. However, the distinction is not one that Congress is willing to recognize.

What Is the Popular Image of American Indian Elders?

My own feeling is that contemporary American Indian elders are rarely portrayed in any of the mass media, so that it would be very difficult for most Americans to form any kind of stereotype about contemporary American Indian elders. Historically, there probably is a stereotype of an American Indian elder who is wise, sage, learned and dispenses that wisdom to others as a moderating and calmative factor. This image can be compared to the other stereotype, that of the young Indian hot headed warrior. The elder steeped in Indian culture who knows the language and knows the tradition is now rare in particular groups as a result of the impact of acculturation. Even among a more intact society such as the Navaho, there is concern that an insufficient number of people are learning the culture and the traditions, so that the ceremonies are dying out or are being greatly reduced.

What Divisions Exist among American Indian Elderly?

There are basically two large divisions within the American Indian population as I see it. The first division is a rural/urban distinction. The urban Indian population is quite distinct from the rural-reservation population in terms of status and characteristics. In addition, people can be placed along a continuum from completely assimilated, sharing largely White values, all the way to the other end of the continuum where you have Indians who pursue and adhere to traditional values.

How Do American Indian Elders Feel about Aging?

There is a very common attitude toward the aging process among the American Indians, which cuts across all groups regardless of acculturation. They are very philosophical about the aging process, meaning that they accept it wholeheartedly. It's a natural process and anything that is a natural process is something that is to be embraced and readily accepted. Unlike whites, American Indians have no problem defining themselves as elders. There are people among whites who refuse to consider themselves "old" or accept the label of "senior citizen" or "elder" until advanced old age, 80s or so. Among American Indians, on the other hand, the culture values age and associates age with wisdom, so there is a tendency for people to emphasize their age and take on the identity of an elder.

What Is the Primary Social Role of the American Indian Elder?

American Indian elders have a social role in the culture and in ceremony that cannot be displaced. However, in other areas of everyday life (e.g., the politics of the tribe, the direction of the tribe, or the business of the tribe or nation), many elders feel left out. In part, that's because American Indian elders today have relatively low educational achievement and most of the business and political activities of the tribe have to be directed by people with a relatively high educational achievement. Within the family structures elders have a very important role that really holds the family together. One of the very common things that you see in rural reservation areas among elders is that the grandparental generation is raising grandchildren or even great-grandchildren.

The study of American Indian aging is barely 15 years old. There are very few works prior to 1975. The early work was based primarily in an anthropological model that viewed American Indians tribes as representatives of "primitive culture." One of the overriding issues (reflecting the interest of anthropologists at the time) was whether elders were performing material or spiritual functions as the basis of their status. Generally, anthropologists came to the conclusion that it was the spiritual or symbolic functions of elders that led to their status. But, more recent scholarship shows that elders' economic or material contributions to the well-being of American Indian nations or tribes is equally important.

What Theories Best Describe How American Indians Respond to the Aging Process?

Of the different theories of aging there are very few that come close to explaining in any comprehensive fashion the experience of aging in the United States. Of all the competing theories, the one that I think comes closest to explaining some of the outcomes is the political economy perspective, which states that where people end up in old age is a function of their experience during the life course within the political economy of the United States. If one looks at American Indians' experience of intermittent employment in young adulthood and middle age, it is not surprising to find that old age is apt to be accompanied by inadequate economic resources.

What Special Challenges Are Faced by Today's American Indian Elders?

Based on my research, the Indian elders' greatest challenge today is to have a lifestyle that assures them of the kinds of things that contribute to well-being in old age. What American Indian elders need and what they struggle with is primarily the consequence of not having the basic necessities of life. Their greatest needs are for financial assistance, for food assistance, and for better information and referral services so that they can use the social services that are currently available.

American Indian elders also have a great need for adequate medical care. Since 1955 the Indian Health Service has focused its resources on treating infectious and acute diseases, which typically occur in infancy or adolescence or young adulthood. Very few resources have been dedicated to treating chronic diseases, which are more typical among elderly populations. There is some sign that IHS is shifting its focus to deal more effectively with the health problems of old age, but it hasn't fully occurred yet.

Over the last 20 years, the morbidity and mortality profiles of American Indians and the general population have become more alike. The diseases that afflict elders in the general population are, more and more, diseases that afflict American Indian elders in old age. Cardiovascular disease is the greatest health risk for older Indians. For the frail elderly the single most important issue that we will be dealing with over the next decade is nursing home placement.

How health is perceived among elderly Indians is an important consideration. As Stephen Kunitz describes in *Navajo Aging*, there are two different ways of measuring functionality in old age: as illness and as disability. The clinical diagnosis may not have anything to do with elder's perceptions of his or her ability to carry on activities. Someone who is considered to be quite disabled may still manage to deal with problems effectively and maintain independence. There is substantial difference between what can be objectively documented and how people actually live their everyday lives. Moreover, among American Indians, as among Blacks, there is a mortality-crossover phenomenon at approximately age 65. Indians who are younger than age 65 die at higher rates than the general population, whereas Indians older than 65 have less risk of mortality compared to the general population.

What Is the Role of the Family in Providing Support to American Indian Elders?

American Indian values suggest that elders should be honored and taken care of within an extended family context. There are very dramatic changes going on within American Indian families in rural reservation environments and in urban areas. First of all, there has been a decline in fertility, resulting in a shrinking pool of potential caregivers. The caregiver pool in rural-reservation areas is also shrinking because of limited job opportunities. Middle-aged and young adults move to urban areas, some for only a temporary period, others for the rest of their lives. A third change that's occurring in the American Indian family, as with other groups in our society, is the rise in the percentage of families that are headed by a female. A fairly common family form in both urban and rural environments is a middle-aged female who has responsibility for bringing up young children (perhaps her own, perhaps her grandchildren) while also being called upon to give assistance to an elderly generation. With the American Indian caregiver pool shrinking, the extended family is going to become less and less able to provide long term care to American

Indian elders. Therefore, we need to develop a formal long term care system that can assist family members when they exceed their capability of taking care of their elders. This seems to be the challenge for the next decade.

In What Areas is Further Research Needed?

The one issue that I think we need to investigate immediately is the reason why American Indian elders don't seem to utilize social services in proportion to their needs. A lot of different things that have been suggested as "barriers to service use," but I am unaware of any study that has ever fully documented those perceived and objective barriers. An example of a perceived barrier could be the amount of paper work you have to do to receive benefits. An actual barrier might be that an elder does not have a car, or lives 50 miles from the nearest health care facility, or perhaps lives ten miles from the nearest paved road. We need to understand the reasons for the under-utilization of social and medical services and then develop a way to get the elder the services that are needed.

Beyond that, I think that a larger issue concerns the characteristics of a culturally sensitive long term care system for American Indian elders. I have no doubt that the system will not be predominantly institutional, but instead will be based upon the development of comprehensive community based services. We also need to understand more about caregiving among elders in order to reduce the strain experienced by caregiving family members.

What Do People Most Need to Understand about American Indian Elders?

I think that Americans need to develop an understanding about American Indian cultures, and elders as the primary bearers of those cultures. Understanding the situation of Indian elders requires that one think about the cultural differences between the culture in which the average person was raised and the culture in which American Indians live today. Only then can the service needs of American Indian elders be placed in the proper context.

Suggested Readings: Native American Elderly

Cuellar, Jose. (1990). *Aging and Health: American Indian/ Alaska Native Elders.* **Stanford, CA: Stanford Geriatric Education Center.**

This monograph provides a concise but comprehensive overview of existing knowledge regarding the physical and mental health of older Native Americans, including information regarding demographic characteristics, morbidity and mortality, cultural traditions and values, and health practices. While intended for health care providers and trainees, this review is an excellent resource for all people interested in understanding health-related issues affecting this population.

John, Robert. (1991). "The State of Research on American Indian Elder's Health, Income Security and Social Support Networks." In *Minority Elders: Longevity, Economics, and Health* (pp. 38-50). Washington, DC: Gerontological Society of America.

An overview of current issues relating to both urban and reservation Native Americans elders.

Kramer, B. Josea. (1991). "Urban American Indian Aging." *Journal of Cross-Cultural Gerontology*, 6, 205-218.

An up-to-date overview of major issues relating to the conditions, social service needs and policies affecting urban Native Americans elders.

Manson, Spero M., & Callaway, Donald G. (1990). "Health and Aging Among American Indians: Issues and Challenges for the Geriatric Sciences." In Mary S. Harper (Ed.), *Minority Aging: Essential Curricula Content for Selected Health and Allied Health Professions* (pp. 63-120). Health Resources and Services. DHHS Publication No. HRS (P-DV-90-4). Washington, DC: U.S. Government Printing Office.

A summary of 1980 U.S. Census data and reports of the Indian Health Service relating to the health and service needs of Native Americans, particularly those residing on reservations.

Schweitzer, Marjorie. (1987). "The Elders: Cultural Dimensions of Aging in Two American Indian Communities." In Jay Sokolovsky (Ed.), *Growing Old in Different Societies: Cross-Cultural Perspectives* (pp. 168-178). Acton, MA: Copley Press.

Indian elders retain power in the family and public domain through traditional roles in rural Native American communities. Schweitzer overviews information on the family and political role of the aged

Native American from the 1940's until the present day. From an anthropological perspective, she gives an overview of the perceptions, interactions and roles of elders in two rural American Indian communities.

Stuart, Paul, & Rathbone-McCuan, Eloise. (1988). "Indian Elderly in the U.S." In Eloise Rathbone-McCuan and B. Havens (Eds.), *North American Elders: United States and Canadian Perspectives* (pp. 235-253). New York: Greenwood.

Overview of the history of Native Americans in relation to the demography, geographic distribution, historical developments in Federal policy and current policy issues and service needs for older Native Americans.

Weibel-Orlando, Joan. (1990). "Grandparenting Styles: Native American Perspectives." In Jay Sokolovsky, *The Cultural Context of Aging*. New York: Bergin and Garvey Publishers.

An anthropological examination of five styles of grandparenting among Native Americans: the distanced grandparent, the ceremonial grandparent, the fictive grandparent, the custodial grandparent, and the cultural conservative grandparent. Ideal for promoting discussion of the family lives of Native American elders.

Williams, G. (1980). "Warriors No More: A Study of American Indian Elderly." In Christine Fry (Ed.), *Aging in Culture and Society: Comparative Viewpoints and Strategies* (pp. 101-111). New York: Bergin.

While not necessarily retaining political power in the public domain of the tribe, Indian elders remain essential to cultural transmission in rural American Indian communities. Definition as elderly typically is related to ability and social role, rather than chronological age.

Audiovisual Resources

Older American Indians
Running time: 13 minutes/video
Public Health Foundation
Attn: Josea Kramer
1102 Crenshaw
Los Angeles, CA 90019
(212) 857-6447

Documents the lives of urban American Indian elderly who were identified through the County of Los Angeles' Urban American Indian Elders Outreach Project. In the work, Older American Indians living in L.A. County describe their own lives and needs as they age in an urban environment.

Understanding and Working With Native American Elderly
Running time: 38 minutes/video
Weber State College
Attn: Jerry Borup
Ogden, UT 84408

A training module developed as part of an AoA grant, dealing with the knowledge and skill development necessary for working with Native American elderly. The video focuses on the knowledge and skills that are needed to enhance the ability of service providers who work with Native American Elderly.

— by Andrew E. Scharlach, Ph.D.,
Esme Fuller-Thomson, MSW, Ph.D.,
B. Josea Kramer, Ph.D.

Chapter 9

Putting Aging on Hold

"We have not directed enough serious attention to the concept of postponement and the enormous benefits to be accrued. Most of the fatal diseases and all of the nonfatal diseases ... increase exponentially with age. Postponing, therefore, has a magnified effect since delaying a process by one doubling will reduce by half the future incidence. We are living too long not to direct more of our efforts toward diseases which make aging a burdensome process."

—Jacob A. Brody, M.D.
Professor of Epidemiology and Research Medicine
School of Public Health, University Of Illinois at Chicago[1]

"Let's say we could develop a way to delay the need for nursing home care for one month. That delay would save $3,000 for a single patient. And if we can delay institutionalization by just one month for 100,000 people a year, that represents savings equal to all the money the government invests each year in basic research for Alzheimer's disease."

—Carl Cotman, Ph.D.
Psychobiologist
University of California at lrvine[2]

Excerpted from *Putting Aging on Hold: Delaying the Diseases of Old Age.* Reprinted with permission from Alliance for Aging Research, 2021 K. Street, N.W., Suite 305, Washington, D.C. 20006, (202)- 293-2856, 1995.

Americans are living longer and healthier than ever. This should come as welcome news. Unfortunately, even with improved health and longevity, the longer people live the greater the chances they will experience a geriatric problem—incontinence, immobility, memory loss, and other chronic disabilities—which could strip away their independence.

The common response by health care systems both public and private is to spend more money on nursing homes and other forms of "sick care." However, a more humane and cost-effective option is to invest more in research which could cure, prevent, or especially delay dysfunctions in later life. This research option—an investment in improving health and enhancing independence for millions of Americans—could remove much of the pressure from an already overtaxed U.S. health care system.

It is a central and powerful fact of life that from youth to old age, a person's chances of surviving twelve additional months steadily decline with the passing of years. In the sense of being biologically fit, a ten year old is practically indestructible. The statistical odds are that for every 10,000 ten year olds, only two will not live to see eleven. Beyond age ten, however, mortality rates double at regular intervals until even the oldest of the old succumb. In all the world there is only one known human, Jeanne Marie Calment of France, who is still alive after 120 years. Demographers and insurance actuaries call this doubling trend the force of mortality.

Health experts in aging research see another force at work, which might be called the force of morbidity. It is the clock, like regularity by which risks of chronic aging-related disease also double approximately every five years after middle age. Except for the rare and pitiable exceptions, including the accelerated progeric conditions such as Down syndrome and Werner's disease, occurrences of Alzheimer's-like dementias, osteoporosis and stroke are nearly unheard of in people younger than 40. But beginning in middle age, the risks double every five to seven years for a wide variety of incurable and chronic afflictions. While most of these infirmities, such as arthritis, frailty and memory loss, are not directly life-threatening, the consequences of a mounting force of morbidity are aging-related health problems on a mass scale. These conditions rob individuals of quality of life in their later years, and they present an aging society with a daunting financial, social and ethical challenge.

The generals in a would-be war on aging-related disability now see a determined strategy of delay against the rising risks to chronic disease as both plausible and highly effective. Delaying the diseases of aging is a relatively new idea, but one with great potential.

Either by delaying the onset by five years or by effecting a five-year "time out" in the progression of these aging related diseases, the exponential portion of the curve would have one less doubling near the end of life. This would eliminate half of all cases of the disease and half of the attendant costs and misery.

Even a brief delay can translate into dramatic savings. For example, it is estimated that postponing physical dependency for older Americans in the aggregate by just one month would save the nation $5 billion in health care and custodial costs. Postponing the onset of Alzheimer's disease by five years would, in the course of time, reduce incidence by half, thus saving half the cost of this terrible, terminal illness, currently estimated at $ 100 billion annually. Similarly, if hip fractures could be delayed five years, the exponential increases would have one less doubling. Ultimately, we would achieve a 50 percent reduction in the number of hip fractures and their costs. Hip fracture is one of the leading causes of hospitalization and one hip fracture alone costs an estimated $40,000 in medical and long-term care costs. Clearly, postponement could cut these high costs and dramatically extend older Americans' active and independent later years.

The best way to postpone the diseases and conditions of aging is to nurture research that will demonstrate who is most vulnerable to these problems and how their risk can be reduced.

This chapter describes the "Longevity Revolution" and its implications for America. It looks at current and projected health care spending and how these amounts might be trimmed by making a greater investment in aging research. The report examines the critical role of research in delaying, preventing and treating the diseases and conditions of aging. It analyzes trends in research funding for aging, both public and private. It puts the leading illnesses and conditions of aging "under the microscope," discussing the number of cases, the total overall costs of the illness, recent breakthroughs in treatments and therapies, and promising directions for future research. The findings of this report include the following:

- The number of Americans 65 and over, currently 33.6 million, will more than double, reaching 70.2 million by 2030;

- The "oldest old," age 85 and older, is the fastest growing segment of the population and will rise from 3.3 million (1994) to 9 million (2030) and possibly as high as 48 million by some estimates (2050). This is the age group most likely to need long-term care;

131

- In 1992, older Americans over the age of 65 accounted for nearly 38 percent of the national health care bill of $800 billion;

- The National Institutes of Health will spend only 7 percent of its 1995 budget on aging-related research, although older Americans account for more than one-third of health care spending;

- Under the President's proposed budget for fiscal year 1996, spending at the National Institute on Aging will actually decrease by $4.4 million from 1995 after adjusting for inflation;

- The growing gap between basic research sponsored by the federal government and applied research and development by private industry could produce diminishing opportunities for the development of new therapeutic agents for older patients;

- Postponing the diseases and conditions of aging can result in dramatic cost savings:

  a five-year delay in onset of Alzheimer's disease could ultimately cut the number estimated $50 billion dollars annually.

  a five-year delay in occurrence of hip fracture annually could cut the number of events by 140,000 annually and save an estimated $5 billion annually;

  a five-year delay in onset of urinary incontinence could save an estimated $8 billion annually; and

  a five-year delay in onset of cardiovascular disease could save an estimated $69 billion annually.

To suggest how a greater investment in aging research can help put aging on hold, this chapter contains a series of policy recommendations. Foremost among these is a call for a stronger national commitment to accelerate research in human aging and to alleviate aging-related diseases. This effort would go well beyond the traditional single disease focus that drives Congressional appropriations for national biomedical research. It calls instead for a national research effort aimed at a whole class of diseases of aging, which, if left unsolved, will be the main driver of U.S. health care costs for at least the next 100 years. It also calls for implementing a comprehensive agenda for aging research that would range from understanding the basic biologic mechanisms of aging to clinical studies, studies of the behavioral, social and psychological aspects of aging, health services research and bioethics research.

What would such an all-out effort for aging research cost? About 1 billion annually. This was the figure cited by the U.S. Bipartisan Commission on Comprehensive Health Care ("The Pepper Commission") in 1990, the Institute of Medicine's National Research Agenda on Aging in 1991 and, annually since 1989, by the Task Force for Aging Research Funding, an ad hoc committee of over 70 nonprofit aging and health groups. The federal Task Force on Aging Research (TFAR) recently released its blueprint for aging research in America, calling for $ 1.1 billion in funding over the next five years to augment the $841 million currently being spent annually by the U.S. Department of Health and Human Services and the Department of Veterans' Affairs. This sum is needed to adequately address all forms of research on aging issues, including biologic, medical, health services, psychological, social, economic, and demographic research.

Knowledge gained from such a strategic aging research effort would benefit the nation's economy and bolster productivity. Increasing the health and activity of older Americans is both socially desirable and economically necessary. The United States will save billions of dollars by keeping older people out of hospitals, out of operating rooms and out of nursing homes. Just as importantly, a coordinated and well-funded aging research effort would hold out hope to current and future generations that long life can be healthy and productive to the end, with the force of morbidity compressed to an irreducible minimum.

The Longevity Revolution and Its Impact

"We need a massive effort to reduce and, for many of the elderly, eliminate the chief threats to their independence... The more independent the elderly are, the less expensive nursing home and institutional care they require. Independence is what the elderly want most."

—Former Health, Education and Welfare Secretary,
Joseph A. Califano, Jr.

The United States is in the midst of an unprecedented demographic revolution. This "Longevity Revolution" is dramatically changing the fabric of American society. For a growing number of seniors, growing older is not an idle time of rest and looking backward, but a productive period where new careers, interests and activities are pursued with vitality. Signs of this cultural shift are everywhere. Mandatory retirement is a thing of the past. Travel plans are aggressively marketed to older consumers. Movies and television shows, as well as commercials, portray older people in active, vital roles. With increasing health, vigor and independence among the older population comes a natural human desire to enjoy all of these commodities for as long as possible.

The Older Population

Longevity has increased at an astonishing rate in the 20th century. Dr. Robert N. Butler, chairman of geriatric medicine at Mount Sinai Medical School in New York, notes that there has been a greater increase in average life expectancy at birth during this century than there was from the time of ancient Rome to the year 1900. Medical and scientific breakthroughs, improved health habits and rising standards of living have combined to raise the average life expectancy from 47 years in 1900 to 72.3 for men and 79.1 for women in 1992.

Currently, Americans age 65 and older constitute 13 percent of the population, or 33.6 million persons. Because of longer life expectancy and the large number of people reaching the oldest ages, Americans age 85 and older represent the fastest growing segment of the population.

Future Growth

But this Longevity Revolution is still in its infancy. The next major factor contributing to the growth in older Americans will be the aging of the post-World War II "Baby Boom," defined by demographers as those born from 1946 to 1964. This is the largest single generation in American history, and its oldest members will begin turning 65 in 2011, ushering in a "Senior Boom." Their numbers will skyrocket, from 40.1 million elderly persons in 2011 to at least 70.2 million by 2030.

The over-85 population—those most likely to need long-term care—will continue to grow especially fast. The "oldest old" are conservatively projected to more than triple from three million (1 percent) in 1993 to nine million (3 percent) in 2030, and to more than double again in size from 2030 to 2050 (to almost 19 million people or 5 percent of the population), according to midrange data from the U.S. Bureau of the Census. Others, including Duke University demographer Dr. Kenneth Manton, using sound methodology, forecast more than twice the Census Bureau's estimated numbers of oldest old: by mid-century, as many as 48 million Americans over age 85.

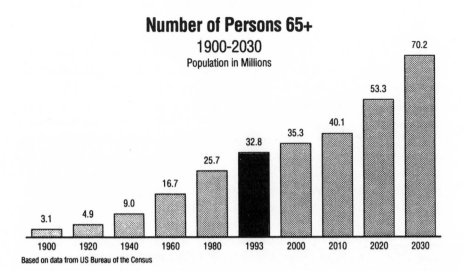

Figure 9.1.

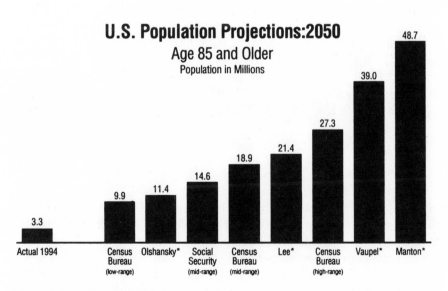

Figure 9.2

135

Health and Long-Term Care Needs of the Older Population

Chronic illnesses that most frequently strike in late life are now the most common forms of illness in the United States. Aging dependent conditions such as Alzheimer's disease, heart disease, adult-onset diabetes and Parkinson's disease are degenerative and often require long periods of care without much hope of full recovery. Many older people are afflicted with numerous other chronic illnesses and debilitating conditions for which we currently lack the ability to effectively prevent or cure. These include arthritis, osteoporosis, urinary incontinence and aging-related losses of sight and hearing. While seldom a cause of death, these problems are the cause of much dependent care and a greatly diminished quality of life for millions of Americans.

From 2010 forward, as the over 85 population expands rapidly, the incidence of illness and dependency could prove crippling to the American health care system. For example, Alzheimer's disease is predicted to afflict some 14 million Americans by 2050—a number equivalent to the total population of Texas.

Understandably, long-term care needs will grow as the population ages. In 1990, there were approximately seven million older people needing long-term care. By 2005, that number is projected to rise to nine million, and to 12 million by 2020.

In sum, longer life expectancy across the population carries the high risk of more people suffering from chronic diseases. These problems will accelerate the demand for long-term care, particularly after 2010. In the absence of research breakthroughs, a six-fold increase in health care costs among our oldest citizens, not counting inflation, is expected with the aging of the Baby Boom.[4]

The High Cost of Health Care

This year, health care spending in the U.S. will pass the trillion dollar mark for the first time, with public and private health care expenditures expected to total $1.007 trillion. More than one-third of this amount will be spent on Americans 65 and over, a rate expected to rise with the growth of that age group unless we find better ways to cure, prevent or postpone the diseases of aging. Each year the nation devotes more of its resources to health care. In 1960, health care expenditures were 5.2 percent of the gross national product (GNP); by 1990, health care expenditures had reached 12.2 percent of the GNP or $696.6 billion. If current trends continue, the Health Care

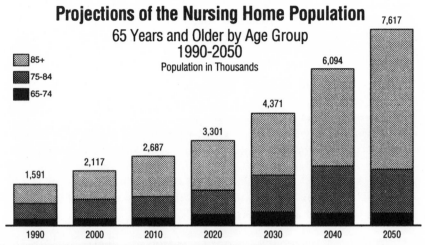

Figure 9.3.

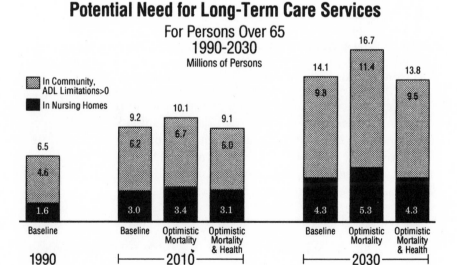

Figure 9.4.

Financing Administration projects that health care could consume 31.5 percent of the GNP in 2020. If expenditures actually reach this level, they would place an unacceptable strain on us as individuals and on society.

Health Care Costs of the Elderly

- The 1992 per capita health care expenditure for people 65 and older was nearly four times what was spent for individuals under 65—$9,125 for older Americans and $2,349 for those under 65;

- By 2004, the cost of health care for those over 65 is projected to constitute 50 percent of the total national health care bill, expected to exceed $2 trillion;

- Unless cures, better means of prevention or effective means to delay the diseases of aging are discovered, Medicare costs for the oldest old could increase six-fold by 2040.

The price of medical and custodial care, coupled with indirect costs such as the burden on caregivers, is a hardship borne by individuals, families, private insurers and the federal government.

A few figures are listed here to suggest the magnitude of their costs, today and in the future:

(All numbers refer to direct and indirect costs)

- Cardiovascular diseases cost $138 billion annually;

- Cancer alone accounts for 10 percent of the total cost of disease in the U.S., coming in at $104 billion annually. While all types of cancer do not follow the exponential growth patterns exhibited by other diseases of aging, some types, such as breast and prostate cancer, are much more common in elderly patients, and the risk increases dramatically with age;

- Alzheimer's disease costs are estimated at $100 billion annually;

- Strokes among older people result in health care costs of almost $30 billion annually;

- By conservative estimates, managing urinary incontinence costs more than $16 billion annually. As the population ages, the annual price tag may rise as high as $30 billion;

- The cost to the nation of osteoporosis was estimated in 1988 to be $ 10 billion annually. Without intervention, these costs may rise during the next 25 years to between $30 and $60 billion. Hip fractures alone account for more than $7 billion annually.

The health care costs associated with our demographic future are staggering. How can America meet the health care cost challenge of our aging population?

The options are to:

1. pay the bills—over $300 billion a year and rising;

2. ration health care and deny lifesaving medical attention to some people over age 65;

3. ignore the problem until a later Congress or a later generation is overwhelmed by these problems; or

4. invest a fraction of the health care costs in scientific research that could lead to prevention, postponement or cure of the major diseases of aging.

Unless the U.S. can mount a successful effort to slow or stop the incidence of these debilitating problems, older Americans will soon represent as much as one-half of a growing national health care bill. Aging research plays a pivotal role in improving the health and enhancing the independence of older persons, and thus curbing costs.

The Importance of Aging Research

"Biomedical research has proven to be one of our nation's wisest investments. It saves lives and money, while creating new jobs across the country. Our success in this vital field has made the United States a world leader in promoting health and in preventing disease and disability."

—President Bill Clinton[5]

Americans are proud of their health care system. They demand and expect the best health care in the world. They believe the United States' scientific community will continue to lead the world in biomedical innovation and will provide the cures and interventions that they need.

But a crisis is brewing. Dwindling financial support for medical research threatens the nations ability to remain a leader in medical innovation. Once the "pipeline" of basic scientific research starts drying up, there will be little left for the private sector to translate into new products and technologies that save and improve lives.

Medical innovation is vital to providing quality and access to health care for all Americans. However, the road to breakthroughs in medical research is not always short or smooth. It can require a significant investment of time and resources.

In the field of aging research in particular, the investment is well worth it. Alzheimer's disease, osteoporosis, urinary incontinence and others are not an inevitable part of the aging process. They are diseases and medical conditions that can be researched, better understood, treated, and ultimately reduced as a major threat.

"Science offers the best hope to improve the older person's quality of life. Research that is directed and supported properly can provide the means to reduce disability and dependence in old age, and can decrease the burdens on a health care system strained to its limits."

—The Institute of Medicine[6]

At its core, aging research emphasizes strategies for maintaining health and independence, improving quality of life and preventing or postponing disabilities during the later years.

The Role of the Federal Government

"Only three cents of every health care dollar is spent on medical research. Without more support, new discoveries will just have to wait. The treatments of today cannot be those of tomorrow."

—C. Everett Koop, M.D.
Former Surgeon General, U.S. Public Health Service

Despite sharply rising health care costs, the aging of the population and the increased incidence of chronic illnesses, the federal government has not yet given healthy aging the attention it deserves as a major national health objective. Regrettably, funding for aging research has flatlined and declined in recent years, placing opportunities for enhanced health and longevity for the elderly at risk in the United States and lessening the chance of cost containment in the future.

The National Institutes of Health

This year, the U.S. will spend an estimated $375 billion on health care for people over age 65—more than $11,000 per person. Yet, the National Institutes of Health (NIH) will spend only 7 percent of its $11.3 billion medical research budget for aging-related research. This 7 percent includes the entire budget of the National Institute on Aging (NIA) as well as all aging research conducted by the 23 Institutes of Health and research centers at the NIH. This represents a research investment of two-tenths of 1 percent of the health care costs of people over age 65. Considering the certainty of our demographic future, investing such a small sum for research in aging is a gross miscalculation of strategy.

The President's fiscal year 1996 budget calls for a 4.1 percent increase in the NIH budget, to $11.7 billion. However, to offset anticipated increases in defense spending, the budgets for fiscal years 1997 through 2000 divide discretionary spending into "protected" and "unprotected" status.

The protected programs and agencies are projected to remain at Fiscal Year (FY) 1996 levels, while the unprotected programs and agencies would be cut by 3 percent in FY 1997, 5 percent in FY 1998, 7 percent in FY 1999 and 9 percent in FY 2000. As part of the "unprotected" group, the NIH budget is projected to drop by $1 billion in FY 2000.

The National Institute on Aging

The NIA leads the federal aging research effort. NIA officials report that federally funded research efforts are already making strides in identifying genetic and environmental factors associated with the aging process. Scientists are isolating genes believed responsible for the onset of aging-related diseases, as well as those conferring health and longevity. They are working diligently to find the best ways of preventing frailty and disability, and of rehabilitating seniors who experience those conditions.

Regrettably, funds for the NIA have grown an average of just 4 percent a year since 1992. Adjusting for inflation, the 1995 NIA budget actually constitutes a $3.2 million reduction in funding, and similarly, the President's budget for 1996, although a 3 percent increase on paper, in practical terms, amounts to a $4.4 million reduction from 1995.

The Need to Do More, Not Less

Federal retreat in research support comes at a time of rapidly expanding research opportunities in aging. New advances—from the characterization of telomerase, the enzyme believed responsible for the immortality of cancer cells, to locating one of the genes known to trigger breast cancer, the use of fetal tissue transplantation for treatment of Parkinson's disease and the developing understanding of the role of nutrition in preventing the chronic diseases of aging—all are generating an increased number of excellent research grant applications. Budget restrictions, however, necessitate that a limited number of new and competing awards can be made at the NIA. In fact, for investigator-initiated projects, which are the backbone of NIH research, fewer than one in five applications in aging research will receive funding in 1995.

The Department of Veterans' Affairs

Outside of the Department of Health and Human Services, the U.S. Department of Veterans' Affairs (VA) is the most active federal agency conducting aging research nationwide. The VA has achieved major advances in the fields of geriatrics and geriatric training. Many medical advances that have benefited all of the elderly in the U.S.—pacemakers, CAT scans, MRI techniques and prosthetic devices—have been pioneered through VA research.

Like the U.S. public at large, the VA patient population is aging. According to sources at the VA, the number of cases of Alzheimer's

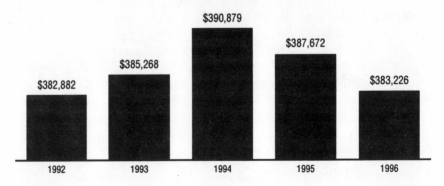

National Institute on Aging Budget
Adjusting for Inflation (1992 Dollars)
Dollars in Thousands

Figure 9.5.

disease and other dementias alone has risen from 200,000 in 1980 to twice that amount in 1990. They project there will be 600,000 dementia patients in VA institutions by the end of the decade.

The VA allots less than 10 percent of its medical research budget for aging studies, although by the end of this century, two-thirds of all men in the U.S. age 65 and over will be veterans.

Severely limited budgets for almost all the NIH and the VA aging research programs point to the need to enlarge the nation's entire health research enterprise. Any substantial boost to aging research should not be made at the expense of other areas of health research. Rather, the importance of a vigorous research effort in aging should highlight the greater goal of a concerted national effort to increase investment in biomedical research and development.

The Role of the Private Sector

"The [pharmaceutical] industry is one of the most research-oriented in the United States. In 1991, it spent almost three times as much on research and development (as a percentage of sales) as the average from all U.S. manufacturers."

—Congressional Budget Office[9]

"Today and in the 21st century, medical progress will depend largely on the growth and profitability of biopharmaceutical industries and the support of clinical experimentation with new drugs."

—Robert M. Goldberg, Ph.D.
Senior Research Fellow, Gordon Public Policy Center
Brandeis University[10]

By capitalizing on the research findings of the NIH, the VA and other federal health research agencies, private companies can apply their resources to developing new treatments, cures and methods of delaying illness. But if this essential government pipeline of laboratory research slows to a trickle due to cutbacks and regulatory roadblocks to technology transfer, even the most well-endowed and productive private industry will have little to work with.

A growing trend in the United States is to rely less on government for solutions to social problems and to rely more on public-private partnerships. Certainly a robust working relationship between government and industry is essential for delaying the illnesses of aging. Private foundations and corporations, which have become increasingly interested in supporting aging research and in developing the careers of researchers, also play a part. The federal government is uniquely positioned to conduct high-caliber biomedical research around the nation. Pharmaceutical companies, biotechnology firms, medical device manufacturers and others depend upon this resource for their very existence. However, government also has a responsibility to allow the marketplace to reward these companies for developing effective new products, or they may choose to spend their money promoting current products, rather than in risky research and development, which may be able to delay aging.

The Public-Private R&D Link

An important link in the development of new medical interventions to delay the diseases of aging is private sector research and develop-

Table 9.1. Pharmaceutical Industry and NIH Research and Development Expenditures in Billions

	Total* Pharm. R&D	NIH R&D	Difference in Pharm. and NIH R&D Spending	Percent More or Less Spent by Pharm.
1982	2.8	3.4	-0.7	-19%
1983	3.2	3.8	-0.6	-15%
1984	3.6	4.3	-0.7	-16%
1985	4.1	4.8	-0.7	-15%
1986	4.7	5.0	-0.3	-5%
1987	5.5	5.9	-0.4	-7%
1988	6.5	6.3	0.2	4%
1989	7.3	6.8	0.5	8%
1990	8.4	7.1	1.3	18%
1991	9.7	7.7	2.0	26%
1992	11.5	8.4	3.1	37%
1993	12.7	9.8	2.9	30%
1994*	13.8	10.3	3.5	34%
1995*	14.9	11.3	3.6	32%

*Note: Pharmaceutical Industry R&D includes amount spent by U.S.-owned subsidiaries in foreign countries and amount spent by foreign-owned companies within the United States
Source: 1. Pharmaceutical Research Manufacturers of America (PhRMA) Annual Survey
2. NIH Data Book
3. NIH Budget Office, FY 1995 Appropriations

ment. New scientific findings developed through government-sponsored research are translated into products such as vaccines, technologies and other therapeutic agents.

The Role of Pharmaceuticals in Controlling Disease

Life expectancy increases and disease incidence and death rate declines are due in significant part to pharmaceutical discoveries over the past three decades.

Of the top 20 killer diseases of the 1960s, six experienced death rate reductions of over 50 percent by 1990, and an additional six improved 25 percent to 50 percent. Many of these, including cardiovascular conditions, diabetes and pneumonia, are aging-related disorders. Of the ten diseases that showed the greatest improvement, pharmaceuticals played an important role in eight.

Pharmaceutical innovations have historically been driven by a cycle of basic research followed by breakthroughs in treatment. As innovations occur, the ability to treat a disease typically evolves from palliation of symptoms to control of fundamental disease mechanisms, to cure and possible prevention. The mix of treatments available is expected to continue to shift toward cure and prevention in the future.

The Biotechnology Industry

There is also growing concern over the health of the biotechnology industry, which has focused on developing novel therapeutics through recombinant DNA technology. Biotechnology was one of the most bullish industries of the 1980s, but several unsuccessful drug trials and other problems have caused investments in the field to dwindle. Analysts predict a wave of bankruptcies and consolidations, which may whittle the number of U.S. biotech firms from 265 publicly-traded companies in 1994 to less than half that number by the end of 1997. According to *Science* magazine (February 3, 1995, p. 618), "The loss of confidence hits the undercapitalized industry where it hurts. According to a 1994 report from the accounting firm Ernst & Young LLP of Palo Alto, California, one half of all biotech companies have less than 2 years' funding in their coffers—far below the 5 to 12 years that's needed to get a drug to the market." As one industry observer points out, however, many biotechnology companies are seeking other sources of funding, including foreign investors, to stay in business.

The Role of Private Foundations

In addition to the important contributions of the pharmaceutical and biotechnology industries, non-profit, private and corporate foundations support aging research and, in particular, help aging researchers to develop their careers. For example, both the Brookdale Foundations National Fellowship Program and the grant programs of the American Federation for Aging Research (AFAR) provide funding to new investigators who need preliminary data to then go on to compete for larger government grants in aging research. Throughout

Table 9.2. Top Illnesses Causing Death

Top 20 Disease Killers	Death rates per 100,000			
	1965	1990	Change 1965-1990	Lives Saved (000)
Ischemic heart disease	309.4	195.1	114.3	285.1
Malignancies (all types)	153.5	201.7	-48.2	-120.2
Cerebrovascular diseases	103.7	57.9	45.8	114.2
Influenza and pneumonia	31.9	31.3	0.6	1.5
Early infancy diseases	28.6	7.0	21.6	53.9
Hypertensive heart disease	28.4	9.4	19.0	47.4
Arteriosclerosis	19.7	3.6	16.1	40.2
Diabetes mellitus	17.1	19.5	-2.4	-6.0
Other heart diseases	15.1	77.1	-62.0	-154.6
Other cardiovascular diseases	14.1	9.7	4.4	11.0
Cirrhosis of the liver	12.8	10.2	2.6	6.5
Ill-defined symptoms	12.1	10.5	1.6	4.0
Congenital anomalies	10.1	5.3	4.8	12.0
Emphysema	9.6	6.6	3.0	7.5
Active rheumatic fever	8.0	2.5	5.5	13.7
Chronic diseases of the endocardium	6.6	4.9	1.7	4.2
Nephritis and nephrosis	6.2	8.3	-2.1	-5.2
Hypertension	6.0	3.7	2.3	5.7
Peptic ulcer	5.4	2.5	2.9	7.2
Hernia and intestinal obstruction	5.2	2.2	3.0	7.5
Total	803.5	669.0	134.5	335.4
Total other diseases*	74.6	133.1	-58.6	-146.0
Population (100,000)	1935.0	2494.0		

* Does not include deaths from accidents, suicides and homicides; 1965 is an extrapolated figure.
Sources: Statistical Abstracts of United States, BCG analysis.
If the U.S. population experienced 1965 death rates today, there would be 335,000 additional deaths per year from the top 20 killers of 1965.

the 1980s and 90s, these programs have grown significantly, raising their total grant-making by more than 1,000 percent.

Several other private and corporate foundations have played pivotal roles in building the private "pot" for aging research. For example, the John A. Hartford Foundation recently committed more than $8 million to establish the Paul Beeson Physician Faculty Scholars Program in Aging Research. The Beeson Program will recognize 30 junior faculty over the next three years and form a core of elite academic geriatricians, ready to train our nation's medical students in the complexities of aging-dependent diseases and conditions. The Commonwealth Fund and donors to the Alliance for Aging Research have contributed an additional $6 million to the Beeson Program, making it the largest aging research scholarship in the nation.

In other, no less important areas, the Glenn Foundation for Medical Research, the Ambrose Monell Foundation and The Starr Foundation, and corporate supporters like Goldman, Sachs & Co. and AlliedSignal Foundation, Inc., have provided significant funds for the field.

While the corporate and private foundation sector has begun to recognize the importance of aging research, there is a great deal more it can do. For example, just as the NIA can only support one-quarter of the qualified applicants in its annual pool, the Brookdale Foundation and AFAR report that they can only support one-fifth of the excellent proposals they receive. Clearly, additional funds would deepen the numbers of people working in the field considerably.

In general, private sector monies—while smaller in absolute terms than those allocated by government and industry—have important long-term effects. First, they can point grant support toward innovative, burgeoning aspects of research that may not attract government or industry support, but that may eventually yield important results. Second, and perhaps most importantly, these funds can provide critical incentives for new investigators to consider and pursue careers in aging research. Often, a seed grant of $30,000 or $40,000 can transform a recent Ph.D. into a scientist who spends three to four decades in pursuit of the scientific information needed to prevent, delay, or even cure what today is an intractable, aging-dependent condition. These are modest investments, well worth taking.

Summary

Dramatic breakthroughs in the private sector must continue if the nation aims to delay, prevent and cure the illnesses of old age. The federal government can encourage these developments by providing private industry with incentives for innovation.

The United States is second to none in the development of new medical treatments, devices and core technologies. To maintain that status, a favorable economic climate is needed for greater research and development in aging-related diseases.

Implementing the Delay Strategy: Policy Recommendations

Treating dependency and disability in older Americans is exacting high financial and human costs on the elderly, on their families, and on both public and private institutions. To date, our nations response to mounting health bills is to add more money for "sick care" and try to figure out who will pay the bills and how. A different approach is seeking ways of preventing these bills.

The most promising remedy is biomedical and behavioral research to delay the diseases and conditions of aging, enhance the independence of older Americans and slow rising health care costs. As policymakers grapple with health care costs and other mounting pressures of a far larger number of older Americans, they should demand new answers from science. With a vigorous research effort in the public and private sectors, embued with the goal of delaying chronic aging-related disease, the U.S. can lead the way to enrich the universal human experience of aging.

Postponing the diseases and conditions of aging must be pursued on several fronts.

A Greater National Commitment to Aging Research

"The federal government should move aggressively to contain costs and mitigate human suffering by funding a research and development program aimed at preventing, delaying and dealing with long-term illnesses and disabilities."

—Final Report of The Pepper Commission 1990

Today, our nations research and development investment in aging research is seriously underfunded. Only a fraction of what the nation devotes to health care is spent on research into human aging. According to recommendations by the U.S. Bipartisan Commission on Comprehensive Health Care ("The Pepper Commission") in 1990, a $1 billion annual research investment is warranted. In 1991, the Institute of Medicine suggested a $913 million annual investment in aging research, along with a one-time construction expenditure of $110 million. The Federal Task Force on Aging Research (TFAR), in its 1995 report, *Threshold of Discovery: Future Directions for Aging Research*, recommends that $ 1.1 billion in the next five years be spent over and above the $841 million currently spent annually on aging research by the Department of Health and Human Services and the Department of VA.

The funds from such an expanded research effort should be applied to aging research at the NIH, the VA and other federal agencies involved in research, which will increase independence for older Americans. As the focal point for aging research at the NIH, the NIA should receive the majority of new funds earmarked for aging research. Other institutes and centers under the direction of the Public Health Service should receive increased funding in proportion to their current spending levels on aging research.

Encouraging Development of New Therapies by the Private Sector

Realizing the very best that research has to offer will require nurturing the current structure of basic research so it can be translated into innovative clinical therapies. A vigorous technology transfer is critical if the breakthroughs of the laboratory are to be transformed into new pharmaceuticals, biotechnology-related therapies, behavioral interventions, medical technologies and better means of disease prevention.

A New Commitment to Geriatric Training

There is currently a shortage of trained geriatricians to meet the needs of the growing number of elderly Americans. The 33.6 million Americans who are 65 and older make up 13 percent of the population, but account for 44 percent of all days spent in the hospital, 40 percent of all visits to internists, and more than one-third of the nation's health care expenditures. Yet only 13 of America's 126 medical schools require either a course or a clinical rotation in geriatrics, and fewer than 4 percent of medical students take an elective course in geriatrics during medical school. As a result, only a small fraction of the more than 550,000 physicians in this country are trained to meet the special needs of older patients.

One promising new private-sector initiative is the $14.3 million Paul Beeson Physician Faculty Scholars in Aging Research program.

This program will support outstanding junior faculty committed to careers in geriatric teaching and practice.

But Congress, too, must increase training opportunities in geriatric medicine nationwide, so that health care professionals can diagnose the health problems of the elderly more effectively, ensure the most appropriate and efficient treatments, extend seniors' independence as long as possible and, by their specialized care, achieve cost savings.

The government should also standardize reimbursement for and support the use of geriatric assessments, to help determine appropriate health care and social services for seniors. Geriatric assessments are conducted by a multidisciplinary team which may include a doctor, a nurse, a physical therapist, an occupational therapist and a social worker, among others. Together they perform a thorough exam to assess the patient's physical and mental health, family life, income, living arrangements, access to community services and ability to perform daily tasks.

A New Commitment to Delaying Aging

The federal government should move aggressively to contain costs and mitigate human suffering by funding a strategic research and development program aimed at delaying long-term illnesses and disabilities that affect the elderly.

This effort should also examine the best treatments for these conditions once they do strike, and include research on outcome measures and national practice guidelines for long-term care.

Unfortunately, impediments can arise to block the progress of any new initiative. Different groups performing aging research within the federal government may have different agendas for and perspectives on unlocking the secrets of aging and may not coalesce behind a "delay" strategy. Public and private funding for aging research has plateaued in recent years and may decline in the future. Without a renewed national commitment to advancing aging research, the delay strategy, with its tremendous potential for cost savings, may itself be delayed or, worse, abandoned.

Conclusion

The United States is at a crossroads. We can choose to make an increased investment in finding new ways to prevent, cure, treat and delay aging-related illnesses today or we can choose to wait and pay later for an unparalleled increase in the cost of caring for our oldest citizens.

We must do better if this country is truly committed to improving the quality of health care. If Congress does not act to reverse the decline in NIH funding, we risk losing many opportunities in the quest to find cures and prevention for debilitating, aging-related diseases.

Aging research helps all Americans. By shedding light on the basic aging process, demonstrating the difference between normal aging and disease and developing ways to slow deterioration in various body systems, researchers in aging can help us add years to our lives and quality to those years.

Most importantly, aging research yields information that can prevent or postpone health problems. Research and innovation remain our best, most cost effective way to stop or slow the incidence of our toughest health challenges—chronic conditions such as Alzheimer's disease, arthritis and stroke.

Research breakthroughs in aging will offer new hope for many older Americans who would otherwise be dependent on others for care. Delaying the diseases and conditions of aging is a new approach, and it has huge potential. Excellent efforts are already underway to learn the best ways of spotting those at risk for these health problems, and postponing their predicament. These and other high-quality efforts merit the nations strongest support.

Footnotes

1. *Strategies to Delay Dysfunction in Later Life*, Springer Publishing Company, New York, New York, 1995, J.A. Brody and R.N. Butler, editors.

2. AARP Bulletin, January 1995.

3. *LIFESPAN: Who Lives Longer—And Why*. Thomas J. Moore. Simon & Schuster, New York, New York, 1993.

4. *Journal of the American Medical Association*, Volume 263, Number 17, May 2, 1990, pp. 2335-2340.

5. In a letter to the National Health Council.

6. *Extending life, Enhancing Life: A National Research Agenda on Aging*, National Academy Press, Washington, DC, 1991.

9. *How Healthcare Reform Affects Pharmaceutical Research and Development*, June 1994.

10. From materials issued by the National Health Council.

Chapter 10

Aging Well

Americans are living longer and their transition into the ranks of old age will not simply be a matter of greater numbers and higher proportions of older Americans living within the policies, institutions, and economic and social contexts of today. The average age of the U.S. population has been increasing throughout this century. A 1997 longevity and retirement study revealed that 41 percent of people now working feel it is at least somewhat likely that they will live to age 85, 23 percent feel somewhat likely they will live to age 90, and even 15 percent feel it is at least somewhat likely they will live to age 95. America is on the brink of massive social change.

As we approach the 21st century, these demographic realities require all Americans to take stock of what an aging America means to them. Policymakers at all levels need to ensure that there are resources, programs and policies in place to provide much-needed support and information for an increasingly older population. Also, it is critical for each American to understand the importance of comprehensive planning for their own longevity.

Many people view aging with both optimism and worry. This need not be the case. The keys to enjoying later life are understanding and planning for what lies ahead. It is never too early or too late to begin. Aging well and leading a quality life depends on much more than what an individual has in the bank, although that is certainly an important consideration. It is also dictated in great part by personal

U.S. Department of Health and Human Services, Administration on Aging, April 1998.

health and well-being as well as lifestyle issues such as housing, leisure activities, volunteerism and life-long learning.

It is important for all Americans to understand that today's choices do have consequences in later life. Leading a quality life as Americans grow older is actually a three-legged stool that, if left unbalanced, will topple over and leave the individual open to negative consequences that can affect their whole sense of well-being. Health, financial and lifestyle choices can enhance the quality of an individual's later years.

Financial

Adequate income and assets are of critical importance to virtually all dimensions of well-being in later life. Experts estimate that retirees will need, on average, 70 percent of their pre-retirement income, lower earners, 90 percent, or more to maintain their standard of living when they stop working. Social Security pays the average retiree about 40 percent of pre-retirement earnings if you retire at age 65. How well you understand your options for managing money and how well you have planned will be the most critical factors in determining your financial well-being as you grow older.

Health

Great improvements in medicine, science and technology have enabled today's older Americans to live longer and healthier lives than any previous generation. Yet, many Americans fail to make the connection between undertaking healthy behaviors today and the impact of these choices later in life. Research has established that there are distinct advantages to physical exercise, both aerobic and weight-bearing. Individuals should design a program which is right for them. Moreover, screening programs can lead to preventive measures, and early treatment interventions that can substantially reduce the impact of illnesses among older people. Just as important is diet. Nutritional status influences the progress of many diseases, and studies have shown that good nutritional status can reduce length of hospital stay.

Lifestyle

Living quality lives as Americans grow older is defined almost entirely by individual financial planning followed by some level of acknowledgment of good health practices, but other lifestyle issues are rarely included in discussions related to longevity. Lifelong learning, volunteerism, caregiving, leisure pursuits, second and third careers, and transportation involve issues which routinely impact on the lives of many Americans. However, most people do not readily identify that decisions made in these areas are an integral part of preparing for their future.

Americans should understand the importance of planning for later life. By gathering information and developing strategies to ensure the best quality of life possible, individuals can ensure that as they live longer, they are also growing stronger.

As the leading advocate for older people and their families at the federal level, the Administration on Aging (AoA) is concerned with the issues facing current and future older Americans. Our advocacy efforts for the rest of this century and into the next millennium will include working to promote the concepts of self-preparation and personal responsibility with regard to aging well.

Chapter 11

Extended Life Spans

It won't be long before life-spans of 120, 150, or even 200 years are possible. Both individuals and society need to plan for the consequences.

In the summer of 1995, several popular books told readers of a remarkable advance in the study of aging. A hormone called melatonin, they proclaimed, might have the power to hold time itself at bay. Mice receiving this natural, harmless substance survived to the human equivalent of 115 years. To the end of their very long lives, the mice retained all the health and vigor of youth. Just conceivably, people who used melatonin also might live far beyond their allotted span without ever growing old.

A furor greeted this announcement. Scientists debated the hormone's effects and squabbled about who deserved credit for the discovery of its age-fighting power. Doctors warned that melatonin might cause unknown harm. Skeptics denied that the results of experiments in mice could be applied to human beings. And in the United States, where melatonin is readily available, tens of thousands of ordinary people began to use this latest miracle drug. Some merely wanted a good night's sleep, for melatonin is a powerful sedative. Many others dreamed of taking a first step toward immortality.

Yet amid the hope and controversy, the true significance of this research was overlooked. What matters is not whether melatonin

Reprinted with permission from *The Futurist*, April 1998 v32 n3 p17(7). © 1998 World Future Society.

itself extends human life. It may well not. But discoveries related to melatonin have given scientists their first handle on aging. For decades, they struggled to figure out why we grow old. Now they can concentrate on developing a cure. And because the cause of aging has turned out to be relatively simple—a pinpoint failure in one biological system, rather than a general "wearing out"—a successful treatment should be much easier to find than, for example, the proverbial cure for cancer.

And if melatonin seems to be a pivotal clue to the nature of aging, it is not the only lead that scientists have discovered in the last few years. Many others stem from genetic engineering, and the Human Genome Project now promises to reveal every detail of our biology, including the mechanisms by which we grow old and die. Even if melatonin itself is not the final answer, it is clear that research has at last built up a critical mass of information about aging. Today's discoveries almost inevitably will trigger, further breakthroughs in our understanding of senescence. After millennia of dreams and decades of hard work, it has at last become reasonable to believe that a practical remedy for aging is not far off.

This presents important problems. Individuals need to start planning for the additional decades of life that they suddenly can expect. Nations must figure out how to support extra generations of healthy, vigorous, but chronologically ancient people who have no established role in society. The world as a whole must find ways to share the benefits of aging research without undermining less flexible cultures or overcrowding our fragile planet. These and many other challenges could require answers in the next five years and almost surely will demand them in less than 20.

What Causes Aging? What Prevents It?

As a technical problem, aging is one of the most complex and elusive phenomena that scientists have ever studied. As early as World War I, Nobel Prize-winning physician Alexis Carrel observed that the wounds of older patients healed more slowly than those of the young. In the following years, he and his colleague P. Lecomte du Nouy discovered that some element in blood plasma caused the difference. Yet, whether healing was promoted by a factor in the blood of the young or delayed by something in the blood of the old, they never were able to learn. It was the first of many such puzzles.

A few years later, Clive McCay of Cornell University found that putting rats on a diet that was nutritious but so low in calories that it could barely sustain life dramatically extended their survival. In one typical study, rats that ordinarily live for only 600 days survived to an average age of 1,100 days, and some reached 1,800 days. Hundreds of scientists have confirmed this phenomenon in many different species.

These extreme calorie-restricted diets confer other benefits as well. Mice and rats are prone to all the diseases that afflict aging men and women. However, when scientists cut their calorie intake by 30% to 50%, animals rarely become ill. Several years ago, scientists at Philadelphia's Institute for Cancer Research studied a kind of rat that always suffers from diseases of the heart, kidney, lung, and prostate, as well as several forms of cancer. When placed on a strict diet, only one animal in 10 developed cancer. Just 2% suffered heart problems. None had kidney disease. Again, scientists have seen much the same reduction in disease in many different species.

In more than 70 years of careful work, no one has ever been able to explain how calorie restriction works its miracles. The trouble is that aging changes almost every aspect of the body's workings. Hormone levels, blood proteins, energy production, genetic activity—all these factors and many more vary with time, and there is no way to tell which might cause us to grow biologically "old" and which is merely an effect of aging. Scientists have proposed nearly 50 distinct theories to account for these observations. Experiments based on many of them have delayed the symptoms of aging, improved health, and extended the lives of laboratory animals.

For instance, hematologist W. Donner Denkla of the National Institutes of Health studied the possibility that an unknown "death hormone" caused aging by shutting down energy production in the cell. To test this idea, he took aged rats and carefully removed their pituitary gland, the presumed source of the fatal hormone. Those animals grew younger, lived longer, and rarely showed any sign of disease. "We were never able to identify the cause of death," says Denkla. "They appeared to be in perfect health right up to the end."

Although such results have puzzled biologists for decades, the explanation turns out to be simple. Many of the changes wrought by time weaken the body and thereby promote further decay. Thus, preventing any of them slows the cumulative erosion that we know as growing old. However, all the early theories of aging, such as Denkla's "death hormone," dealt with secondary factors. Hidden behind them, there lies a more fundamental source of aging.

This root cause has now been identified.

A Crucial Breakthrough

In the mid-1980s, Walter Pierpaoli, a medical researcher trained in immunology and endocrinology and the founder of the Institute for Integrative Biomedical Research in Switzerland, had grown increasingly interested in the role of an obscure hormone called melatonin.

Though little known then outside a small research community, melatonin already had proved to be remarkably versatile. Melatonin floods our bloodstream in childhood. When our supply wanes, we enter puberty. This is more than coincidence. Melatonin actively restrains sexual maturation until our bodies are well developed enough to support reproduction. Melatonin levels also vary on a daily cycle, rising in the evening and falling toward morning; this governs our sleep patterns, hormone levels, and many other basic bodily functions.

Pierpaoli and other scientists found that melatonin also bolsters our defenses against disease. As he pondered what he knew about this hormone, Pierpaoli found an intriguing connection: Melatonin seemed uniquely involved with time. It controlled maturation. It regulated our daily cycle. It was needed for many of the functions that decline as we grow old. Might it somehow govern aging itself?

He tested this notion by giving mice doses of melatonin each night, when their natural supply was at its peak. The animals lived much longer than normal. It was his public announcement of this discovery, in a best-seller entitled *The Melatonin Miracle* (Simon & Schuster, 1995), that triggered the current wave of interest in this hormone.

Subsequent studies proved even more revealing. Pierpaoli then turned to the gland that manufactures melatonin. Known as the pineal, it is a small structure, about the size and shape of a kidney bean, located deep within the brain. Since the late 1980s, Pierpaoli and his colleagues have been transplanting pineals between mice. They removed the pineals from old mice and replaced them with glands from young animals. This is an enormously delicate, stressful operation, and one-fourth of the mice died in surgery. Yet the survivors enjoyed longer lives than even melatonin could provide, the human equivalent of 125 years. (This suggests that, while melatonin is important in aging, it is not the only substance whose loss contributes to growing old. Some other pineal factor, yet unidentified, may also be involved.) As surgical techniques improve, Pierpaoli's mice are living longer. In his most recent experiments, old mice given young pineals have survived to the equivalent of 140 years—approximately double their natural span.

Even if melatonin itself turns out not to extend human lives, the lessons from this decade-plus of painstaking work are clear: Aging begins in the pineal, with a specific change that disrupts the daily cycle of melatonin and perhaps other hormones. Now that scientists know where to look, they can find that change and prevent it, fix it, or compensate for it. And once science can chart its way to new knowledge, the discovery is sure to follow. If practical human life extension has not arrived already, it lies only a few years off.

There is a good chance that longer lives will also bring better health: Pierpaoli's mice rarely fall ill. Instead, they appear young and healthy to the end of their lives, then die with no warning or obvious cause. When science does extend our lives, we may no longer have to fear a long, painful death from cancer, heart disease, emphysema, or any of the other disorders that now routinely strike us down as we age.

There is one more implication here as well. If we live, for instance, 40 years longer than nature would have allowed, as some scientists think possible, then we have four more decades in which science can seek to extend our lives still further. Before the baby-boom generation reaches 115 or 120, new treatments very likely will push death back to age 150 or 200, or even into the indefinite future. The world may not be literally postmortal, but our deaths are not likely to arrive on schedule.

Impacts of "Agelessness" On Society

Extended life-spans are likely to produce significant economic impacts, even an end to retirement as we know it. In the United States, Social Security already is in trouble. Contrary to popular belief, we do not live out our retirement years on the money that we and our employers contributed to the Social Security pension fund while we were still on the job. All that we put into the system is exhausted within a few years. Instead, we live on the contributions of those still in the work force, as they in turn will exist on the generosity of workers yet unborn. This system functioned well at first, because relatively few people lived for more than a year or two after they became full-time consumers. Age 65 was chosen as the retirement age specifically for that reason. In the 1880s, when Otto von Bismarck established a pension system for employees of the German government, only one worker in 20 survived long enough to collect his first payment. In the 1930s, there were five American workers to support each retiree. Today, there are only two, and as medicine stretches our average lifespan, the number continues to decline. By 2030, under current rules, the Social Security system will be bankrupt. Some estimates place the date as early as 2012.

Other countries face similar predicaments. Italy, saddled with what is widely regarded as the most unstable pension system in the world, is finding it difficult to support its retirees. Even in wealthy Japan, planners worry about how their retirement system will fare as modern health care has stretched life expectancies for the current generation to 80 years. In Russia, pensions seldom are enough to pay for a small apartment, utilities, and a livable diet. Often, pensions do not arrive at all. In any city, hungry retirees can be seen at informal bazaars trying to sell handicrafts, surplus furniture, even their old clothes in order to buy food. Throughout much of the developed world, the elderly could face a future as bleak as Russia's present if they must depend on government pensions to support their old age.

Life extension can only make the prospect of retirement more daunting still. No social security program in the world, and few private pension plans, can provide for the needs of pure consumers who can expect to live to the age of 115 or 120. We find it difficult to envision any traditional system of retirement that could cope with lives so prolonged as those the baby-boom generation and its heirs are likely to enjoy.

Almost inevitably, this means that most baby boomers are unlikely to retire by age 65. They may never be able to retire completely. Instead, they will remain in the job market or, if the anti-aging revolution is delayed slightly longer than we expect, will return to it. They will compete for jobs with younger workers, and by remaining in place for years beyond their original time of retirement, they will make it difficult or impossible for their successors to move from entry-level jobs into positions of authority.

Impacts on Business

Certain businesses will be particularly affected by the transition to extended life. For example, the longer people remain healthy and active, the larger the market for sports equipment and clothing. And if older people can make do with part-time employment, many of them are likely to travel, bringing new growth to the hospitality industry. On the other hand, how many people will feel the need for life and health insurance if they can expect to live far beyond their natural span with little fear of major illness?

Life extension will transform one industry above all: health care. In the late 1990s, hospitals, clinics, medical laboratories, and related services represent fully 14% of the U.S. economy. Health care employs some 10.4 million Americans and pays out more than $283 billion per year in salaries. It is one of the fastest-growing industries in the national economy. As of 1994, the most recent year for which final results are available, health care grew by 12.5%, behind space commerce (a much smaller industry), data processing, and electronic information services. Most observers believe that this remarkable growth will continue, thanks in large part to the fact that people are now living longer—into the years when they become subject to chronic illness and require more care.

But this rapid growth is unlikely to continue. Fully half of the money now devoted to health care in the United States is spent during the last six months of the patient's life, combating illnesses that doctor and victim alike know will prove terminal. As healthy life-spans stretch out, any final decline almost surely will be compressed from months or years to weeks. Very possibly, like Denkla's rats, we will simply pass out of life without warning or obvious cause, in good health to the last—and demanding little health care.

True, we will continue to suffer broken legs, colds, auto accidents, and life's other random afflictions. Hereditary diseases will take their toll, at least until genetic research eliminates them. But these will not make up for the removal of heart disease, cancer, diabetes, arthritis, and the many other "markets" for health care that could all but disappear with successful anti-aging therapy. Hundreds of thousands of health-related jobs now expected to appear in the coming decades will never arrive. Hundreds of thousands of the jobs that now exist could vanish in the next 15 years. The effects will ripple throughout the economy. Unemployment will rise. Wages will fall. Canada, Europe, and Japan face much the same economic shock as will occur in the United States. Thus, growth will slow around the world. It could be many years before the global economy expands enough to give its unexpectedly large population the standard of living it once enjoyed.

Living Well While Living Longer

The key to financial survival for life-extended boomers will be a kind of flexibility the World War II generation never needed. The best job for you is not the one with the highest salary or richest benefits, but the one that offers the best chance to broaden your skills. It may be within the same company, in which case you will have to apply for it just like any outsider. It may be with the competition, or in a different industry altogether. Or it may be whatever make-do job will keep you afloat while you take graduate-level courses or professional training. No option can be overlooked. No plan can go unrevised whenever an opportunity beckons or a new idea dawns.

Here are the rules for coping with extended longevity:

- Give up the notion of a traditional retirement at or before age 65. Unless your economic position is rock-solid, you could eventually be forced back to work. And it turns out that the penalty for a few years of retirement is much too severe. Economist Charles Brown of the University of Michigan once surveyed a group of men who had taken early retirement and then returned to work. Most were skilled white-collar workers, and none was older than 63 when these men went job-hunting. Yet they had been forced to accept pay cuts that averaged 40% of their previous salaries. Better to remain on the job, if possible, until you are absolutely certain that you will never have to return.

  There are alternatives, however. You may decide to start your own business; "retire" to a farm like the one you grew up on and work 60 hours a week for yourself instead of 40 or so for someone else; become a teacher and pass your hard-won skills on to a new generation. Or you may find, just before you qualify for one of those rare pensions, that your longtime employer no longer needs you and you have no choice but to scramble for a living at an age when you hoped leisure would be at hand. What you are not likely to do is play golf and putter around the house.

- If you are not already saving for the future, it is long past time to begin. If you are saving, then try to save more. Financial planners advise that everyone should have savings equal to a year's living expenses before he or she even begins to worry about a retirement fund. Even in today's tight job market, it can take that long for a displaced executive to find another position. Sickness, legal problems, or other unforeseen costs can easily drain the equivalent of a year's salary.

  Now let's set a reasonable savings target. Assume that you will manage to invest your "retirement" nest egg wisely enough so that you can eventually siphon off 10% per year for living expenses without touching the principal. (Few achieve even that level of profit, year in and year out, good times and bad.) In that case, you need to save 10 times as much in investment capital as you hope to spend each year. If your family income is $60,000—a fairly modest sum these days—and you want a post-career income equal to 80% of that, you will need to save up $480,000 to meet your goal. Bank fully 25% of your current income, and it still will take you 32 years to build your retirement fund! With a bit of luck, investment profits could speed the process, but figure on at least 20 years of scrimping before you can begin to collect your reward. Even that is unlikely to support the kind of retirement that you probably hoped for—you will have to pay your own way for many years longer than previous generations did—but at least it is a start.

Here are some other suggestions. No one of them will offer a complete solution for your circumstances and goals. Yet most of these prescriptions apply to everyone. Some combination of them should see you through.

• Keep learning. It does not matter how secure your current job or business appears to be. As the twenty-first century ticks away, the number of people seeking a living will grow much faster than the economy. Competition for every niche will tighten for the next 40 years, as the baby boomers vie with their children and grandchildren for a place in the job market. The only way to survive is to remain on the cutting edge in your core specialty and to build ancillary skills to supplement it. It is not enough to be a competent accountant; you also need experience in marketing, manufacturing, team management, and many similar fields. The most successful salesman will have to master the other skills of running a business. Even artists and writers, whose unique personal vision differentiates them from their competition, will have to be proficient at public speaking, the use of graphics and layout software, and Web-page design, just for a start. In any field, constant training is the only way to compete.

Learning is even more important for those who lack a well-paid career and work instead in the blue-collar fields. The most recent employment projections from the Bureau of Labor Statistics extend only to 2005, but they show trends that will continue for many years to come. Manufacturing jobs have vanished by the millions over the last 20 years; another 12% of the remainder will have disappeared in the decade ending in 2005. Professional specialty jobs are the fastest-growing group and also will add the most new jobs during the period, some 5 million in all. Job growth will be over 14% in all categories that require an associate's degree or better, but less than 14% in any category open to someone with only a high-school diploma. Jobs that demand a master's degree or doctorate will grow by 29%. Fields requiring a year or less of on-the-job training will grow by only 5%, the slowest of any category.

At the same time, too many schools have not been doing their job. Though U.S. educational performance is finally improving, dropout rates remain at about 25% overall, and only half of high-school graduates go on to college. Thus three-fourths of the people entering the job market in the coming years will be looking for work in the slowest-growing fields. In short, the competition for tomorrow's jobs will be greatest exactly where opportunities are hardest to find. A poor general education and the lack of marketable job skills will guarantee a life of poverty and frustration. The only way for today's blue-collar workers to find even minimal security is to train for a new career in the white-collar world. Tomorrow morning would not be too soon to begin.

- Cultivate multiple revenue sources. Even when you have a solid career, secondary income can come in handy. One software designer we know is a part-time woodworker. For him, the tactile experience of wielding century-old hand tools on rich wood surfaces provides a welcome break from the abstractions of his high-pressure workplace. The hobby also produces classic New England furniture that sells well to tourists in the shops of his New Hampshire hometown. His wife, a medical secretary, also writes for the local newspaper. If either of them loses his or her job, this secondary income will cushion the blow. Until then, the profits— nearly $10,000 in an average year—are divided between their daughter's college fund and their investment portfolio. Neither of them is covered by a pension plan, and neither intends to retire. But 20 years from now, they expect to leave their primary occupations and pursue woodworking and writing full time. Unlike full retirement, it is a goal they should have no trouble accomplishing.

- Consider self-employment. For many executives displaced late in their careers, building their own business has proved the only way to keep going. However difficult the transition, they have discovered the advantages of taking their livelihood into their hands. Chief among them: The only boss who can never fire you without warning looks back at you from the mirror.

An acquaintance of ours spent almost 30 years testing small computers, working in the same laboratory while his division passed repeatedly from one corporate owner to another. Eventually, the latest owner closed the test lab, and he and his colleagues found themselves on the street. Now he consults part time for his erstwhile co-workers, who bought their former employer's equipment and set up their own testing service. He and his wife also purchased a coffee-and-bagel shop in their hometown. He gets up at 4:00 a.m. each day to pick up fresh bagels from a specialty baker. She abandoned a long string of dead-end secretarial jobs to run the operation. Of self-employment, he comments ironically: "We have more money now than we ever did, but neither of us has time to spend it." Being unable to retire does not disappoint him, however. He was raised on a Maine potato farm, where his 90-year-old father still puts in a full day's work. To him, the idea of complete leisure never seemed entirely real. As it turns out, he was right.

- Plan to retire in stages, and perhaps earlier than we have advised. Although retirement at 65 seems a lost cause, you eventually may have little choice but to end your career. As the working population explodes and unemployment figures begin to mount, Americans will call on their government to solve the problem. At first, Washington is likely to offer training programs in an attempt to give the jobless career skills that can earn them a living. In the end, it will turn out that there are not enough openings for all who need them. At that point, all those held-over boomers will come under fire. Congress may enact high taxes on the incomes of seniors who work more than, say, 20 hours per week. It might offer incentives for those who leave a full-time career for semi-retirement. Just conceivably, it could find more subtle ways to accomplish its goal. The effect will be to make it easier to leave work, even with a significant loss of income, than to remain on the job. If boomers still dominate the business world, legislation will be the only way to provide opportunities for their juniors.

The way to avoid this, and to have a pleasanter life in the process, is to cut back voluntarily. Whenever you can afford it, forget work weeks that stretch beyond 40 hours and instead work part time. Flexible working schedules are becoming commonplace these days. Well before 2010, most companies will offer job sharing, permitting one part-time employee to split duties with another. Anyone so inclined can use the new hours of freedom to develop a hobby into a small business. Otherwise, partial retirement will prove a valuable transition, inoculating habitual workers against the shock of retiring only to find that they have nothing to do.

- Consider alternative living arrangements. Almost everyone prefers to remain in his or her own home so long as health permits. Yet at both ends of the age spectrum, people are living in multi-generational and group homes at a rate not seen in decades. The reason is money. With real earnings far below those once available to their parents, many workers in their 20s and 30s cannot afford to buy a house or rent an apartment on their own. So they move back in with their parents or band together in shared housing. Many seniors are strapped for cash, despite Social Security, Medicare, and often a pension. So they move in with their offspring. Three-generation households are so common that there even is a magazine dedicated to boomers struggling to cope with having their parents and children underfoot.

Many life-extended boomers will find themselves in the same position. Bereft of pensions, with scant government benefits, and with too little invested, they will find that life is better in comfortable surroundings, even if that means sharing with relatives or strangers. For some boomers, this will be just a return to their youth, when communes and "crash pads" were commonplace. Others will find that the idea takes some getting used to. But simple arithmetic will convince many of tomorrow's long-lived seniors that housing shared is housing they can afford. This is one more option to bear in mind.

To Live Long and Prosper

We will be the first generation to enjoy the benefits of aging research. Because this change is so novel and so unexpected, preparing for extended life will be one of the greatest challenges we ever face. Future generations will know how long a life to plan. They will have developed mechanisms for allocating society's resources among those who need them. But we can only take it on faith that science will deliver what it now so clearly promises. By the time we know for certain that our own lives will be longer than nature intended, many of us will have entered our traditional retirement years, when our preparations for an extended life should be well under way. Society will not yet have adjusted itself to ease our transition.

Given the alternative, most people are likely to feel that extra decades of healthy, vital life are well worth the trouble it will take to make them comfortable and secure. But reshaping our personal futures will be difficult, and the penalty for being unprepared will be long years of poverty and stagnation. Already, it is time to begin.

Issues for a Postmortal World

Like all great liberations, the anti-aging revolution will uproot much of what has gone before. In this case, the change affects the single most important fact of existence. Psychology, government, social expectations—almost everything we believe or do—is based on the understanding that we will grow old and die on nature's schedule. When this ancient truth changes, we can expect dislocations on an epic scale.

In this chapter, we have dealt with only a few of the practical issues most closely related to our everyday lives. Many more questions will require our attention:

- How can we provide a decent living for all who need it?

- How will Third World extremists, who often perceive other lifestyles as an affront to their God, react when rich Westerners not only live in comfort, but live far longer than nature allows?

- How can we control population in a world where death may soon be optional?

- How will life extension affect a global environment that already seems burdened by too many people.

- Above all, what personal and societal values can sustain us through the most profound transition humanity has ever known? Will God be as obsolete as mortality, or will the promise of longer, healthier lives give us more time and incentive to develop our spirituality?

We consider these and other issues at length in *Cheating Death*.

Telomerase Discovery

A breakthrough to stop aging at the chromosome level was announced in January by researchers at the University of Texas Southwestern Medical Center and Genron Corporation. The work involves telomerase, a natural enzyme found in young human cells. The chemical rebuilds telomeres—protective caps on each end of a chromosome that normally shorten after the cell divides. [See "Reversing Human Aging" by Michael Fossel, THE FUTURIST, July-August 1997.]

As adults age, their natural supply of telomerase disappears, so the telomeres grow progressively shorter with each cell division, until the cell dies. What scientists have now done is to resupply older cells with telomerase to see if doing so would restore youthfulness to the cell and extend its life. The technique appears to work.

A potential drawback is that anything that promotes cell division could also promote cancer. At the same time, an understanding of telomerase therapy could show how to stop cancer as well. Researchers are now exploring these possibilities.

—by Marvin Cetron and Owen Davies.

Marvin Cetron is president of Forecasting International Ltd., 3612 Boat Dock Drive, Falls Church, Virginia 22041. Telephone 1-703-379-9033; fax 1-703-379-1999.

Owen Davies is a former senior editor at Omni magazine and is a freelance writer specializing in science, technology, and the future. He lives in New Hampshire.

This article is adapted from their new book *Cheating Death: The Promise and the Future Impact of Trying to Live Forever*, [C] 1998 by Marvin Cetron and Owen Davies. Reprinted by arrangement with St. Martin's Press, Inc.

Part Two

Midlife Issues and the Retirement Years

Chapter 12

Women at Midlife

With the exceptions of investigations of estrogen replacement therapy (ERT), menopause, the "empty nest," and other topics related to a woman's fertility or care of others, women's midlife aging experience has been understudied. The major studies of midlife development have been by male investigators looking at male subjects. The results of these studies, like those of research on heart disease, have been applied to women with the assumption that what was true for the gander was true for the goose. Another source of information for many women searching for understanding about midlife has been popular literature, such as Gail Sheehey's (1992) *The Silent Passage* and Germaine Greer's (1992) *The Change*. Not only were these works not research based, but they focused on menopause, leading to more constructions of a woman's midlife experience that are biologically oriented.

Several other factors limit the value of earlier research. First, the experience of midlife for women is changing rapidly. The generation of women now entering midlife differs from previous generations. Raised "traditionally," they have lived through the historical shift to a feminist self-view in adulthood. They gained control of reproduction, and they are the first generation in which so many have worked outside of the home and built identities based on value in the workplace.

Beyond this, most of the few research studies of women in midlife focus on "problems" women face at midlife (for example, physical changes, children leaving home) and how women "cope" with them.

But midlife is not just about mortality, crumbling bones, and hot flashes. Most studies of mental health implicitly, at least, define "wellness" as not being sick and as an absence of anxiety, depression, or other mental disorders.

New conceptions of psychological well-being emphasize positive characteristics of growth and development, such as caring and trusting ties with others, a purpose in life, self-acceptance, and personal growth. The distinction is not trivial; although mental health research using a psychopathology model has often documented a higher incidence of psychological problems among women than among men, when positive well-being is the focus, women often show higher scores than men (Ryff, 1995). Identifying factors related to a woman's midlife satisfaction can provide a guide for women, as well as goals. The profile of a woman at midlife who feels satisfied with her life provides a role model to any woman who wishes to transcend the negative stereotypes of her culture.

Research into women's midlife experience is clearly needed. From the perspective of the individual woman, the invisibility of women in midlife in the research literature leaves a woman at the mercy of cultural stereotypes and media portrayals, or lack of portrayals. Negative images of aging women abound and, without alternative images, serve to elicit a woman's own internalized ageism and sexism. Images of miserable empty nesters, women being left for younger women, menopausal madness, and dowager's humps can become self-fulfilling prophecies. A woman without alternative models and images may see her future in a limited way.

The lack of positive images of women in midlife affects others as well. For instance, without images to contradict the over-the-hill image of aging women, employers are more likely to pass over these women for employment or promotions. Add age discrimination to sex and color discrimination, and the challenge of having a purposeful vision of the future becomes enormous. Women at midlife, if kept invisible and isolated because their stories are not heard and their experiences are not researched, will be disadvantaged in a competitive labor market.

A need for sociologically and psychologically oriented research on woman at midlife exists. Social workers working with midlife women need to know not only what may aid in the prevention of osteoporosis, but also what factors are associated with midlife psychological well-being and with prevention of the marginality that can result from aging in an ageist, sexist society—a problem that women of all economic strata face.

It is also important for women to have accurate images of what a woman's experience of midlife is. Just what, if anything, do women like about midlife? What do they dislike? What are their stereotypical images of midlife women? What do midlife women see as their strengths and vulnerabilities? The participants in the study discussed in this article were eager to share their experiences and hear what other women were going through. They were eager to construct new images and build new knowledge. Not only will their stories help women struggling in isolation with the emotional, psychological, social, and physical changes that they feel no one talks about, they will help women enter the next stage of adulthood in a more confident, validated way.

Literature Review

The most influential theorists in conceptualizing midlife transitions have been Jung, Jaques (who coined the term "midlife crisis"), Erikson, Vaillant, and Levinson—all men writing about men. Their writings suggest that midlife satisfaction is related to having a sense of generativity and giving to future generations (Erikson, 1950); to being able to accept one's age, find meaning and purpose, and not yearn for the activities of youth (Jung, 1933/1983); to having resolved the fear of death (Jaques, 1965); to loosening up and seizing one more chance of rebirth (Vaillant, 1977); and to forming a realistic picture of oneself and the world (Levinson, 1978).

The theoretical and empirical literature focusing specifically on the midlife experiences of women is much thinner. Heilbrun (1988) contended that meaningful work is critical to a woman's well-being as she ages. Apter (1995), one of the few scholars to examine the actual experience of midlife women, found the greatest challenge for a woman was integrating the images formed in adolescence of being female with that of being a woman in midlife. In addition, she found that a woman's most important insight was that she could at last listen to her own voice.

The literature on resilience and on coping with stress also provides potential insights into factors that might be associated with successful passage through midlife. Pearlin and Schooler (1978) pointed to a correlation between coping well and low self-denigration, high self-esteem, and high self-effectance. Self-in-relation theorists (Miller, 1976) emphasized the importance to a woman's identity of having connections with others. Other researchers have identified the importance of a friendship network and a confidante to women's emotional health (Baruch & Brooks-Gunn, 1984). Studies of temperament indicate that certain traits are stable and consistent over the life cycle. The existence of temperamental traits associated with resilience and vulnerability (Wolin & Wolin, 1993) suggests that personality factors contribute to women's midlife satisfaction.

Hypotheses

The theoretical suggestions discussed, as well as clinical experience with a large number of midlife women, led me to make several hypotheses about psychological sources of well-being in midlife for women (see McQuaide, 1996a). I hypothesized that a woman who was experiencing midlife (defined as ages 40 to 60) as a period of well-being would be more likely:

- to have the ability to grieve and let go of the past

- to have the ability to construct a new midlife self

- to believe in a protective, spiritual force outside of her self

- to have the ability to find purpose and meaning in her life and to have a vision for the future

- to believe that she has a right to a life and is not obligated to a life of self-sacrifice

- to be accepting of herself, self-forgiving, and have a benign (not harsh) superego

- to be accepting of her own body.

This chapter describes the results of a research study testing these hypotheses and identifying the demographic, situational, and psychological factors associated with midlife well-being for women.

Method

A questionnaire on attitudes, beliefs, and feelings about midlife was distributed by mail to midlife respondents recruited through posters in doctors' offices and university buildings, announcements in organizational bulletins, and advertisements in local newspapers; 103 women, ranging in age from 40 to 59, completed the survey. All of the women were white and lived in the New York City area. Detailed characteristics of the sample are given in Table 12.1.

The questionnaire had three parts. First, respondents were asked to describe their current psychological state in several ways: They were asked to rate themselves on a five-point Likert-type scale with regard to how happy or unhappy they were feeling at this time in their life, whether they were having an easy or difficult time coping, and whether they were finding this time in their life confusing or not. They were also asked to give themselves a grade from A (excellent) to F (very poor) in terms of 17 areas of life: having friends, dealing with fear and anxiety, dealing with depression, dealing with anger, dealing with guilt, family relationships, job and career, spirituality, intimacy, money management, creativity, leisure time, finding satisfaction, finding contentment, self-acceptance, acceptance of their body, and coping with this stage of life. The scores on the 17 areas were summed to provide an average grade or index of well-being reflecting their overall rating of themselves at this time in their life. Finally they were asked to indicate the current and recent sources of stress in their lives.

Second, the women were asked to indicate their level of agreement with 122 statements about themselves, using a five-point Likert-type scale, ranging from 1=strongly agree to 5=strongly disagree. Over half of the items made up 10 scales designed to measure the various psychological constructs that I had hypothesized would be relevant to midlife well-being. These included self-esteem, lack of self-denigration, self-effectance, optimism, the ability to grieve, the belief that one has a right to a life, having a vision or goal and a sense of meaning in one's life, being aware of constructing a new identity in midlife, having a positive narrative about one's life, and having a benign (not overly harsh) superego. Additional scales measured such issues as the women's sense of their own spirituality, their feelings about their own appearance, the degree to which they felt marginal, whether or not they had positive images of midlife, feelings about their sex life, and feelings about their ability to manage their finances. I developed the scales on a rational-empirical basis. For each construct, a number of items were written that, on their face, appeared to reflect that construct. (The items for the initial self-esteem, self-denigration, and self-effectance scales were derived from those presented in Pearlin & Schooler, 1978.) After gathering data on 50 women, the responses to the items provisionally making up each scale were factor analyzed. Items were then eliminated so the remaining items on each scale constituted a monofactorial scale, with all items having loadings of at least 0.60 on a single factor.

Third, the questionnaire contained a series of qualitative questions. The participants were asked what they liked and disliked about

Table 12.1. Characteristics of the Sample

Characteristic	%
Health	
Good or excellent	94.1
Other categories	5.9
Menopausal status	
Postmenopausal	44.3
Premenopausal	55.7
Education	
Four years of college	58.3
Less than four years of college	33.0
High school	8.7
Marital status	
Married	67.6
Living with significant other	6.7
Separated or divorced	18.6
Widowed	1.0
Single	5.9
Family income ($)	
<30,000	9.1
30,000-49,999	18.4
50,000-99,999	41.8
$\geq$ 100,000	30.6
Reported sexual orientation	
Heterosexual	97.1
Homosexual or bisexual	2.9
Labor force status	
Full-time paid employment	59.4
Part-time paid employment	20.8
Homemaker	6.9
Student	4.0
Disabled, unemployed, or involuntarily retired	8.9
Occupational status[a]	
Managerial, professional, and technical	67.7
Skilled or semiskilled blue-collar	6.3
Clerical, sales, or other white-collar	26.0
Family responsibilities	
Taking care of own or spouse's parents	11.9
Children still living at home	35.0
Attitude toward feminism	
Describe self as a feminist	17.6
Describe self as a "traditional" woman	5.9
Describe self as a mix of both	76.5

Age: M=49.82
Range: 40-59 years; SD=4.87

[a] Of those in paid labor force.

midlife, how they saw themselves as changing in midlife, what their images of "typical" and "ideal" midlife women were, what the best times in their own lives had been, what their weaknesses and strengths in dealing with life were, and when they felt strongest or most vulnerable. They were also asked about how well understood they had felt as they were going through midlife, what their emotional needs were at this time, and what areas they would like to see more midlife research on; they then had space for open-ended comments.

Quantitative Findings

Overall Well-Being at Midlife

In general, the women surveyed expressed high degrees of well-being: 72.5 percent (n=74) indicated that at this time in their life they felt "very happy" or "happy," and 64.3 percent (n=65) felt that they were finding this time in their life "not very confusing" or "not confusing at all." By contrast, only 13.7 percent (n=14) of the women indicated that they were "unhappy" or "very unhappy," and a somewhat larger number, although still a clear minority, 27.7 percent (n=28), indicated that they were finding this period "confusing" or "very confusing." Being happy and unconfused did not necessarily mean that they were not finding midlife a time of turmoil and struggle: Only 41.2 percent (n=42), far fewer than the number reporting happiness, wrote that they were having a "very easy time" or "easy time" coping, whereas 39.2 percent (n=40) reported a "difficult" or "somewhat difficult" time coping. The same pattern appears with respect to how the respondents rated themselves on specific areas of their lives. On the "report card," more than half the 103 respondents (56.2 percent) gave themselves an overall grade of B (good) or better. Only 9.7 percent gave themselves a C (fair) or lower.

The several measures of well-being measured by the survey were highly intercorrelated (for example, for the aggregate grade on the 17 areas of a respondent's life and the average of the respondent's self-ratings with respect to happiness, ease of coping, and confusion, r=.78, p < .01). In the analyses reported below, the aggregate grade was used as an index of well-being.

Demographic and Situational Correlates of Well-Being

The responses of the women were first analyzed by separate one-way analyses of variance (ANOVAs) for each of the demographic and situational variables: health, income, having a confidante, having a group of friends, employment status, menopausal status, education level, occupational group, marital status, sexual orientation, and feminist versus traditional orientation. The ANOVAs indicated that women who reported high levels of well-being at midlife were distinguished from those who reported lower levels of satisfaction by several demographic and situational variables: good health, annual family income above $30,000, having a confidante or group of friends, and being employed or a homemaker were good predictors of well-being. The better a woman's health, the more likely she was to report high levels of well-being [F(3, 98)=7.183, p=.0002]. Menopausal status was not related to well-being, however [F(1, 95)=.586, p=.4459]. Whether or not a woman reported menopausal symptoms (for example, hot flashes) was also not related to well-being [F(1, 98)=.919, p=.3401].

Low family income was associated with low levels of well-being [F(3, 94)=3.594, p=.0165], because of the problems faced by women at the bottom of the income scale. As long as family income was above $30,000 per year, income made no difference, but those with incomes below $30,000 were less satisfied than the other income groups. Occupational group had no effect [F(3, 98)=1.371, p=.2563], and women who were homemakers or who were students and not in the paid labor force were no more and no less likely to express satisfaction than women who worked in the paid labor force. However, being out of the paid labor force involuntarily (for example, because of being laid off, forced into early retirement, or because of physical disability) was associated with lower levels of well-being [F(4, 96)=3.766, p=.0069]. Educational level was not associated with differences in level of satisfaction [F(4, 97)=1.462, p=.2197].

Marital status [F(5, 96)=.443, p=.8169], whether or not a woman had children living at home [F(1, 91)=.062, p=.8044], whether she had children at all [F(1,100)=3.082, p=.0822), and her sexual orientation [F(2, 100)=.394, p=.6748] had no significant effect on well-being, nor did whether or not a woman perceived herself as a feminist, a traditional woman, or a mix of the two [F(2, 99)=1.421, p=.2464]. However, women who responded positively to the question, Do you have a confidante to whom you can speak freely and honestly about yourself? were significantly more likely to express a positive sense of well-being than women who did not [F(1, 101)=6.029, p=.0158], and women who reported having a group of women friends with whom they were close also reported significantly greater satisfaction with their lives [F(1,101)=13.843, p=.0003]. Finally, the number of current and recent sources of stress was negatively correlated with well-being (r=-.42).

To explore the significance of the situational and demographic variables further, a multiple regression analysis was undertaken. A model comprising four variables—the number of stressors, health status, family income (below or above $30,000 per year), and whether or not a woman had social supports (having either a confidante or a group of friends or both)—accounts for 38.9 percent of the variance in well-being associated with demographic and situational factors (Table 12.2.). Distinguishing between whether a woman has an intimate, a close group of friends, or both does not appreciably change the amount of explained variance. Labor force status also failed to explain additional variance, despite its first-order association with well-being. The latter situation appears to result from the fact that being involuntarily out of the labor force is often caused by having health problems and results in low family income. Hence, adding labor force status to health and family income does not add to the explanation of well-being. An alternative model using stress, labor force status, and social supports alone (and omitting health and income) explains somewhat less of the overall variance in well-being (30.1 percent) than the stress, health, income, and social support model, however.

Psychological Correlates of Well-Being

A woman's score on several of the measures of psychological function was, as was hypothesized, strongly related to whether or not she reported high levels of well-being. High self-esteem, lack of self-denigration, and a benign superego showed the highest correlations with the overall self-rating ($r=.70$ to $r=.73$). (With the exceptions specifically noted below, all correlation coefficients were significant at $p < .0001$.) Having the ability to grieve one's past, having a vision of the future and being able to create meaning in one's life, being able to construct a positive self-narrative, having a high sense of self-effectance, being optimistic, and believing one had a right to a life also predicted well-being, although not as strongly ($r=.56$ to $r=.64$). However, contrary to my hypothesis, feeling one was constructing a new identity in midlife was only weakly related to well-being ($r=.27$, $p=.005$).

Women who reported doing well at midlife also reported that they had a sense of their own relevance. They did not feel marginal or useless ($r=.61$). There was a less strong although significant correlation between well-being and positive feelings about one's own appearance ($r=.54$) or having positive images of midlife women ($r=.44$). Satisfaction with one's sex life was also moderately associated with well-being

181

Table 12.2. Multiple Regression Analysis: Demographic Variables

Independent Variable	ß	SE	t	r
Stress	-1.6208	.4452	-3.641	.0005
Health	-4.2005	1.2468	-3.369	.0005
Income	2.4980	.8356	2.9894	.0036
Social support	-6.9358	2.6037	-2.6602	.0093

Dependent variable: Index of well-being (grade)
Constant: 74.1268. Multiple R=.6172; $F(4, 89)$=13.5354, $p < .0001$

(r=.47). Confidence in one's ability to manage finances was not, however (r=.22, p=.0269). Surprisingly, a sense of spirituality was completely irrelevant to feelings of well-being (r=-.06, p=.6623).

To further elucidate factors associated with well-being, a multiple regression analysis was undertaken. A model containing four psychological variables—lack of self-denigration, having a vision of the future and being able to create meaning in one's life, being able to construct a positive self-narrative, and not feeling marginal or useless—accounts for the largest proportion of variance in well-being (Table 12.3.). Together these four variables explained 62.9 percent of the variance, a substantially larger proportion than the 38.9 percent explained by the situational and demographic variables.

The failure of the other psychological variables to add appreciably to the prediction of well-being is the consequence of the high degree of correlation among these variables. To take the most extreme

Table 12.3. Multiple Regression Analysis: Psychological Characteristics

Independent Variable	ß	SE	t	r
Self-denigration	-.4035	.1054	-3.8302	.0002
Vision of future	-.3651	.1679	2.1741	.0321
Positive narrative	.4061	.1538	2.6402	.0097
Lack of marginality	-.6810	.2812	-2.4217	.0173

Dependent variable: Index of well-being (grade)
Constant: 59.1811. Multiple R=.7931 $F(4, 97)$=41.1276, $p < .0001$

example, lack of self-denigration, a benign superego, and self-esteem all have correlations with each other above r=.85. Reflecting this, a number of other models, almost as good at explaining well-being as the optimal model, can be constructed by substituting, for instance, having a benign superego or good self-esteem for lack of self-denigration, a high sense of self-effectance for having a vision of the future, and a sense of optimism or the ability to grieve one's past for having a positive self-narrative. A model combining even some of the relatively poorer predictors of well-being, such as feeling one has the right to a life, having positive images of midlife, having positive feelings about one's appearance, and being satisfied with one's sex life, can explain over half of the variance in well-being, although the contribution of these variables to explaining well-being is drowned out when they are combined with the better predictors with which they are correlated.

From a clinical and a theoretical perspective, the significance of such psychological constructs as superego strength and self-esteem should not be discounted because they are pushed out of the regression model by the marginally more powerful ability of lack of self-denigration (with which superego strength and self-esteem are correlated) to predict well-being. The different constructs reflect different underlying theoretical explanations, each of which would appear to be effective as a tool for understanding midlife well-being. The superego construct reflects, of course, a psychodynamic perspective, whereas the self-esteem construct may reflect more of a phenomenological viewpoint and the lack of self-denigration construct more of a cognitive viewpoint. Having goals and a vision of the future, having a sense of self-effectance, being able to grieve the past, and being able to construct a meaningful narrative may reflect more of a cognitive constructivist viewpoint. The present study was not systematically designed to test the adequacy of models of midlife well-being coming explicitly from the differing theoretical perspectives, but it suggests the potential value of doing so.

Qualitative Findings

The qualitative responses to the questionnaire of the 10 women who had the highest overall self-rating of well-being (the aggregate score on the 17 areas of functioning) and those with the 10 lowest were compared impressionistically.

Both the group scoring highest in midlife satisfaction and the group scoring lowest in satisfaction were unanimous in reporting that what they liked best about midlife was increased independence and freedom—freedom from worrying about what others think, from responsibility for children, and from menstrual periods and freedom to develop an identity based on pursuing their own and not others' interests. High scorers were more likely to feel freedom "to" do something new (for example, develop relationships with women friends, build a career) whereas low scorers were more likely to report freedom "from" (for example, menstruation, pregnancy, and appearance worries). Low scorers were also more likely to report enjoying watching their children and grandchildren grow; high scorers more frequently reported that they most enjoyed doing things in a larger world beyond the family. All high scorers reported feeling their physical and emotional changes were understood by those around them, whereas not a single low scorer felt understood.

Both high and low scorers disliked the physical changes of midlife the most, especially the decrease in energy and in the ability to do things they once could do. Also frequently mentioned by both groups were gray hair, wrinkles, memory difficulties, and extra weight. The high scorers were more likely to mention disliking the discrepancy between how they saw themselves (very positively) and how they imagined society saw them (as unattractive). Low scorers were more likely to mention that they disliked the sense of life winding down, mortality, fear of the future and being alone, and mood swings. One woman reported feeling like midlife was the neglected middle child of adulthood: she felt she was too old to get hired for a job with benefits, yet too young for Medicare. Both groups noted that men do not lose social value as they age the way women do, and that gray hair and wrinkles are not seen as unattractive in men. They saw the double standard of aging as unfair.

High scorers had generally positive images of midlife (for example, less stress caused by children, open-mindedness and positive anticipation of the future, confidence in their potential to grow and contribute to the world), although these were often mixed with some negative images (depression, loss of libido, fatigue, and overweight). Low scorers reported predominantly negative images (a tired has-been, a woman struggling with a job she does not like, depression), although they saw the typical midlife woman as finding pleasure in children and grandchildren.

The high scorers were more task oriented and saw their weaknesses as traits such as procrastination, disorganization, and over-extending themselves. The low scorers were more aware of issues related to self-esteem, fear, and being ruled by others' wishes. Doubting the self and not valuing the self were mentioned by every woman who reported low satisfaction with midlife. Both groups mentioned perfectionism—with parenting, career, or being a woman—as being a problem.

Both high and low scorers saw perseverance as their greatest strength. High scorers emphasized traits that enabled them to move forward (learning from mistakes, letting go of negatives that they could not change, self-forgiveness). Low scorers emphasized survival ("taking care of myself because no one else will," "I can appear in control even when I'm going to pieces," "I'm there for others in a crisis").

High scorers saw themselves as feeling strongest when they felt challenged and had a sense of high self-effectance. Low scorers also felt strongest when accomplishing something independently; however, they also mentioned feeling strongest when not beset by doubts, when not in the presence of a negative. Both groups felt most vulnerable when in love, when they or someone they loved was sick, and when there were financial problems. Both high and low scorers saw the most important psychological needs at midlife as being valued, productive, loved, accepted, understood, attractive, and independent, and as having inner resources to replace the losses of midlife.

Respondents with high satisfaction and those with low satisfaction identified similar kinds of research as being potentially helpful for midlife women. Women were most interested in research on hormone replacement—especially "natural" sources of estrogen—and on ways that modern women are going through midlife that differ from the ways their mothers and previous generations negotiated "the change." Several women wondered whether research could help identify whether all the changes stereotypically associated with menopause and midlife were real or whether they occurred because they were "supposed" to happen and thus were just a self-fulfilling prophecy. One woman stated emphatically that what was needed was not midlife research but midlife PR! Changing society's outdated attitudes toward aging was reflected in most subjects' enthusiasm for research on women.

Conclusions and Implications for Social Work Practice

Society's Attitudes

First, social workers working with midlife clients should not adopt the negative stereotypes that currently prevail because of the lack of positive images of midlife women. To assume that midlife women are developmentally programmed to experience menopausal instability and depression or empty nest loneliness would be inaccurate and may lead to a self-fulfilling prophecy. Results of this study indicate, for instance, that menopausal symptoms and the empty nest are irrelevant to well-being in midlife for certain women. Midlife, for white middle-class and upper middle-class women, at least, is not a time of torment. Most of the women participating in this study were satisfied with themselves and their lives. Despite their happiness, they did find it a challenging stage of life. Almost three-quarters reported that they were happy, yet barely half that number reported that they were having an easy time coping. For some people, having stressors to cope with does not prevent them from being happy.

The women who reported most satisfaction with the 17 areas of their lives examined differed from those with the least satisfaction in a number of ways. Their annual family income was above $30,000 (how much above $30,000 did not seem to matter), they were healthy, and they were not involuntarily out of the labor force. Menopausal status and symptoms, caring for parents, an emptied nest, educational level, marital status, occupation, and feminism were not correlated to midlife well-being. It seemed that it was not so much what the women had but what they did with it that made the biggest difference to their well-being. If the woman was "blocked from being in the world" (through disability, poor health, involuntary unemployment, limited spending power), then she was less likely to be happy. "Being a player" seems to be critical to well-being. On a macro level, social work interventions that help women maintain their health and employment, avoid marginality, and maintain an adequate income would benefit midlife women.

The most satisfied women unanimously reported that this was the best or happiest time of life. They were actively participating in what the world has to offer and looking forward to a future filled with new opportunities as enjoyable as the opportunities of the past. Women not doing well yearned for earlier days when there was a sense of possibility—for a happy marriage, wonderful children, an exciting career. The present lacked a comparable sense of wonderful possibility. Opportunities in midlife were either invisible or inferior to those of earlier days. The women lacked positive images for vision building or meaning making, and they were finding dreams from the past an ineffective solace. Social workers can help women by enabling their active participation in the world and helping them find a sense of meaning and opportunity in the world.

Involvement with Others

Being able to participate in a social world by having a confidante or a group of women friends, as well as having positive models, was also predictive of midlife satisfaction. The women who reported doing well were involved with others and felt that the changes they were going through were understood by others. The women doing poorly felt isolated and were angry about being misunderstood. Social workers' ability to offer empathic individual and group treatment to help strengthen a woman's connection to a social network has the potential to offer precisely the help struggling midlife women need.

Women doing well and those not doing well reported feeling vulnerable under similar circumstances (when in love or when sick), and they reported their emotional needs as being the same (wanting to be loved, valued, respected), but their responses to vulnerability differed. Women doing well responded to vulnerability and emotional need by being challenged and becoming active in the world, resulting in increased self-effectance and power. Women having a more difficult time responded by feeling self-doubt rather than challenge, and they were frustrated in their attempts to get their needs met. For them the most rewarding aspect of the social world was children and grandchildren, a kind of vicarious enjoyment of the sense of possibility.

The Self

Women doing well were aware of a troubling discrepancy between the positive way they saw themselves and the social devaluation they perceived, and they felt challenged to live lives that contradicted the "over the hill" stereotype. Their sense of "personhood" was stronger than ever, yet society and the media were fading them into an invisibility that does not sit well with the baby boomer generation. They were aware of dissonance between the increased freedom and power they felt and negative cultural stereotypes and media portrayals. Women not doing well reported less dissonance, seeming to comply with cultural messages about obsolescence. Unlike women with greater satisfaction, they lacked alternative images of midlife aging.

All the women bemoaned the loss of physical capabilities and attractiveness and, to varying degrees, were astonished that so many areas of life were actually changing. Feeling more freedom yet more physical limitations was a source of frustration. Women doing well did not turn against the self. They reported being able to grieve old images of themselves (a constructive grief), value who they were becoming, construct a life story that was balanced toward the positive, feel positive about their appearance, and feel like important contributors in the world. They had a dream and were pursuing it armed with feelings of self-effectance, self-acceptance, and self-esteem. They reported believing that they had a right to a life, or a right to have power. They did not have to live vicariously or wait until everyone else was taken care of before their own needs mattered. Hopefully these research findings can guide social work practitioners in their collaborative treatment planning with clients who come for help during midlife.

On a micro level, social workers can help midlife women enormously. The clinical interventions in which social workers are trained are precisely the interventions that would develop characteristics associated with midlife well-being. Women who feel that the changes they are going through are empathetically understood and who have a group or individual to confide in have some protection against midlife dissatisfaction, according to the results of this study. Social workers, using group or individual treatment skills, can help women raise self-esteem, break the habit of self-denigration, develop goals for the future, grieve the past, and compose a positive life narrative.

One surprising result of this study was that spirituality did not correlate highly with high midlife coping for this sample. My guess would be that this is because, although for a subgroup of women spirituality contributes to well-being, there is another group, which cancels out the effects of the first group, for whom spirituality is either neutrally unimportant or actively rejected.

This investigation has examined characteristics of women who are doing well at midlife. Both for social policy and for clinical work with women, these observations suggest some of the goals that would facilitate midlife well-being (for clinical examples of individual and group approaches see McQuaide, 1996a, 1996b). This current study focused on middle-class white women. Whether these findings also apply to women from other racial or ethnic groups or to poorer women remains a topic for future research and is currently being investigated.

What we have learned is that a woman needs a decent job and a decent income. She needs to stay actively involved in the world, not just the social world, and she needs to keep herself challenged. More than ever, having a supportive social environment and not denigrating oneself are critical. For social workers involved politically and clinically with the midlife woman these issues are central.

References

Apter, T. (1995). *Secret Paths: Women in the New Midlife*. New York: W. W. Norton.

Baruch, G., & Brooks-Gunn, J. (Eds.). (1984). *Women in Midlife*. New York: Plenum.

Erikson, E. H. (1950). *Childhood and Society*. New York: W. W. Norton.

Greet, G. (1992). *The Change: Women, Aging, and the Menopause*. New York: Alfred A. Knopf.

Heilbrun, C. G. (1988). *Writing a Woman's Life*. New York: Ballantine Books.

Jaques, E. (1965). Death and the mid-life crisis. *International Journal of Psychoanalysis*, 46, 502-514.

Jung, C. G. (1933/1983). The stages of life. In A. Storr (Ed.), *The Essential Jung*. Princeton, NJ: Princeton University Press.

Levinson, D. J. (1978). *The Seasons of a Man's Life*. (with C. Darrow, E. Klein, M. Levinson, & B. McKee). New York: Alfred A. Knopf.

McQuaide, S. (1996a). Keeping the wise blood: The construction of images in a mid life women's group. *Social Work with Groups*, 19, 131-145.

McQuaide, S. (1996b). Self hatred, the right to a life, and the tasks of midlife. *Clinical Social Work* Journal, 24, 35-47.

Miller, J. B. (1976). *Toward a New Psychology of Women*. Boston: Beacon Press.

Pearlin, L. I., & Schooler, C. (1978). The structure of coping. *Journal of Health and Social Behavior*, 19, 2-21.

Ryff, C. (1995). Psychological well-being in adult life. *Current Directions in Psychological Science*, 4, 99-105.

Sheehey, G. (1992). *The Silent Passage*. New York: Random House.

Vaillant, G. E. (1977). *Adaptation to Life*. Boston: Little, Brown.

Wolin, S. J., & Wolin, S. (1993). *The Resilient Self: How Survivors of Troubled Families Rise above Adversity*. New York: Ullard Books.

—by Sharon McQuaide

Sharon McQuaide, PhD, is assistant professor, Graduate School of Social Service, Fordham University, 113 West 60th Street, New York, NY 10023. The author thanks John Ehrenreich for his statistical assistance.

Chapter 13

Decisions about Retirement Living

There really is no place like home. When asked about their preference for housing, most seniors answer, "What l would really like to do is to stay right here." The person's own home represents security and independence to most Americans.

Most housing, however, is designed for young, active, and mobile people. To live at home, a person must, at the very least, be able to drive, go shopping, cook. and do household chores. Many of us will lose one or more of these abilities as we grow older.

One option is to purchase in-home services, to cope with declining abilities. For a fee, an army of workers will appear to cut your grass, wash your windows, cook your meals, do the shopping, and even provide personal care and/or skilled nursing care. This may be the option for you, depending on the amount of help you need. However, this can be expensive and will require a lot of management and coordination.

For people willing to relocate, there are plenty of options, although there may be some confusion about what all the terms mean. You may hear about "board and care homes," "personal care homes," "life care" and "continuing care retirement facilities." All refer 'to some type of "assisted living" or service-oriented housing.

Housing options generally fail into three categories, based on level of services and/or care provided:

Administration on Aging (AoA), July 1995, *Elder Action: Action Ideas for Older Persons and Their Families*. This Elder Action was developed by the National Eldercare Institute on Long Term Care and Alzheimer's Disease at the Suncoast Gerontology Center University of South Florida.

- independent retirement housing, providing meals, activities, house-keeping and maintenance to more active seniors;

- "assisted living," providing housing along with supportive services for seniors needing assistance with personal care or medication taking;

- housing providing nursing care services for seniors who become temporarily ill or who require long term health care.

Some examples of these retirement options are:

Independent Living Retirement Communities

These complexes are for seniors who are able to live on their own, but want the convenience of a comprehensive service package. Meals, housekeeping, activities, transportation and security are provided to active older adults.

"Assisted Living" Facilities

In addition to the services mentioned above, these facilities provide personal care assistance to residents. This means that, in addition to housekeeping services, residents receive assistance in managing their medications. and a helping hand with bathing, grooming and dressing.

"Assisted Living" facilities come in all shapes and sizes. Settings can range from three or more older people in a homelike setting, to dozens of residents in an institutional environment.

Nursing Homes

For individuals already disabled to the point of requiring daily nursing care as well as other support services, nursing homes provide comprehensive care services in a single setting. While most older persons and their families see nursing home care only as a last resort, they may in fact be the best setting for disabled persons with multiple problems and requiring multiple types of services.

Continuing Care Retirement Communities

Continuing Care Retirement Communities, sometimes also called Life Care Communities, combine all three levels of care independent living, assisted living and nursing home care in a single setting. Traditionally, such communities required a sizeable entry fee, plus monthly maintenance fees, in exchange for a living unit, meals, and eventual health care coverage, up to the nursing home level. More recently, such communities have also begun to make their services available on a pure rental basis, rather than on the shared risk basis of the traditional life care endowment. In short, CCRCs provide residents with the independence of retirement home living and the security of long term care.

Some Other Housing Options:

- Group Homes provide independent, private living in a house shared by several senior citizens who split the cost of rent, housekeeping services, utilities, and meals.

- Shared Housing is offered by home owners who are willing to share their house with others. Service provision must be negotiated on a case by case basis.

- Adult Foster Care involves a family caring for a dependent person in their home. Meals, housekeeping and help with dressing, eating, bathing, and other personal care are provided. Ask the local social services department if adult foster care is available in your area.

To Move or Not to Move

The main advantage of living in some type of congregate housing is security. The presence of others provides continued monitoring of health care. Another big draw of such facilities, especially for those with limited mobility, are the built-in social contacts and activities. Experts agree that social contacts increase satisfaction with life and have a positive impact on physical health. Other seniors report relief at relinquishing housekeeping tasks.

Weighing the advantages of service oriented housing against the independence offered by a single family home is a complicated task. Timing is all-important. The most useful way to approach such decisions is to begin early by getting all the information possible on one's various options.

Chapter 14

Confronting the Question of Moving

Moving from one residence to another is an event familiar to most people. Every year millions of households change from one residence to another. In 1993, about 17 million moves occurred, nearly 18 percent of all U.S. households. Nearly a million of these moves were by persons 65 or over.

For most middle-aged and older persons, the decision to move may have more significant consequences than for younger persons. At later ages, it is often more difficult for people to change their situation again if the move turns out to be unsatisfactory. For example, the decision to sell one's home and move to a rental unit is a big decision at any age but can be especially difficult at later ages. Alternatively, moving in with an adult child may result in a big reduction in privacy. And it may be difficult to change the situation once the move is made.

Today there are many new options for older people. Have you been thinking about moving? If so, plan ahead! This chapter provides information on things to do and consider.

Why People Move

People move for many reasons. The most common reasons vary by age. For people later in life, the reason is more commonly associated with changing family situations and economic circumstances.

Reprinted with permission from the *National Policy and Resource Center on Women and Aging Letter*, Volume 2 Number 1, March 1997.

More people "age in place" than move. In fact, statistics indicate that the longer you live in a particular residence, the less likely it is that you will move.

Table 14.1. The Top Three Reasons for Moving

All Americans	Older Americans
To be near(er) a new (old) job or school	Moving in with or near to family or another person
Need a larger place	To reduce living costs
To create an independent living situation ("own home")	Dealing with becoming widowed, divorced, or separated

Source: U.S. Department of Commerce. *American Housing Survey for the United States in 1993.* Washington, DC: General Printing Office, 1995.

Table 14.2. Why Older People Moved in 1992

Wanted to move closer to family	15%
Wanted to change locations	10
Could not afford to stay in prior home	9
New home purchase or upgrade	9
Health reasons	9
Different residence but same town	8
Home unsuitable to needs (too big, etc.)	8
Death of spouse or because of divorce	7
Retired	7
Transferred jobs or moved closer to work	6
Seeking a different climate	6
Other	9
Total	100*

Source: A representative national survey (American Association of Retired Persons. Understanding Senior Housing for the 1990s. AARP, 1993.)

*Column does not add to 100 due to rounding.

Studies show that when the decision to move is made, it is often done quickly. A 1993 survey by AARP found that while 46 percent of older movers spend a year or more planning a move, 54 percent decide to move within a one year period. In fact, 42 percent plan for less than six months.

Unanticipated events (changing family situation, economic issues, health change) often create an incentive or need to make quick changes. Federal cutbacks in housing programs are creating new uncertainties. Table 14.2. gives a more detailed list of the reasons why older people move. While moving closer to family is the top reason, the list is long and quite diverse.

These and other data suggest that even if one currently plans to stay put, it is a good idea to think ahead and not ignore the possibility of a future move.

Plan in Advance: Factors to Consider

There are some important questions you can ask yourself when thinking about whether to stay put or to move:

- What lifestyle?
- How important are certain family members and friends?
- What type of neighborhood do I/we want to live in?
- What particular setting will my health require?
- Is it affordable?

Lifestyle considerations include the extent to which you may want to live with other older persons out of sight and sound of children. If currently a homeowner, how will you manage (and do you want) to continue to mow lawns, shovel snow, and do heavy house-cleaning? Are you an active person who wants to walk, swim, or play sports? Or would you rather spend most of your time at home with friends close by? Whatever the choice, it is a good idea to make a conscious decision about the kind of life you want to live and then decide whether to move or stay put.

Wanting to be close to family members is a good reason to stay put if they live in the area. It is also a good reason to move if they are far away. In fact, this is the major reason that older people move today.

However, you may currently have a network of friends providing social and supportive activities that is unlikely to be duplicated if you move. Sometimes networks of friends can be more supportive than younger family members who are busy with their children and careers.

The neighborhood is a source of services and familiarity. Do you need or prefer a neighborhood where you can walk to shop for food, medicine, and other goods? Or are you able to travel by car or public transport to more distant stores and malls?

Increasing numbers of special service programs are offered to individuals as they grow older. But availability varies widely by state and locality.

Of course, current and future health is a big consideration. Does increasing frailty mean that you need more supportive services—as found, for example, in an assisted living facility or a continuing care retirement community?

No matter what choice you would like to make, it will be shaped by your economic situation. For some there will be the opportunity to sell a home and invest in a life care community. For others, rising housing costs will force a move to less expensive housing.

A home is often an elder's largest asset. But as the saying goes, "you can't eat bricks and mortar." Fortunately, it has become easier to find banks that will let you borrow against your home equity while you are living in the home. These are called "reverse annuities." One thing is certain: an abrupt decision on what to do about one's home should be avoided.

Getting About

Having a nice residence isn't enough. One's ability to get around often changes with age. One needs to shop, visit family and friends, see the doctor, etc. Access to transportation is an important component of the decision to stay put or to move. Statistics indicate that older Americans make 90 percent of their trips in private automobiles, often driven by themselves. But many people find it appropriate to stop driving at later ages.

Some communities have specialized transportation services for older and disabled persons. These include medical transportation, regularly scheduled bus routes, taxi vouchers, and on-demand van service. Any plan to move should include an assessment of what transportation resources are available.

So You've Decided to Move . . .

Romantic thinking is not just a hazard of youth. At times we all see only the merits and not the imperfections of a situation. A desired living location can give rise to this kind of thinking—the memory of happy summers spent, the sight of newly finished floors, scenes of couples hard at play, the expectation of frequent visits by family. But moving is a major change and, for some older people, irreversible. It pays to make a reasoned assessment before deciding to move.

First, get as much information as you can about the city/town where you plan to move. Better yet, live there for a week, month, or year—especially at the less attractive times (e.g., summer in Florida). Visit the city/ town's library, city hall, and chamber of commerce to seek information. Talk to retired persons who live there (a senior center is one place to meet them).

Second, especially if you cannot spend much time there, use your eyes and ears. Subscribe to the local newspapers. Call the senior center and ask for people you can telephone. If you are computer "plugged in," use the internet.

Third, check out the climate. How hot does it get, how cold, for how long? Is it rainy, snowy, humid, dry? Decide whether or not you will be comfortable in this particular climate. What chores are likely to be created by the weather: snow shoveling, watering, etc.?

Fourth, be realistic about the cost of living. Check into food costs, housing, taxes (sales, income, inheritance, and property), transportation, and health care. Is it an area likely to become more expensive in the future?

Fifth, what health care resources are available? Can you exercise your choice of managed care or fee-for-service care? Do you have ready access to emergency care and a good general hospital?

Sixth, are desirable recreational and cultural resources available-movies, walking areas, museums, lakes or ocean, walking areas, gardens, sports facilities, etc.?

Seventh, determine whether the area has the type of housing you desire. Many people do not realize the wide range of housing options currently available. Table 14.3 lists some of the major alternatives.

Finally, one of the first things you should do is to start the stressful and difficult job of deciding what will go with you and what must be sold, given away, or discarded.

Special Issues for Women

When married couples consider moving, women must have a decisive voice in the deliberations. Remember, married women outlive their spouses on average by about seven years. If you become widowed, will you be able to sustain the lifestyle established as a couple? Will you have to move again and, if so, at what cost? Will the initial

Table 14.3. A Guide to Housing Options in Later Life

	Advantages	Disadvantages
Single Family Home	Privacy Ownership An equity asset	Expense Upkeep and maintenance Design (e.g., stairs)
Single Apartment	Few upkeep concerns Shared services Design (e.g., one floor)	Other tenants Lack of equity Restricted space
Condominium	An equity asset Same as apartment	Other tenants Financial obligations
Apartment added to a single family home	Additional owner income Companionship and security Increases affordable rentals Possibility of trading services for rent	Initial construction cost Neighborhood opposition Zoning restrictions Building code compliance
Homes providing both board and some care	Homelike environment Interaction with others Economical	Usually not licensed Operators may lack training Few social activities
Elderly congregate housing with meals taken together	Extends independent living Reduces social isolation Provides physical and emotional security	May promote dependency Expensive to build and operate Some lack kitchen facilities Expensive for most elderly
Facilities providing housing and some "care for life" (life care communities)	Offer prepaid health care Financial/medical cost security Social activities/support systems Need not move from the community if more care needed	Too expensive for many What protection if they close? Usually no property deed Monthly payments could rise Often rural and isolated
Housing shared with a housing unit owner	Less expensive/shared costs Companionship and security Intergenerational cooperation Uses existing housing Program inexpensive to operate	Who selects house mates? Less privacy Doesn't meet medical needs May affect benefit eligibility Zoning ordinances

Adapted from Phyllis H. Mutschler. "Where Elders Live." In J. J. Callahan, Jr., ed. *Aging in Place.* Amityville, NY: Baywood Publishing Co., Inc., 1993.

move consume savings that should be available to support you as a single person?

Women who are (or may be) suddenly living on their own must confront a new set of tasks related to home maintenance: heavy chores and housecleaning, car repair, and driving—jobs you may not have assumed primary responsibility for in the past. And jobs that you may find increasingly difficult as you grow older.

Knowledge is crucial about home systems (e.g., heating and plumbing), home and auto maintenance and repairs, and other tasks historically managed by men.

Also important are a willingness to rely on outside help (whether from family and friends or purchased) and assertiveness skills (to ensure that helpers listen and do tasks according to your preferences).

Fortunately, AARP, some senior centers, adult education programs, and other organizations conduct workshops or courses and offer materials to help women with these concerns.

Resources

J. Howells, *Where to Retire*. Oakland, CA: Gateway Books, 1995.

J. Martindale & M. Moses, *Creating Your Own Future: A Woman's Guide to Retirement Planning*. Naperville, IL: Sourcebooks Trade, 1991.

W. Wasch, *Home Planning for Your Later Years*. (new designs, living options, smart decisions, financing). Wilton, CT: Beverly Cracom, 1996.

Consumer Reports magazine, August, 1990. Information regarding moving and moving companies.

The Women & Aging Letter is a project of Brandeis University, in cooperation with the American Society on Aging, the National Black Women's Health Project, and the Coalition of Labor Union Women. The Center is located at the Heller School, Brandeis University, Waltham, MA 02254-9110, tel: 800-929-1995. For information about subscribing to the Women and Aging letter, contact the Center as noted above.

Chapter 15

Volunteering Is Linked to Well-Being during Retirement

Volunteering boosts self-esteem and energy and gives Americans a sense of mastery over their lives, particularly in later midlife, says a new Cornell University study.

That may be why Americans in a smaller, preliminary Cornell study said they would like to spend as much time doing volunteer work as they now spend on leisure activities

Yet most people, the new study finds, don't seek out community involvement. Of those who volunteer, 44 percent do so because someone asked them, says Phyllis Moen, the Ferris Family Professor in Life Course Studies in human development and sociology and the director of the Bronfenbrenner Life Course Center at Cornell.

Moen reported her findings to national volunteering experts at the "National Forum on Life Cycles and Volunteering: The Impact of Work, Family and Mid-Life Issues" April 30 at Cornell. The forum examined the latest research and trends in volunteerism and how life-course factors affect volunteering

The benefits of volunteering affect not only those currently working as volunteers but also people who have ever volunteered, especially those in formal volunteering capacities, such as serving on boards of directors and working with service and religious groups, says Moen, who points out that a greater proportion of Americans volunteer regularly than do citizens of any other country.

"Community commitments, especially formal participation, help enhance our sense of identity, promote on-going networks of social relationships and foster expectations of what to do when we wake up in the morning, much like paid work," Moen told participants at the forum, sponsored by the College of Human Ecology. "Except volunteering has one huge advantage over paid work: You can quit if you don't like it," she said

Moen pointed out that "we become what we do—volunteering gives us a sense of ourselves as engaged in meaningful, productive activities that help change the world and a wider view of our possibilities, which benefit our psychological well-being."

She stressed that volunteering should become more of a public issue with institutional support and greater societal value and recognition, in the way paid work is now.

Specifically, she found:

1. In focus groups, employees in midlife, ages 30 to 60, describe themselves as spending about 8 percent of their time volunteering and 13 percent in leisure. Ideally, they say they would like to spend 14 percent of their time volunteering and 24 percent in leisure.

2. People who volunteer early in life are much more likely to volunteer later in life, when the personal benefits are particularly acute. "If individuals don't volunteer while they are employed, it is unlikely they will volunteer after retirement," said Moen, in an interview. "That lack of participation takes on an important significance for retirees and doesn't bode well for their psychological well-being."

3. Volunteerism is particularly beneficial to men, urbanites, those with less income, and in poor health, and retirees who don't work.

4. About one-third of all American men and the same proportion of women participate in community service work, though men tend to put in more hours on average. For those between 35 and 54 years of age, for example, men spend almost 6 hours weekly compared with 4.5 hours for women. That is because many men between these ages participate in community service to enhance their careers while women are spending more time raising their families, Moen explained.

Moen is the director of the Cornell Retirement and Well-Being Study of a random sample of 762 men and women, between ages 50 and 72, that examines the retirement transition. It is being conducted with Vivian Fields, a researcher in the Department of Human Development, and it is funded as part of the Cornell Applied Gerontology Research Institute by the National Institute on Aging.

Moen also draws on in-depth interview data from workers in upstate New York as part of the Cornell Family and Careers Institute, a Sloan Center on Working Families that addresses the challenges and strategies of working families, such as their decisions, stresses, beliefs and expectations and their coping strategies for parenting, child care and financial decisions. Her findings emerge from both projects.

Contact Susan S. Lang
Office (607) 255-3613
E-Mail: SSL4@cornell.edu

Chapter 16

A Grandparents' Guide for Family Nurturing and Safety

The most exciting thing about being a grandparent is watching your own child become nurturing. The miracle of a new baby is overwhelming, but to watch your son or daughter becoming a parent is just as miraculous. We watch with awe, pride and, sometimes, trepidation as our sons and daughters do their best to raise strong and healthy offspring. We know how demanding a job that is. We want to help. We should help. And we do.

We want to keep our grandchildren safe and sound. We want to make our homes and theirs safe havens where nothing bad can happen to them. We want to share with our own children the lessons we learned—and learn a few new tips ourselves.

The contributions grandparents make to their families are extraordinary. Some, like baby-sitting or giving them safe cribs or strollers, are tangible. Others, like providing a role model for grandchildren, are intangible but just as powerful and real. We do know that virtually every study of child development shows that youngsters lucky enough to have loving grandparents are destined to be winners. All research on single parents shows that the future of the children is correlated with support from grandparents.

We also know that grandparents can make their children's job of parenting a lot easier. When you lend a sympathetic ear to an upset parent you provide a safe outlet for often difficult emotions. When you

The U.S. Consumer Product Safety Commission (CPSC), 1997. For more information, call CPSC's toll-free hotline at 800-638-2772 or visit its web site at http://www.cpsc.gov.

give your children a night off by baby-sitting, you give them and your grandchild a much-needed break from the inevitable strains of the nuclear family. When your children know that, in a pinch, there is someone to step in to love their children and keep them safe, you give them the most valuable kind of support.

More and more, we see grandparents providing reliable and dedicated child care. In fact, the U.S. Census Bureau estimates that about 1.3 million children are entrusted to their grandparents every day. That same 1994 study says another 2.4 million children live in households headed by a grandparent. It means that numbers of grandparents make it possible for the young ones to grow up in stable homes and communities.

But it's the daily acknowledgment that we get from our children and grandchildren that inspires us to develop and maintain those loving connections. What fun to watch their eyes widen and sparkle when you tell your grandchildren about how their mommy was as a small child! We know it's not always easy, that it takes thought, finesse and devotion. It requires us to be emotionally flexible and nurturing. We have to be vigilant and make our homes safe for children. We need to take our role modeling seriously—for our children and grandchildren.

We hope we can help. Because when grandparenting works, there's nothing better. We know. We're grandparents too.

Sincerely,

Dr. T. Berry Brazelton
Clinical Professor Emeritus of Pediatrics at Harvard Medical School
and Chairman, Pampers Parenting Institute

Ann Brown
Chairman, U.S. Consumer Product Safety Commission

Bridging the Generations and Building the Bonds

Take your role seriously—you have a lot to give. With babies and toddlers, you can be an additional source of love and care. For school-age children, you can teach family values and history. You can inspire older children and adolescents to want to grow up to be like you. To do that, you have to be a consistent presence in their lives. If you can, offer to baby-sit regularly or when needed. That allows you to lavish all your special attention on your grandchildren. At the same time, you'll win the eternal gratitude of your children, who need downtime.

- In between visits, fill in the gaps with a weekly phone call to the child at a pre-arranged time. Encourage each child to share a "news" item with you, something only he or she can reveal. That way a phone call becomes an event that everyone looks forward to.

- Videotapes are another wonderful way of keeping up with your grandchildren's everyday experiences and milestones. Of course, exchange letters or e-mail and ask for packages of drawings and schoolwork. They give you insight into how they're developing and what interests them. Your positive-feedback-praise helps to build self-esteem they'll need to get along in the world.

- Read a story or conjure up a fantasy for them on videotape. Let them hear it at bedtime. That way, they'll remember you between visits.

- Your active participation instills a sense of family and continuity that adds to your grandchildren's feeling of belonging and security. You can magnify that by sharing your family history. Children love stories about when their parents were young—the time Mommy fell out of the apple tree and didn't break a bone, or when Daddy woke up at 3:00 in the morning because he couldn't wait for his birthday presents.

- Holidays are another opportunity to bring the family tradition to children and create memories that help make your family close. Encourage everyone to celebrate them at your house. When that's not possible, link up by phone and take time to talk about family beliefs and rituals. Even when there is resistance about getting together, it is worth it. They never forget rituals. We need values for our children and grandchildren, and this is a way to perpetuate them.

- For those of us who live too far away, or are not able to baby-sit, there are lots of other ways to stay close. Arrange for regular visits with your grandchildren and have them visit you. See each grandchild separately if you can. The kind of individual attention you give is key.

- Making rituals out of meeting with your grandchildren, having things that you do only with them, makes them feel unique. Besides, taking them to the zoo or to a special restaurant is fun for you, too.

- One of the things I have always loved doing with my grandchildren is taking them to the nearby playground. It's a wonderful place for children to have fun and run off steam.

But, as caretakers of our grandchildren, even for an afternoon, we need to be careful. Most serious injuries on playgrounds come from falls onto hard surfaces. In fact, grass is one of the worst surfaces because it can become hard, packed dirt.

Checking for playground surfacing that "gives" is extremely important. Wood chips, mulch, sand, pea gravel, or rubber matting are all good choices. After all, you want your time together to be full of fun, not tears. Even today, I have scars on my knees from falls on my old neighborhood playground.

- The constant contact with your grandchildren teaches you how to really listen to them, to understand what they mean to say, not just the words they use. There was a time I brought my granddaughter Lil to my office for the annual "Take Our Daughters To Work Day." I asked all the girls, "Who wears a bike helmet?" Almost all of them except Lil raised their hands. I asked her why, and she said, "Gramma Ann, I look like a dork." I figured if she felt that way, so must hundreds of others who would rather go without protection than look unhip. A project we did with the Automobile Association of America confirmed the fear. So we went to the bike helmet manufacturers who redesigned them—put in bright colors and sparkle. Now my granddaughter tells me, "You know, Gramma Ann, they're awesome."

- When we take our grandchildren's words seriously and respect their opinions, they do let us know what's going on. That strengthens the growing bonds between you and your grandchild.

Making It Work

Even with all the advantages of an extended family, the course of those relationships doesn't always run smooth. Parents and grandparents are bound to disagree over child-rearing choices. The trick is in knowing how to cool the friction before the fire gets out of hand.

- What most young parents need from their own parents is sympathetic support, not advice and criticism. While it's sometimes painful to watch your children go through the trial-and-error of parenthood, it's part of their learning curve. It's best to let them know you're there for them, that you're willing and eager to listen and that you'd be glad to offer the wisdom of your own experience if and when they want it. A regular "date" with them to let your child unload is a sure way of keeping in touch.

- Occasionally, our children or grandchildren will do something we feel so strongly about, we'll want to intervene right then and there. Resist temptation. It only undermines the parents in front of the children and sets up tensions. The time to talk about the problem is calmly and reasonably and privately. Even if you ultimately disagree, it inspires trust when you accept their parenting decisions. Remind your children of their own childhood crises and how they handled them.

Grandparents must respect their children as the parents. Grandparents are notorious for overindulging their young charges, and parents often worry that this will undercut their own child-rearing efforts. However, Grandma and Grandpa's treats, no matter how frequent, are just one more sign to children that they are cherished. Grandparents can be tolerant, loving and supportive, without having to discipline and instruct the way parents must. They can afford to see all the good things in a child and ignore the bad. That's a wonderful mirror into which a child can look.

- Children always know that their parents' insistence on proper nutrition and a sensible bedtime is good and loving in the most profound sense. So when it comes to major issues, grandparents should always abide by the limits set by the parents to avoid confusion and bad feeling on all sides.

- One of the great gifts we have is our ability to influence young children. Removed from the power struggles of the immediate family, a grandparent isn't likely to meet with as much resistance as a parent would in suggesting a child do some homework or set the table. It is one way grandparents help parents by reinforcing the values that parents want to instill.

Let your children know that you made more than your share of mistakes when they were little, and that, just as they do now, you had to learn how to take good care of them. I will never forget the time when my baby daughter Laura was about to swallow something that looked to her like a piece of cherry candy. It wasn't candy. It was a bright-red glue pellet from a craft set. That is how I learned the importance of baby-proofing our home.

- Then my grown-up daughter had the fun of reminding me of those lessons when my own grandchildren were little and she brought them to visit me. She went around my house to be sure I had put all the peanuts and candies up high—and locked away the pills—and put safety plugs on the electrical outlets.

- Where babies are concerned, we can all use good advice. But as a grandparent, I try hard not to give it unless I'm asked. It's much better if I wait until I hear, "Mom, I need advice."

- It may be our privilege as grandparents to indulge and maybe even spoil our grandchildren a bit. For example, I may buy more toys or treats for my grandchildren than I did for my daughters. But you need to be careful, too. A friend of mine, a new grandmother, proudly showed me the toy she bought for her two-year-old grandson. The age label on the toy was for an older child. Like me, she thought she had the smartest grandchild imaginable, and the toy would challenge him. But those age labels on toys are often safety recommendations, not measures of skill or ability. By providing appropriate playthings, you can spoil your grandchildren and keep them safe at the same time.

- We're there with the power of example. Try not to force your beliefs. Rather, in a loving and conversational way, set a good example. For instance, my grandchildren see me in my job giving back to society. They've got the idea that's a good thing from watching what I do and how much I care about child safety. They've become safety ambassadors, very interested in safety for themselves and for their friends. It's your very presence that affects them. You're a grandparent figure. If you're informal, loving, friendly and casual, and you set a good example, it's the best way to encourage learning, values and connection that go beyond your family to the community and society at large.

Making your home safe for your grandchildren is an ongoing project that changes with each stage of his or her development. What works for a newborn isn't going to be enough for a crawling, alert 8-month-old, and certainly not for an inquisitive toddler. Daunting as it seems now, I can assure you, it'll seem less so as you grow along with your grandchild. It's an effort that will make you, your grandchildren and their parents feel relaxed and secure.

- Maintain an "emergency procedure" that allows you to quickly contact your grandchild's doctor, hospital emergency room and poison control center. Keep these phone numbers by every phone in the house when your grandchild is visiting.

- One way that will help you see potential hazards to your grand-children is to get down on your hands and knees and see a room from their perspective.

- Never underestimate your grandchild's ability to climb, explore or move furniture to reach something high up. Follow the U.S. Consumer Product Safety Commission's Grandchild Safety Checklist to ensure your home will be safe for your grandchild.

It's important to keep in close touch with your children and respect the way they raise their own children. While you have considerably more experience in child-rearing, there are still things your children can teach you. For example, when I was a young mother, I thought I was keeping my daughters safe by putting them to sleep on their stomachs. Well, parents today are putting infants to sleep on their backs—which has dramatically reduced the risk of Sudden Infant Death Syndrome (SIDS). We've also learned that putting babies to sleep on top of comforters or pillows, no matter how beautiful, may be associated with infant suffocation. Even that special old crib you've kept for your long-awaited grandchild may be dangerous because it doesn't meet current safety standards. As grandparents, then, it's important for us to be attuned to changes in child-rearing and safety practices.

Here is a practical, no-frills, easy-to-use checklist from the U.S. Consumer Product Safety Commission to get you started. Use these tips to keep your grandchildren safe. (Please note: Many of these safety tips apply to children of all ages from infants to preschoolers, but have been broken down into age ranges for easier reference.)

Grandchild Safety Checklist

Young Infants

Young infants follow objects with their eyes. They explore with their hands, feet and mouths. They begin sitting and crawling.

213

- Put your grandchild to sleep on his or her back in a crib with a firm, flat mattress and no soft bedding underneath.

- Make sure your crib is sturdy, with no loose or missing hardware; used cribs may not meet current safety standards.

- Don't give grandchildren toys or other items with small parts, or tie toys around their necks.

- In a car, always buckle your grandchild in a child safety seat on the back seat.

Older Infants

Older infants crawl and learn to walk. They enjoy bath play and explore objects by banging and poking.

- Never leave your grandchild alone for a moment near any water or in the bathtub, even with a bath seat; check bath water with your wrist or elbow to be sure it is not too hot.

- Don't leave a baby unattended on a changing table or other nursery equipment; always use all safety straps.

- If you use a baby walker for your grandchild, make sure it has special safety features to prevent falls down stairs, or use a stationary activity center instead.

- Keep window blind and curtain cords out of reach of grandchildren; dress grandchildren in clothing without drawstrings.

Toddlers

Toddlers have lots of energy and curiosity. They like exploring, climbing and playing with small objects.

- Keep all medicines in containers with safety caps; be sure medicines, cleaning products, and other household chemicals are out of reach and locked away from children.

- Use safety gates for stairs, safety plugs for electrical outlets, and safety latches for drawers and cabinets.

- Buy toys labeled for children under age 3; these are often safety recommendations, not measures of a child's skill or ability.

- Never leave your grandchildren alone in or near swimming pools.

Preschoolers

Preschoolers are very active. They run, jump and climb.

- Keep children—and furniture they can climb on—away from windows.

- At playgrounds, look for protective surfacing under equipment.

- Be sure your grandchildren wear helmets when riding tricycles or bicycles.

- At all ages, make sure your smoke detectors work; keep matches and lighters away from children.

About the Authors

T. Berry Brazelton, M.D. may be most recognized by parents and health professionals alike for his many books on family and child development and for his television show What Every Baby Knows. But Dr. Brazelton is also renowned for his pioneering scientific work and his pediatric practice, which led him to believe that a newborn baby arrives in a family with a strong individuality. He found that a baby's behavior gives wonderful clues for parents and strengthens the bond between baby and parents. He has also focused on cross-cultural differences in parenting and child behavior, and on the importance of early intervention for at-risk infants and their families.

Dr. Brazelton is currently Chairman of the Pampers Parenting Institute, a one-stop resource center for parents seeking advice from experts.

His classic book, *Infants and Mothers*, has reached nearly one million families in this country and is translated into 18 languages. *Touchpoints* is his most recent book for parents, and is reaching half a million families to date.

In 1972, Dr. Brazelton helped establish the Child Development Unit at Children's Hospital in Boston. There, Dr. Brazelton also oversees the Touchpoints Project and The Brazelton Institute. His interest in children and families has also led him into the halls of the U.S. Congress, where he has testified on the importance of the Family and Medical Leave Act and of child care and support for all working parents. In 1989, Congress appointed him to the National Commission on Children. He is a parent advocate. His research establishes the baby's contribution through the Neonatal Behavioral Assessment and is used all over the world to reach parents.

Ann Brown was sworn in as Chairman of the U.S. Consumer Product Safety Commission (CPSC) on March 10, 1994. She was nominated by President Clinton and confirmed by the U.S. Senate as a Commissioner and the seventh Chairman of the CPSC.

As Chairman, Ann Brown's goal is to keep families—especially children safe in their homes. She has frequently cited the equal responsibility of consumers, industry and the CPSC in promoting consumer safety. Her actions on behalf of children have earned Chairman Brown the "Champion of Safe Kids Award" from the National Safe Kids Campaign, the "Humanitarian of the Year" award from the Danny Foundation, and the "Clarion Award" from the National Parents Day Coalition. In 1995, Chairman Brown received the "Government Communicator of the Year Award," and in 1996, the "Golden Trumpet Award" from the Publicity Club of Chicago.

Her leadership of agency efforts to provide better customer service has been honored with three awards for reinventing government from Vice President Al Gore, including an award for outstanding improvement of CPSC's toll-free hotline, its most direct link to the public.

For more than two decades prior to her appointment, Mrs. Brown was a consumer advocate. She served as vice president of the Consumer Federation of America for nearly 15 years, and was chairman of the board of the consumer advocacy group Public Voice from 1983 to 1994. In 1989, Mrs. Brown was named "Washingtonian of the Year," by Washingtonian magazine.

For more information on child and parenting topics, visit Dr. Brazelton's home page on the Internet.

Part Three

Caring for the Aging Body

Chapter 17

Growing Older, Eating Better

Whether it happens at age 65 or 85, older people eventually face one or more problems that interfere with their ability to eat well.

When Bernadette Harkins, 89, of Rockville, Md., could no longer feed herself properly, she moved to an assisted-living residence. Today, she can enjoy three meals a day served to her and about 30 other people in their home-like communal dining room.

When Harry, 85, of Moscow, Pa., could no longer feed himself properly, he moved in with his daughter and her family. Today, with her guidance, he's eating six times a day, snacking on high-calorie, high-protein foods, and maintaining a near-normal weight.

Harry, who asked that his last name not be used, and Harkins typify many of today's older generation. Living alone in most cases, they often are unable to meet their dietary needs and are forced to make compromises.

Harry didn't know how to cook. He developed cancer, which made it even more important that he eat a well-balanced diet. Harkins knew how to cook but didn't take time to prepare adequate meals for herself.

"I would snack is what I'd do," she said. "I would think about getting a meal and then just have a cup of tea and toast. I knew I wasn't doing the right thing as far as nutrition was concerned."

Their eating problems stemmed from loneliness and lack of desire or skill to cook. Other older people may eat poorly for other reasons, ranging from financial difficulties to physical problems.

U.S. Department of Health and Human Services, Food and Drug Administration (FDA), *FDA Consumer*, March 1996, revised December 1996.

The solutions can be just as varied, from finding alternative living arrangements to accepting home-delivered meals to using the food label recently revised by the Food and Drug Administration and the U.S. Department of Agriculture. Physical activity also is important in maintaining a healthy lifestyle.

Why the Concern

Nutrition remains important throughout life. Many chronic diseases that develop late in life, such as osteoporosis, can be influenced by earlier poor habits. Insufficient exercise and calcium intake, especially during adolescence and early adulthood, can significantly increase the risk of osteoporosis, a disease that causes bones to become brittle and crack or break.

But good nutrition in the later years still can help lessen the effects of diseases prevalent among older Americans or improve the quality of life in people who have such diseases. They include osteoporosis, obesity, high blood pressure, heart disease, certain cancers, gastrointestinal problems, and chronic undernutrition.

Studies show that a good diet in later years helps both in reducing the risk of these diseases and in managing the diseases' signs and symptoms. This contributes to a higher quality of life, enabling older people to maintain their independence by continuing to perform basic daily activities, such as bathing, dressing and eating.

Poor nutrition, on the other hand, can prolong recovery from illnesses, increase the costs and incidence of institutionalization, and lead to a poorer quality of life.

The Single Life

Whether it happens at age 65 or 85, older people eventually face one or more problems that interfere with their ability to eat well.

Social isolation is a common one. Older people who find themselves single after many years of living with another person may find it difficult to be alone, especially at mealtimes. They may become depressed and lose interest in preparing or eating regular meals, or they may eat only sparingly.

In a study published in the July 1993 *Journals of Gerontology*, researchers found that newly widowed people, most of whom were women, were less likely to say they enjoy mealtimes, less likely to report good appetites, and less likely to report good eating behaviors than their married counterparts. Nearly 85 percent of widowed subjects reported a weight change during the two years following their spouse's death, as compared with 30 percent of married subjects. The widowed group was more likely to report an average weight loss of 7.6 pounds (17 kilograms).

According to the study, most of the women said they had enjoyed cooking and eating when they were married, but, as widows, they found those activities "a chore," especially since there was no one to appreciate their cooking efforts.

For many widowed men who may have left the cooking to their wives, the problem may extend even further: They may not know how to cook and prepare foods. Instead, they may snack or eat out a lot, both of which may lead people to eat too much fat and cholesterol and not get enough vitamins and minerals.

Special Diets

At the same time, many older people, because of chronic medical problems, may require special diets: for example, a low-fat, low-cholesterol diet for heart disease, a low-sodium diet for high blood pressure, or a low-calorie diet for weight reduction. Special diets often require extra effort, but older people may instead settle for foods that are quick and easy to prepare, such as frozen dinners, canned foods, lunch meats, and others that may provide too many calories, or contain too much fat and sodium for their needs.

On the other hand, Mona Sutnick, Ed.D., a registered dietitian in private practice in Philadelphia, pointed out that some people may go overboard on their special diets, overly restricting foods that may be more beneficial than detrimental to their health.

"My advice for a 60-year-old person might be 'watch your fat' but for an 80-year-old who's underweight, I'd say, 'eat the fat, get the calories,' " Sutnick said.

Physical Problems

Some older people may overly restrict foods important to good health because of chewing difficulties and gastrointestinal disturbances, such as constipation, diarrhea and heartburn. Because missing teeth and poorly fitting dentures make it hard to chew, older people may forego fresh fruits and vegetables, which are important sources of vitamins, minerals and fiber. Or they may avoid dairy products, believing they cause gas or constipation. By doing so, they miss out on important sources of calcium, protein and some vitamins.

221

Adverse reactions from medications can cause older people to avoid certain foods. Some medications alter the sense of taste, which can adversely affect appetite. This adds to the problem of naturally diminishing senses of taste and smell, common as people age.

Other medical problems, such as arthritis, stroke or Alzheimer's disease, can interfere with good nutrition. It may be difficult, if not impossible, for example, for people with arthritis or who have had a stroke to cook, shop, or even lift a fork to eat. Dementia associated with Alzheimer's and other diseases may cause them to eat poorly or forget to eat altogether.

Money Matters

Lack of money is a particular problem among older Americans who may have no income other than Social Security. According to 1994 U.S. Census Bureau data, nearly 12 percent of people 65 and over are below the average poverty level for their age group. In 1994, the poverty level for a person 65 and over was $7,108 a year.

According to the 1994 data, the mean annual income for people 65 and over was $16,709, almost $10,000 less than what they earned on average between ages 55 and 64.

Lack of money may lead older people to scrimp on important food purchase—for example, perishable items like fresh fruits, vegetables and meat—because of higher costs and fear of waste. They may avoid cooking or baking foods like meats, stews and casseroles because recipes for these foods usually yield large quantities.

Financial problems also may cause older people to delay medical and dental treatments that could correct problems that interfere with good nutrition.

Food Programs

Many older people may find help under the Older Americans Act, which provides nutrition and other services that target older people who are in greatest social and economic need, with particular attention on low-income minorities. According to the U.S. Administration on Aging, which administers the Older Americans Act, the nutrition programs were set up to address the dietary inadequacy and social isolation among older people.

Home-delivered meals and congregate nutrition services are the primary nutrition programs. The congregate meal program allows seniors to gather at a local site, often the local senior citizen center, school or other public building or a restaurant, for a meal and other activities, such as games and lectures on nutrition and other topics of interest to older people.

Available since 1972, these programs, funded by the federal, state and local governments, ensure that senior citizens get at least one nutritious meal five to seven days a week. Under current standards, that meal must comply with the Dietary Guidelines for Americans and provide at least one-third of the Recommended Dietary Allowances for an older person. Often, people receive foods that correspond with their special dietary needs, such as no-added-salt foods for those who need to restrict their sodium intake or ground meat for those who have trouble chewing.

Other nutrition services provided under the Older Americans Act are nutrition education, screening and counseling.

While these nutrition programs target poor people, they are available to other older people regardless of income, according to Jean Lloyd, a registered dietitian and nutrition officer with the Administration on Aging. Although no one is charged for the meals, older people can voluntarily and confidentially donate money, she said.

The meals provide not only good nutrition, but they also give older people a chance to socialize—a key factor in preventing the adverse nutritional effects of social isolation.

For those who qualify, food stamps are another aid for improving nutrition. Under this program, a one-person household can receive up to $115 a month in food stamps to buy most grocery items.

For the homebound, grocery-shopping assistance is available in many areas. Usually provided by non-government organizations, this service shops for and delivers groceries to people at their request. The recipient pays for the groceries and sometimes a service fee.

In some communities, private organizations also sell home-delivered meals.

Other Assistance

Family members and friends can help ensure that older people take advantage of food programs by putting them in touch with the appropriate agencies or organizations and helping them fill out the necessary forms. Some other steps they can take include:

- looking in occasionally to ensure that the older person is eating adequately
- preparing foods for and making them available to the older person
- joining the older person for meals.

In some cases, they may help see that the older person is moved to an environment, such as their home, an assisted-living facility, or a nursing home, that can help ensure that the older person gets proper nutrition.

Whatever an older person's living situation, proper medical and dental treatment is important for treating medical problems, such as gastrointestinal distress and chewing difficulties, that interfere with good nutrition. If a medication seems to ruin an older person's taste and appetite, a switch to another drug may help.

A review of basic diet principles may help improve nutrition. Explaining to older people the importance of good nutrition in the later years may motivate them to make a greater effort to select nutritious foods.

Look to the Label

The food label can help older people select a good diet. Revamped in 1992, the label gives the nutritional content of most foods and enables consumers to see how a food fits in with daily dietary recommendations.

Some of the information appears as claims describing the food's nutritional benefits: for example, "low in cholesterol" or "high in potassium." Understrict government rules, these claims can be used only if the food meets certain criteria. This means that claims can be trusted. For example, a "low-cholesterol" food can provide no more than 20 milligrams (mg) of cholesterol and no more than 2 grams of saturated fat per serving. A high-potassium food must provide at least 700 mg of potassium per serving.

Less common but also helpful are label claims linking a nutrient or food to the risk of a disease or health-related condition. So far, FDA allows only eight of these claims because they are the only ones supported by scientific evidence. One claim links sodium, a nutrient found in salt and used in many processed foods, to high blood pressure. On the food label, this claim would read something like this:

"Diets low in sodium may reduce the risk of high blood pressure, a disease associated with many factors."

More in-depth information is found on the "Nutrition Facts" panel on the side or back of the food label. This information is required on almost all food packages. Unlike before, this nutrition information is easier to read because it appears in bigger type and is usually on a white or other neutral contrasting background, when practical.

Some nutrition information also may be available for many raw meats, poultry and fish and fresh fruits and vegetables at the point of purchase. The information may appear in brochures or on posters or placards.

Physical Activity

Besides diet, physical activity is part of a healthy lifestyle at any age. It can help reduce and control weight by burning calories. Moderate exercise that places weight on bones, such as walking, helps maintain and possibly even increases bone strength in older people. A study published in the Dec. 28, 1994, *Journal of the American Medical Association* found that intensive strength training can help preserve bone density and improve muscle mass, strength and balance in postmenopausal women. In the study, subjects used weight machines for strength training.

Also, scientists looking into the benefits of exercise for older people agree that regular exercise can improve the functioning of the heart and lungs, increase strength and flexibility, and contribute to a feeling of well-being.

Any regular physical activity is good, from brisk walking to light gardening. Common sense is the key. But, before a vigorous exercise program is started or started after a long period of rest, a doctor should be consulted.

Taking time out for exercise, using the food label to help pick nutritious foods, taking advantage of the several assistance programs available, and getting needed medical attention can go a long way in helping older people avoid the nutritional pitfalls of aging and more fully enjoy their senior years.

—Paula Kurtzwell

Paula Kurtzweil is a member of FDA's public affairs staff.

For More Information

To learn more about the food label and nutrition for older people, write for these publications:

- *Using the New Food Label to Choose Healthier Foods.* FDA, 5600 Fishers Lane (HFE-88), Rockville, MD 20857. Ask for publication number (FDA) 94-2276.

- *Healthy Eating for a Healthy Life.* AARP (American Association of Retired Persons) Fulfillment, 601 E. St.5 N.W., Washington,

DC 20049. Ask for publication by title and stock number D15565.

To learn about meal programs for senior citizens in your area, call the Administration on Aging's Elder Care Locator, (1-800) 677-1116.

For information about food stamps, contact your county's food stamp office listed in the blue pages of the telephone book.

To find a registered dietitian in your area, call the National Center for Nutrition and Dietetics Consumer Nutrition Hotline, (1-800) 366-1655.

How to Use Nutrition Facts

The Nutrition Facts panel is the place to go for more complete nutrition information.

Start at the top with serving size information. Serving sizes are:

- given in both household and metric units

- uniform across product lines so you can more easily compare the nutritional qualities of similar foods

- close to the amounts people really eat (although they're not recommended amounts).

Be sure to look at % Daily Values on the right. They show how a serving of food fits in with current recommendations for a healthful diet. A high percentage means the food contains a lot of a nutrient. A low percentage means it contains a little. The goal is to choose foods that together give you about 100 percent a day.

We hope you found this reprint from FDA Consumer magazine useful and informative. *FDA Consumer*, the magazine of the U.S. Food and Drug Administration, provides a wealth of information on FDA-related health issues: food safety, nutrition, drugs, medical devices, cosmetics, radiation protection, vaccines, blood products, and veterinary medicine. For a sample copy of *FDA Consumer* and a subscription order form, write to: Food and Drug Administration, HFI-40, Rockville, MD 20857.

Chapter 18

Eating Well as We Age

Eating Well

Many older people have trouble eating well. This chapter tells why. Then it gives ideas on what you can do about it. Using the food label is one way to eat well. There are others.

Problem: Can't Chew

Do you have trouble chewing? If so, you may have trouble eating foods like meat and fresh fruits and vegetables.

Table 18.1. What to do: Try other foods.

Instead of:	Try:
fresh fruit	fruit juices; soft canned fruits, like applesauce, peaches and pears
raw vegetables	vegetable juices; creamed and mashed cooked vegetables
meat	ground meat; other high-protein foods, like eggs, milk, cheese, and yogurt; and foods made with milk, like pudding and cream soups
sliced bread	cooked cereals, rice, bread pudding, and soft cookies

U.S. Department of Health and Human Service, Food and Drug Administration (FDA), NIH Pub. No. 97-2311, May 1997.

Problem: Upset stomach

Stomach problems, like too much gas, may make you stay away from foods you think cause the problem. This means you could be missing out on important nutrients, like vitamins, calcium, fiber and protein.

Table 18.2. What to do: Try other foods.

Instead of:	Try:
milk	milk foods that may not bother you, like cream soups, pudding, yogurt and cheese
vegetables like cabbage and broccoli	other vegetables, like green beans, carrots and potatoes; vegetable juices
fresh fruit	fruit juices; soft canned fruits

See a doctor about your stomach problems.

Problem: Can't shop

You may have problems shopping for food. Maybe you can't drive anymore. You may have trouble walking or standing for a long time. What to do:

- Ask the local food store to bring groceries to your home. Some stores deliver free. Sometimes there is a charge.

- Ask your church or synagogue for volunteer help. Or sign up for help with a local volunteer center.

- Ask a family member or neighbor to shop for you. Or pay someone to do it.

Some companies let you hire home health workers for a few hours a week. These workers may shop for you, among other things. Look for these companies in the Yellow Pages of the phone book under "Home Health Services."

Problem: Can't cook

You may have problems with cooking. It may be hard for you to hold cooking utensils, and pots and pans. Or you may have trouble standing for a long time.

What to do:

- Use a microwave oven to cook TV dinners, other frozen foods, and foods made up ahead of time by the store.

- Take part in group meal programs offered through senior citizen programs. Or, have meals brought to your home.

- Move to a place where someone else will cook, like a family member's home or a home for senior citizens.

To find out about senior citizen group meals and home-delivered meals, call (1-800) 677-1116. These meals cost little or no money.

Problem: No appetite

Older people who live alone sometimes feel lonely at mealtimes. Loneliness can make you lose your appetite. Or you may not feel like making meals for just yourself. Maybe your food has no flavor or tastes bad. This could be caused by medicines you are taking.
What to do:

- Eat with family and friends.

- Take part in group meal programs, offered through senior citizen programs.

- Ask your doctor if your medicines could be causing appetite or taste problems. If so, ask about changing medicines.

- Increase the flavor of food by adding spices and herbs.

Problem: Short on money

Not having enough money to buy enough food can keep you from eating well.
What to do:

- Buy low-cost foods, like dried beans and peas, rice and pasta. Or buy foods that contain these items, like split pea soup and canned beans and rice.

- Use coupons for money off on foods you like.

- Buy foods on sale. Also buy store-brand foods. They often cost less.

- Find out if your local church or synagogue offers free or low-cost meals.

- Take part in group meal programs offered through local senior citizen programs. Or, have meals brought to your home.

- Get food stamps. Call the food stamp office listed under your county government in the blue pages of the telephone book.

Read the Label

Look for words that say something healthy about the food. Examples are:

- Low Fat
- Cholesterol Free
- Good Source of Fiber

Look for words that tell about the food's relation to a disease. A low-fat food may say: "While many factors affect heart disease, diets low in saturated fat and cholesterol may reduce the risk of this disease."

The words may be on the front or side of the food package. FDA makes sure these words are true.

Look for "Nutrition Facts"

Most food labels tell what kinds and amounts of vitamins, minerals, protein, fat, and other nutrients are in a food. This information is called "Nutrition Facts." You can find it on the side or back of most food labels.

Use "Nutrition Facts"

1. Look at the serving size.

2. Find the %Daily Value. The numbers underneath tell how much of each nutrient listed is in one serving.

3. About 100% of each nutrient each day is usually healthful. If you're on a special diet, like a low-sodium or low-fat diet, use the % numbers to pick low-sodium and low-fat foods.

The 3g (grams) of total fat in one serving of this food provides 5% of fat for the day, leaving 95% more fat allowed that day in a normal diet. The 300 mg (milligrams) of sodium provide 13% for the day, leaving 87% more sodium allowed that day in a normal diet. The "mg" number is much larger than the "g" number because it takes many, many milligrams to equal 1 gram.

Do You Have More Questions About Eating Well As You Age?

Ask your doctor or other health-care worker. And ask FDA. There may be an FDA office near you. Look for the number in the blue pages of the phone book. Or, write a letter to: FDA HFE-88, Rockville, MD 20857.

Chapter 19

When an Older Person Needs Help in the Kitchen

It's widely known that as the years roll on, many elderly people will need help running the kitchen. After all, it's a demanding job— shopping, cleaning out the refrigerator, preparing meals, storing left-overs.

What is not so well understood is that it actually can be danger-ous for an older person who can no longer manage well trying to run a kitchen alone. Why? Because the health of the elderly is often frag-ile. They're highly susceptible to food poisoning and prone to develop nutritional deficiencies. The sensory losses of aging—sight and smell in particular— can cause food handling problems. Also, tight budgets couple with ingrained feelings against "waste" cause many elderly people to hang on to risky food for too long.

Let's take a closer look...

Susceptibility to Food Poisoning

The elderly are much more vulnerable to food poisoning than the general public. For one thing, less stomach acid—which helps digest food and kill microbes in food—is produced as the body ages.

Also, in ways that are not well understood, aging seems to weaken the immune system. A food poisoning illness that simply might make someone else sick for a few days could be devastating for an elderly person. And many elderly people suffer chronic conditions —heart

U.S. Department of Agriculture (USDA), *Food News for Consumers*, Spring 1988.

disease, diabetes—which lower their resistance. Undergoing chemo-therapy for cancer weakens the immune system.

Nutritional Problems

Older people are likely to develop nutritional difficulties. For ease of preparation, they may rely too heavily on canned and frozen foods, which can be over-sugared or salted. Their diets may be lacking in fresh meats, fruits and vegetables. They may suffer calcium deficiencies, a condition which often develops in old age, particularly if they have trouble digesting milk.

Eating and drinking improperly or infrequently also can precipitate serious medical problems, says nurse Liz Weiss, head of Home Care Support at Iona House, Washington, D.C. Weiss explains. "Patients on diuretics for fluid retention can easily become dehydrated if they don't get enough liquids. And diabetics, who must be extra careful to avoid certain foods and eat regularly, can easily get into trouble."

Food Handling Problems Caused by Aging Itself

There are, in addition, the problems attendant to aging itself. Consider sensory loss. Basically, sensory loss means a diminished ability to sense and interpret one's surroundings with sharpness and clarity.

What goes wrong? First, vision dims. Fifty percent of Americans with severe vision problems are over 65. Many older people also have trouble distinguishing between closely related colors, particularly blues and greens. It's not surprising that someone who used to keep an immaculate kitchen now may have spots and spills everywhere, not realize when a fork or pan is still dirty or notice mold on bread or other stored food.

Second, hearing fades. Actually, this is the most common problem of old age. Some 40 percent of those 75 and older suffer hearing loss. Imagine how much more difficult it would be if you couldn't hear the teapot whistle, or if you couldn't hear when something boils over.

Third, taste and smell dim. A recent Duke University study highlights this problem. In a test of common odors like chocolate, cinnamon, coffee, grape, onion, pepper, root beer, soy sauce and tea, college students correctly "named that smell" with 86 percent accuracy. Elderly subjects got only 34 percent of the answers right. The side-effects of taste and smell loss are numerous. Some people lose interest in food and become malnourished. Others over-season food, taking in too much sugar or salt.

But, critical from the food safety standpoint, all those with significant smell loss will have trouble knowing when stored food is spoiled. Most spoilage agents, in addition to making food look bad, give off an unpleasant odor.

Money Problems and Attitudes about Waste

Financial constraints add to the food handling problems of the elderly. Living on a tight budget makes it difficult to throw away food, even things in questionable condition. Plus, today's elderly are depression-survivors, and keenly conscious of "not being wasteful." Consider USDA microbiologist Carl Custer's story about an elderly woman in his family. "The last time we went to Aunt Emma's," says Custer. "I was horrified to find her refrigerator set at about 55°F. For safety, it should run at about 40. When I asked her about it as tactfully as possible, she said, "Hate to waste electricity!"

Now you know some of the things that can go wrong when an elderly person needs help in the kitchen. But how could you tell, in an actual situation, whether someone you are caring for needs more help?

How Would You Know When Someone Needs More Assistance?

Case workers and visiting nurses advise that we should alert to any significant changes in household management. "You may see dishes not cleaned up or things moldering in the refrigerator," says Liz Weiss.

"Food inventories might be off," says Marian Mathur, the nutritionist for the D.C. Visiting Nurse Association. "You know someone brought groceries in four days ago, but nothing's been touched. Maybe they're not eating."

"Sudden weight loss—perhaps again they're forgetting to eat—another bad sign," Mathur adds.

Mental state also should be noted. Are they depressed? "Depressed people may not feel like cooking or eating," says Mathur.

A failure of time-orientation is another red flag. For instance, Mathur explains, "You always drop by at 4 p.m. on Saturday, but the individual seems amazed when you turn up then."

Recognize any of the signs? Perhaps, but don't panic. While an emerging problem of this kind needs prompt attention, it needn't be defeating. See the "tips" chart for coping suggestions and groups that can offer help. And remember that for an individual problem, usually you can find a workable, individual solution.

Tips to Avoid Trouble Before it Starts

1. Be observant—Note any marked change in habits that could mean an elderly person needs more help in the kitchen.

2. Watch nutrition—Make sure they're getting the 4 basic food groups—protein, dairy, cereals and grain, vegetables and fruit. Note: pasta is a tasty, healthful, easy-to-eat food choice.

3. Shopping—Shop for 1 week at a time, favoring single-serving type purchases where feasible. Clear unused leftovers out of the refrigerator every other week.

4. Cooking and storing—Help with cooking batches of several favorite foods. Package portions like TV dinners for later use. For example, a meal tray might include servings of meatloaf, macaroni-and-cheese and green beans.

5. The freezer—Date packages with a marking pen, writing in large letters. Move older packages to the front of the freezer as you add new items.

6. Drinks & snacks—If getting enough liquids is a problem, suggest the use of the microwave for truly "instant" coffee and tea. Keep a basket of fresh, soft, denture-friendly fruit handy too. Grapes, bananas and ripe pears are good.

7. Using an oven timer—For someone who's getting forgetful but still likes to cook, try a brightly colored portable timer. For example, a person could put the casserole in the oven, set the timer for 45 minutes and takes it along to watch the noon news. When the timer sounds, the casserole's done.

8. Jar and bottle opening—If hand strength and dexterity are a problem, you can compensate. Contact your local chapter of the Arthritis Foundation for information on gripper pads, cap poppers and other useful gadgets.

9. Equipment check—Make sure the refrigerator (safe at 40°F) and freezer (safe at 0°F) are running properly. A frosted-over

unit won't cool properly, so defrost every few months as necessary. New microwave? Go over adequate thawing, cooking and reheating times with the older person who'll be using the oven. Thorough cooking is a must for bacterial (food poisoning) control.

10. Lactose problems? Remember, cheese and yogurt, which don't bother most lactose-intolerant people, are good calcium stand-ins for milk. Many large stores now also carry specially treated milk suitable for those with lactose digestion problems.

Other Resources

Write or call the American Association for Retired Persons, 601 E. St.5 N.W. Washington, DC 20049, (202) 872- 4700, for lists of publications and service groups.

Caring for a Cancer Patient? Order free copy of *Eating Hints — Recipes and Tips for Better Nutrition During Cancer Treatment* from the Office of Cancer Communications, National Cancer Institute, Building 31, Room 10A 18, Bethesda, Md. 20892. Phone: 1-800-4-CANCER.

Can that dish of leftover meatloaf be saved? Call USDA's Meat and Poultry Hotline 1-800-535-4555; in the Wash. D.C. area, call 447-3333.

— by Mary Ann Parmley

Chapter 20

Improving Health with Antioxidants

For optimal nutrition, healthy adults should strive to attain diets rich in antioxidants through consumption of fruits and vegetables and the use of nutritional supplements. The Alliance for Aging Research recommends the following ranges of antioxidant consumption for health promotion and disease prevention in an aging population.

Vitamin C: 250-1000mg
Vitamin E: 100-400 international units (IU)
Beta carotene: 17,000-50,000 IU (10-30 mg)

Additional evidence suggests that several other antioxidants, including carotenoids such as lycopene and minerals such as selenium and zinc, also play a role in the prevention of illness. Further research is needed to establish national daily intake levels for these antioxidants and to understand changing nutritional needs with advancing age.

The Alliance for Aging Research is the first national non-profit health organization to issue specific public health guidelines on the benefits of antioxidants in helping prevent some of the leading chronic diseases and causes of death and disability. The Alliance and a scientific advisory panel, comprised of leading researchers in nutrition, aging research and consumer safety, hope these guidelines will provide consumers with up-to-date advice. on optimal nutrition and will

Reprinted with the permission of the Alliance for Aging Research, 2021 K Street, N.W., No. 305, Washington, DC., 20006, (202)-293-2856, undated.

give policy makers a framework to make needed changes in U.S. nutrition policy. The Alliance recommends policies that would expand both public and private sector initiatives to educate consumers about the benefits of antioxidants and the role of nutrition in maintaining good health and independence throughout life.

Aging Research

Scientific interest and understanding of antioxidants in the diet began almost four decades ago with laboratory research into aging and age-related diseases. In 1956, researchers in aging at the University of California, Berkeley proposed that the naturally-occurring byproducts of oxygen use in human cells, called free radicals, were closely related to the incidence of many chronic illnesses associated with aging. Free radicals are normally produced by the body's own metabolism and are necessary for many normal functions like the workings of the brain and the immune and digestive systems. However, these same oxygen free radicals can also cause damage to cells. Research has found that certain nutrients called antioxidants can block the harmful actions of free radicals, thereby controlling cell damage and retarding the progression of normal changes and illness associated with growing older.

The damage to cell membranes and destruction of cells is believed to play a major role in the development of cancer, heart disease and other degenerative illnesses. Many scientists are convinced that the cumulative effects of free radicals are an important underlying cause of the gradual decline that is associated with aging in individuals, healthy and sick. The process of oxidation can also be accelerated by pollution, cigarette smoke, radiation and sunlight. Antioxidants work by helping to neutralize free radical activity and by preventing cellular damage.

While more research is needed to better understand the role of both free radicals and antioxidants in aging, abundant evidence now exists for a link between daily intake of antioxidants and the prevention of illness.

Antioxidants

An impressive amount of research indicates that antioxidants play a significant role in preventing cancer, heart disease, cataracts and other diseases associated with aging. There is now significant epidemiological and clinical evidence that these nutrients, including beta carotene and vitamins C and E, have a direct relationship to the prevention of these and other chronic conditions. While numerous factors, including heredity and overall lifestyle, play a role in the development of chronic age-related illnesses, there is now strong, evidence that increased intake of antioxidants will help prevent numerous life-threatening and costly diseases.

A review of medical journals from the mid-1970's to the present reveals more than 200 epidemiological and clinical studies that have examined the role of fruits and vegetables or the antioxidant nutrients they contain in preventing disease. These studies consistently show a statistically significant protective effect of higher dietary intakes of antioxidant nutrients.

Research by Dr. Gladys Block, one of our panel members, for example, indicates approximately 130 studies that examined the role of fruits and vegetables or antioxidants in preventing numerous types of cancer including lung, larynx, esophagus, oral, pancreas, stomach, cervix, rectum, colon, ovary, endometrium, breast and bladder. Of these major studies, about 120 demonstrated a significant reduction in cancer risk.

Several influential scientific studies have demonstrated the potential for antioxidant nutrients in reducing risk for chronic age-related diseases.

- Nutrition intervention trials in Linxian, China, among 29,584 adults age 40 to 69, indicated that vitamin and mineral supplementation, particularly with the combination of beta carotene, vitamin E and selenium, were associated with a reduced risk of several types of cancers.

- A U.S. study of 87,000 female nurses age 30 to 55 demonstrated a 22% lower risk of heart disease in those with high levels of beta-carotene intake. Those reporting a high intake of vitamin E—almost entirely through supplements—showed a 41 % lower risk of heart disease.

- A U.S. study of 40,000 male health professionals, age 40 to 75, showed similar benefits as the Nurses' Health Study for beta carotene and vitamin E.

- A Canadian study of 96 healthy older adults taking antioxidant-enriched nutrient supplements demonstrated a significant increase in immune responses and a 50% reduction in infectious disease episodes.

- A Canadian study of 175 cataract patients and 175 cataract free people revealed the latter group used significantly more supplementary vitamins C and E; results of the analysis suggested a reduction in the risk of cataract of at least 50% by antioxidant supplementation.

Also, numerous ongoing trials are continuing to further establish the preventive benefits of antioxidants against diseases. The Physicians' Health study is testing beta carotene among more than 22,000 male physicians, and the Women's Health Study is testing vitamin E and beta carotene among approximately 40,000 female health professionals.

Of course, the success of an intervention will depend on the nature of the risk group and the duration and level of antioxidant consumption. Some recent studies have shown that intervening in high risk groups with one or two nutrients, given for a relatively short time, may not be sufficient to overcome a lifetime of accumulated risk.

Sources of Antioxidants

Antioxidants are abundant in many fruits and vegetables. Vitamin C-rich foods include citrus fruits and cabbage family (cruciferous) vegetables among many others. Beta carotene is found in many of the same cruciferous vegetables and dark green leafy vegetables. Several orange-colored fruits are rich in beta carotene. Vitamin E can be found in a variety of grains, nuts, seeds and oils. It is difficult to achieve optimal levels of vitamin E intake through diet alone, especially given the high fat content of the foods in which it is found.

Public Health Issues

The risk of cancer is increasing for many Americans. Heart disease remains the nation's number one killer. Cataract surgery is the most frequently performed medical procedure under the Medicare program. These and other chronic age-related diseases are the health challenges now facing the nation. Any and all public health means which can be used in the prevention of chronic age-related disease should be encouraged by government policy. Increased intake of antioxidants is one such means which can be used safely to improve the health of Americans of all ages. Through government policies encouraging disease prevention, individuals can be empowered to take responsibility for their own health.

242

The National Cancer Institute recommends that Americans consume at least five servings of fruits and vegetables a day. This is consistent with the U.S. Department of Agriculture "Food Pyramid" guide to dietary consumption. Unfortunately, most Americans do not consume the recommended amounts of fruits and vegetables. A 1990 analysis of the National Health and Nutrition Examination Survey (N HANES 11) revealed that less than 10 percent of Americans actually consume two servings of fruits and three servings of vegetables a day.

Older Americans are at increased nutritional risk. In April 1993 the Nutrition Screening Initiative, of which the Alliance is an advisory member, reported that malnourishment is a serious problem among America's older population. The study found that one-half of all hospital patients above age 65 are malnourished, as are more than two in five nursing home residents and an equal number of people receiving home care assistance.

Policy Issues

Despite the overwhelming body of evidence that a diet high in antioxidants can be effective in preventing chronic illnesses associated with aging, the Food and Drug Administration (FDA) has not yet approved an antioxidant health claim. It is hoped that these recommendations will serve as a public health model for the FDA to provide this needed information to help prevent some of the nation's leading causes of death and some of our most costly aging-related diseases.

Americans need to increase consumption of antioxidants beyond levels traditionally defined by the government as Recommended Daily Allowances (RDA). Unfortunately, government nutrition policy is inconsistent. Consumption of even the minimum amounts of fruits and vegetables recommended under the Food Pyramid guide would yield a higher intake of antioxidants than established by the U.S. RDA.

The RDA was developed during World War II to provide a target level of nutrient intakes to guide national policy in planning the food supply for troops and for the civilian population. It has been periodically updated since that time, and is intended to provide sufficient nutrients to avoid deficiencies. However, the RDA does not take into account the currently recognized role of some nutrients in protecting against chronic diseases. The RDA is used as the basis for other guidelines used in nutrition labeling and in other areas of nutrition policy. In 1990, when the FDA attempted to lower the nutrient standards used for nutrition labeling, the Alliance for Aging Research joined with numerous public health advocates, consumer groups and organizations representing low-income people to oppose this recommendation.

An important moment for American consumers and for preventive health care came on October 25, 1994, when the President signed the Dietary Supplement Health and Education Act. For the first time this Act established a rational framework for Food and Drug Administration regulation of vitamins, minerals, herbs, amino acids and other dietary products. The new law is intended to assure that consumers have access to safe dietary supplements and to information about those supplements. It will be important to monitor the implementation of this new law which holds out the promise of improving the American consumer's access to a wide range of safe dietary products and to truthful and non-misleading information about those products.

Beyond improving FDA regulation of dietary supplements and increasing RDAs to ensure protective levels of nutrients, the federal government should provide funding for research which will address the special dietary and nutrient needs of elderly persons, in particular those nutrients capable of delaying or mitigating the degenerative diseases that often accompany aging. *The Threshold of Discovery — Future Directions for Research on Aging* — the final report of the Congressionally-mandated Task Force on Aging Research (TFAR), issued in June, 1995 — cites research on dietary supplementation as an area of "immediate priority" in aging research.

The TFAR report distills some 3,000 recommendations for research in aging down to 192 high priority projects about one-third of which are considered "immediate priority." This report also "costs out" the opportunities for priority research in aging. A total additional federal research expenditure of $13.8 million is recommended for additional research on nutritional supplements over the next five years. The importance of research on dietary supplementation and the role of free radicals and antioxidants in aging is critical, noted the TFAR report: "Any preventive effects of antioxidants would have tremendous potential for forestalling a range of degenerative diseases ... [A]ntioxidants appear to be linked to possible prevention of some cancers, senile dementias, and cardiovascular diseases. With the escalating costs of medical treatment and personal care for an aging population, simple preventive schemes involving dietary supplementation may have tremendous benefits." It is time for U.S. nutritional policy to reflect our nation's changing needs.

The Alliance Specifically Calls on the Federal Government to:

- Expedite approval of an antioxidant health claim by the FDA.

- Increase RDAs to ensure protective levels of nutrients.

- Focus greater attention on research and educational programs for the nutritional needs of older Americans.

- Increase research funding for antioxidants and other potentially protective ingredients in the diet as recommended in the 1995 final report of the Congressionally-mandated Task Force on Aging Research.

- Establish as a priority the development of RDAs for older Americans which take into consideration not only chronological age, but also physiological age and chronic disease status.

- Encourage health and social service professionals serving older persons and their caregivers to routinely evaluate their nutritional status as a part of regular assessment procedures to maintain the health and independence of older Americans.

Chapter 21

A Good Night's Sleep

Few things in life are as eagerly anticipated as a good night's sleep. Yet many older people find that bedtime is the hardest part of the day. Although sleep patterns change as we age, sleep that is disturbed and unrefreshing is not an inevitable part of aging. In fact, troubled sleep may be a sign of emotional or physical disorders and should be carefully evaluated by a doctor or sleep specialist.

Sleep and Aging

The normal sleep cycle consists of two different kinds of sleep: REM (rapid eye movement or dreaming sleep) and non-REM (quiet sleep). Everyone has about four to five cycles of REM and non-REM sleep a night. For older people, the amount of time spent in the deepest stages of non-REM sleep decreases. This may explain why older people are thought of as light sleepers.

Although the amount of sleep each person needs varies widely, the range usually falls between 7 and 8 hours a night. While these individual requirements remain fairly constant throughout adulthood, aging does reduce the amount of sleep you can expect to get at any one time. By age 75, for a variety of reasons, some people may find they are waking up several times each night. However, no matter what your age, talk to a doctor if your sleep patterns change.

National Institute on Aging (NIA) "Age Page," August 1998.

Common Sleep Disorders

At any age insomnia is the most common sleep complaint. Insomnia means taking a long time to fall asleep (more than 30 to 45 minutes), waking up many times each night, or waking up early and being unable to get back to sleep. With rare exceptions, insomnia is a symptom of a problem, not the problem itself.

Insomnia can be coupled with other sleep disorders. Sleep apnea is a common problem that causes breathing to stop for periods of up to 2 minutes, many times each night. Central sleep apnea happens when the respiratory muscles do not function as they should; obstructive sleep apnea happens when something blocks the flow of air through the neck passage. In either case, the sleeper is totally unaware of his or her struggle to breathe. Daytime sleepiness coupled with loud snoring are clues that sleep apnea may be a problem. A doctor specializing in sleep disorders can make a definite diagnosis and recommend treatment. A wide range of treatments are available, including gadgets that help you stay off your back when sleeping, medication, and surgery.

Suggestions for a Good Night's Sleep

Getting a good night's sleep can make a big difference in your quality of life. Here are some suggestions to improve your sleep:

- Follow a regular schedule—go to sleep and get up at the same time each day.

- Try to exercise at regular times each day. Moderate physical activity 2 to 4 hours before bedtime may improve your sleep.

- To adjust your internal sleep clock, try to get some exposure to the natural light in the afternoon each day.

- Be aware of what you eat. Avoid drinking beverages with caffeine late in the day, since caffeine is a stimulant and can keep you awake. Also, if you like a snack before bed, a glass of warm milk may help.

- Don't drink alcohol or smoke cigarettes to help you sleep. Even small amounts of alcohol can make it harder to stay asleep. Smoking is not only dangerous (the hazard of falling asleep with a lit cigarette), but nicotine is a stimulant.

- Create a safe and comfortable sleeping environment. Make sure there are locks on all doors and smoke alarms on each floor. A lamp that's easy to turn on and a telephone by your bedside may be helpful. In addition, the room should be dark, well ventilated, and have all nonessential sounds blocked out.

- Develop a bedtime routine. Do the same things each night to tell your body that it's time to wind down. Some people watch the evening news, read a book, or soak in a warm bath.

- Use your bedroom only for sleeping. After turning off the light, give yourself about 15 minutes of trying to fall asleep. If you are still awake or if you lose your drowsiness, get up and go into another room until you feel sleepy again.

- Try not to worry about your sleep. Some people find that playing mental games is helpful. For example, think black—a black cat on a black velvet pillow on a black corduroy sofa, etc.; or tell yourself it's 5 minutes before you have to get up and you're just trying to get a few extra winks.

Additional Information Sources

If you are so tired during the day that you cannot function normally and if this fatigue lasts for more than 2 to 3 weeks, you should see your family doctor or a sleep disorders specialist for a complete evaluation.

For general information about sleep, contact the Better Sleep Council, P.O. Box 13, Washington, DC 20044. They publish the Sleep Better, Liver Better Guide.

The Wakefulness-Sleep Education and Research Foundation publishes *101 Questions About Sleep and Dreams* ($6.18 includes shipping). Contact the publisher at W-SERF, 4820 Rancho Drive, Del Mar, CA 92014.

The National Sleep Foundation was created by the American Sleep Disorders Association to provide educational materials on sleep. When contacting the Foundation, indicate the specific sleep problems you are interested in knowing more about, and write to 122 South Robertson Boulevard, Los Angeles, CA 90048.

The National Institute of Aging offers a variety of resources on aging. Contact the NIA Information Center, P.O. Box 8057, Gaithersburg, MD 20898-8057.

Chapter 22

Don't Take It Easy—Exercise!

Whether you're 40 or 60 years old, you can exercise and improve your health. Physical activity is good for your heart, mood, and confidence. Exercising has even helped 80 and 90 year old people living in nursing homes to grow stronger and more independent. Older people who become more active—including those with medical problems—may feel better and have more energy than ever before.

Why Should I Exercise?

Staying physically active is key to good health well into later years. Yet only about 1 in 4 older adults exercises regularly. Many older people think they are too old or too frail to exercise.

Nothing could be further from the truth. Physical activity of any kind—from heavy-duty exercises such as jogging or bicycling to easier efforts like walking—is good for you. Vigorous exercise can help strengthen your heart and lungs. Taking a brisk walk regularly can help lower your risk of health problems like heart disease or depression. Climbing stairs, calisthenics, or housework can increase your strength, stamina, and self-confidence. Weight-lifting or strength training is a good way to stop muscle loss and slow down bone loss. Your daily activities will become easier as you feel better.

Researchers now know that:

- Regular, active exercise such as swimming and running, raises your heart rate and may greatly reduce stiffening of the arteries.

National Institute of Aging (NIA) "Age Page," 1995.

251

Stiff arteries are a major cause of high blood pressure, which can lead to heart disease and stroke.

• People who are physically active are less likely to develop adult onset diabetes, or they can control it better if they do have it. Exercise increases the body's ability to control the blood glucose level.

• Regular activity, such as walking or gardening, may lower the risk of severe intestinal bleeding in later life by almost half.

• Strength training, like lifting weights or exercising against resistance, can make bones stronger, improve balance, and increase muscle strength and mass. This can prevent or slow bone-weakening osteoporosis, and may lower the risk of falls, which can cause hip fractures or other injures.

• Strength training can lessen arthritis pain. It doesn't cure arthritis, but stronger muscles may ease the strain and therefore the pain.

• Light exercise may be good for your mental health. A group of healthy, older adults said they felt less anxious or stressful after exercising for one year.

What Kind of Exercise Should I Do?

Physical activity and exercise programs should meet your needs and skills. The amount and type of exercise depends on what you want to do. Different exercises do different things: some may slow bone loss, others may reduce the risk of falls, still others may improve the fitness of your heart and lungs. Some may do all three.

You can exercise at home alone, with a buddy, or as part of a group. Talk to your doctor before you begin, especially if you are over 60 or have a medical problem. Move at your own speed, and don't try to take on too much at first. A class can be a good idea if you haven't exercised for a long time or are just beginning. A qualified teacher will make sure you are doing the exercise in the right way.

It may take a little effort to make exercise a regular part of your life. Once you start, try to stick with it. If you stop exercising, after awhile, the benefits disappear.

One good way to stay active is to make physical activity part of every day. Thirty minutes of moderate activity each day is a good goal. You don't have to exercise for 30 minutes all at once. Short bursts of activity, like taking the stairs instead of the elevator, or walking instead of driving, can add up to 30 minutes of exercise a day. Raking leaves, playing actively with children, gardening, and even doing household chores can all be done in a way that can count toward your daily total.

It's a good idea to include some stretching, strength training, and aerobic or endurance exercise in your exercise plan. People who are weak or frail, and may risk falling, should start slowly. Begin with stretching and strength training; add aerobics later. Aerobics are safer and easier once you feel balanced and your muscles are stronger.

Stretching—improves flexibility, eases movement, and lowers the risk of injury and muscle strain. Stretching increases blood flow and gets your body ready for exercise. A warm-up and cool-down period of 5 to 15 minutes should be done slowly and carefully before and after all types of exercise. Stretching can help loosen muscles in the arms, shoulders, back, chest, stomach, buttocks, thighs, and calves. It's also very relaxing.

Strength training (also called resistance training or weight-lifting)—builds muscle and bone, both of which decline with age. Strengthening exercises for the upper and lower body can be done by lifting weights or working out with machines or an elastic band. It is very important to have an expert teach you how to work with weights. Without help, you can get hurt. With help, older adults can work their way up to many of the same weight-lifting routines as younger adults. Once you know what to do, simple strength training exercises can be done at home. For beginners, household items, such as soup cans or milk jugs filled with water or sand, can be used as weights.

Strength training activities do not have to take a lot of time; 30 to 40 minutes at least two or three times each week is all that's needed. Try not to exercise the same muscles two days in a row.

Sample Strength Training Plan:

1. Start with a weight you can lift without too much effort five times.

2. When you can easily do that, lift it five times, rest a few minutes, then do it again. (This is two sets.)

3. Increase to three sets.

4. When you can easily do that, lift the weight 10 times in each set.

5. When you can easily do that, lift the weight 15 times in each set.

6. Once that's easy, slowly increase the weight.

(Always check with your doctor first. Work with a qualified teacher to make sure you are doing the exercise right.)

Aerobic exercises (also called endurance exercises)—strengthen the heart and improve overall fitness by increasing the body's ability to use oxygen. Swimming, walking, and dancing are "low-impact" aerobic activities. They avoid the muscle and joint pounding of more "high-impact" exercises like jogging and jumping rope.

Aerobic exercises raise the number of heart beats each minute (heart rate). It's best to get your heart rate to a certain point and keep it there for 20 minutes or more. If you have not exercised in awhile, start slowly. As you get stronger, you can try to increase your heart rate. Aerobics should be done for 20 to 40 minutes at least three times each week.

How To Measure Your Heart Rate

Your heart rate tells how many times your heart beats each minute. The maximum heart rate is the fastest your heart can beat. Exercise above 75% of that rate is too much for most people. You can figure out the number of times your heart should beat each minute during exercise (your personal "target" heart rate), with the following guidelines and just a little bit of math.

Look for the age category closest to your age in the table below and read the line across:

Table 22.1.

Age	Target Heart Rate Zone	Average Maximum Heart Rate
55	50%-75%	100%
60	80-120	165
65	83-123	160
70+	75-113	155

For example, if you are 60 years old, your target zone is 80-120 beats per minute.

When you begin your exercise program, choose the lowest level in the zone closest to your age and keep your heart rate at that level for the first few months. As you get into better shape, you can slowly build up to a higher level.

To see if you are within your target heart rate zone, measure your heartbeats right after exercising. One good way is to place the tips of your first two fingers on the inside of your wrist, just below the bottom of your thumb. Count your pulse for 10 seconds and then multiply by six to find the number of beats per minute. If you are below your target zone, you may want to exercise a little harder next time. Slow down if you are above your target zone.

Before starting any aerobics program, check with your doctor and ask about your own target heart rate. Some blood pressure medicines, for example, can affect how you figure out your target heart rate.

Helpful Hints

- Choose activities that you like.

- Make small changes so that physical activity becomes a part of each day.

- Stop and check with your doctor right away if you develop sudden pain, shortness of breath, or feel ill.

- Exercise with a group, with a buddy, or alone. Pick what's easiest and most fun.

- Be realistic about what you can do.

Resources

Local gyms, universities, or hospitals can help you find a teacher or program that works for you. You can also check with local churches or synagogues, senior and civic centers, parks, recreation associations, YMCAs, YWCAs, and even local shopping malls for exercise, wellness, or walking programs. Many community centers also offer programs for older people who may be worried about special health problems like heart disease or falling. Your local library may carry books or tapes about exercise and aging.

For more information, contact:

National Heart, Lung, and Blood Institute Information Center
P.O. Box 30105
Bethesda, MD 20824-0105
(301) 251-1222

National Arthritis and Musculoskeletal and Skin Diseases Information Clearinghouse (NAMSIC)
1 AMS Circle
Bethesda, MD 20892-3675
(301) 495-4484

American Association of Retired Persons (AARP)
Health Promotion Services
601 E. Street, N.W.
Washington, D.C. 20049
(202) 434-2277

American Heart Association
National Center
Public Information Department
7272 Greenville Avenue
Dallas, TX 75231-4596
(214) 373-6300

American College of Sports Medicine
P.O. Box 1440
Indianapolis, IN 46206-1440
(317) 637-9200 ext. 117

The National Institute on Aging (NIA) offers free information on health and aging. For a list of NIA publications call 1-800-222-2225 (1-800-222-4225 TTY) or write:
NIA Information Center
P.O. Box 8057
Gaithersburg, MD 20892-8057

Chapter 23

Walking . . . A Step in the Right Direction

Walking is one of the easiest ways to exercise. You can do it almost anywhere and at any time. Walking is also inexpensive. All you need is a pair of comfortable shoes.

Walking will:

- Give you more energy
- Make you feel good
- Help you to relax
- Reduce stress
- Help you sleep better
- Tone your muscles
- Help control your appetite
- Increase the number of calories your body uses

For all these reasons, people have started walking programs. If you would like to start your own program, read and follow the information provided here.

Is It Okay for Me To Walk?

Answer the following questions before you begin a walking program:

- Has your doctor ever told you that you have heart trouble?

National Institute of Diabetes and Digestive and Kidney Diseases (NIDDK), NIH Pub. No. 97-4155, October 1996. E-text last updated: February 1998.

- When you exercise, do you have pains in your chest or on your left side (neck, shoulder or arm)?

- Do you often feel faint or have dizzy spells?

- Do you feel extremely breathless after mild activity?

- Has your doctor told you that you have high blood pressure?

- Has your doctor told you that you have bone or joint problems, like arthritis, that could get worse if you exercise?

- Are you over 50 years old and not use to a lot of exercise?

- Do you have a condition or physical reason not mentioned here that might interfere with an exercise program?

If you answered yes to any of these questions, please check with your doctor before starting a walking program or other form of exercise.

How Do I Start a Walking Program?

It is important to design a program that will work for you. In planning your walking program, keep the following points in mind:

- Choose a safe place to walk. Find a partner or group of people to walk with you. Your walking partner(s) should be able to walk with you on the same schedule and at the same speed.

- Wear shoes with thick flexible soles that will cushion your feet and absorb shock.

- Wear clothes that are right for the season. Cotton clothes for the summer help to keep you cool by absorbing sweat and allowing it to evaporate. Layer your clothing in the winter, and as you warm up, you can take off some layers.

- Stretch before you walk. See the warm up exercises here.

- Think of your walk in three parts. Walk slowly for 5 minutes. Increase your speed for the next 5 minutes. Finally, to cool down, walk slowly again for 5 minutes.

- Try to walk at least three times per week. Add 2 to 3 minutes per week to the fast walk. If you walk less than three times per week, increase the fast walk more slowly.

- To avoid stiff or sore muscles or joints, start gradually. Over several weeks, begin walking faster, going further, and walking for longer periods of time.

- The more you walk, the better you will feel. You also use more calories.

Safety Tips

Keep safety in mind when you plan your route and the time of your walk.

- Walk in the daytime or at night in well-lighted areas.
- Walk in a group at all times.
- Notify your local police station of your group's walking time and route.
- Do not wear jewelry.
- Do not wear headphones.
- Be aware of your surroundings.

How Do I Warm Up?

Before you start to walk, do the stretching exercises shown here. Remember not to bounce when you stretch. Perform slow movements and stretch only as far as you feel comfortable.

Side Reaches

Reach one arm over your head and to the side. Keep your hips steady and your shoulders straight to the side. Hold for 10 seconds and repeat on the other side.

Wall Push

Lean your hands on a wall with your feet about 3-4 feet away from the wall. Bend one knee and point it toward the wall. Keep your back leg straight with your foot flat and your toes pointed straight ahead. Hold for 10 seconds and repeat with the other leg.

Knee Pull

Lean your back against a wall. Keep your head, hips, and feet in a straight line. Pull one knee to your chest, hold for 10 seconds, then repeat with the other leg.

Leg Curl

Pull your foot to your buttocks with your opposite hand. Keep your knee pointing straight to the ground. Hold for 10 seconds and repeat with the other foot.

Taking the First Step

Walking right is very important.

• Walk with your chin up and your shoulders held slightly back.
• Walk so that the heel of your foot touches the ground first. Roll your weight forward.
• Walk with your toes pointed forward.
• Swing your arms as you walk.

Table 23.1. A Sample Walking Program

	Warm up Time	Fast Walk Time*	Cool Down Time	Total Time
Week 1	Walk slowly 5 min.	Walk briskly 5 min.	Walk slowly 5 min.	15 min.
Week 2	Walk slowly 5 min.	Walk briskly 8 min.	Walk slowly 5 min.	18 min.
Week 3	Walk slowly 5 min.	Walk briskly 11 min.	Walk slowly 5 min.	21 min.
Week 4	Walk slowly 5 min.	Walk briskly 14 min.	Walk slowly 5 min.	24 min.
Week 5	Walk slowly 5 min.	Walk briskly 17 min.	Walk slowly 5 min.	27 min.
Week 6	Walk slowly 5 min.	Walk briskly 20 min.	Walk slowly 5 min.	30 min.
Week 7	Walk slowly 5 min.	Walk briskly 23 min.	Walk slowly 5 min.	33 min.
Week 8	Walk slowly 5 min.	Walk briskly 26 min.	Walk slowly 5 min.	36 min.
Week 9 & Beyond	Walk slowly 5 min.	Walk briskly 30 min.	Walk slowly 5 min.	40 min.

*If you walk less than three times per week, increase the fast walk time more slowly.

Weight-control Information Network
1 Win Way
Bethesda, MD 20892-3665
(301) 984-7378
800-WIN-8098
Fax: (301) 984-7196
E-mail: win@info.niddk.nih.gov
The Weight-control Information Network (WIN) is a service of the National Institute of Diabetes and Digestive and Kidney Diseases (NIDDK), part of the National Institutes of Health, under the U.S. Public Health Service. Authorized by Congress (Public Law 103-43), WIN assembles and disseminates to health professionals and the public information on weight control, obesity, and nutritional disorders. WIN responds to requests for information; develops, reviews, and distributes publications; and develops communications strategies to encourage individuals to achieve and maintain a healthy weight. Publications produced by the clearinghouse are reviewed carefully for scientific accuracy, content, and readability.

Chapter 24

Water Tai Chi

Water tai chi is a combination of the principles of water fitness and the graceful flowing movements of tai chi chuan. Incorporating the slow, powerful exercises of this Chinese martial art into your existing aqua program adds a fresh new dimension to classes that enhance not only the body, but the mind and spirit.

Traditional tai chi, which means "supreme ultimate," has been practiced for six centuries in China. Today it is one of the most practiced exercises in the world. The Chinese perform tai chi for improved health, self defense and spiritual growth. Chi refers to the vital force, or intrinsic energy, that is said to flow through the meridian channels of the body. It is said regular tai chi practice ensures the body's meridians remain open and flowing with chi.

Water tai chi is performed upright in chest depth water. Its movements can be incorporated into the warm-up, conditioning and cool-down phases of an aquatic class. Many find the exercises improve strength, flexibility, balance, coordination and posture. Additionally, participants develop grace and powerful use of the whole body. On a psychological level, reported benefits include increased vitality and energy, improved focus, relaxation and a sense of well-being.

Participants of all ages can enjoy and appreciate the unique, graceful, and flowing movements of tai chi. The mind-body concepts of the ancient martial art of tai chi chuan combined with the gentle qualities

American Fitness, July-August, 1998, v16 n4 p52(3). © 1998 Aerobics and Fitness Association of America.

of water exercise attract people looking for alternative ways to de-stress and bring balance to their lives.

Seniors benefit from water tai chi's emphasis on balance and pos-ture. The Arthritis Foundation, a long time supporter of water exer-cise, recently stated tai chi may be the ideal exercise for arthritis sufferers. Studies are underway concerning possible uses in treating the elderly for loss of balance and frequent falls.

Body Temperature

Introduce tai chi movements only after thoroughly warming up the body. Cooling can occur quickly with slow movements in typical pool temperatures of 80 to 84 degrees, resulting in chilled, uncomfortable participants. Adding power and speed to the movements or alternat-ing between faster and slower movements can help maintain comfort. Therapy pools with temperatures near 90 degrees favor relaxation and are ideal for water tai chi.

Water Depth

Chest depth water allows for total submergence of arms and pro-vide adequate stabilization of feet. Buoyancy is directly affected by the water's depth For example, a body submerged at rib cage depth weighs about 75% less than it would on land, and approximately 90% less when submerged to the neck. Deeper water makes it difficult to overcome the effects of buoyancy.

Aquatic Shoes

Tai chi footwork, including the pivot twist step, side step, and turn back and kick are easier and safer to execute with shoes on. Aquatic shoes improve traction, support and footing, and protect the bottom of the feet. Movements are executed with knees slightly bent, and one or both feet grounded while maintaining a low cen-ter of gravity. The objective is to overcome the effects of buoyancy and remain grounded.

Drag and Viscosity

Water tai chi is different from the traditional land version in that the resistive and supportive qualities of water provide an ideal envi-ronment for slow, rounded, flowing movements. Water provides about

12 times the resistance of air, so the body naturally moves more slowly in the water due to drag forces.

Drag, the resistance encountered as the body moves through water, increases with the length of the limbs, or levers. A long lever is a fully extended arm or leg, while a short lever is a flexed arm or leg. Water tai chi exercises utilize both short and long levers.

The viscosity of water will naturally slow down a moving body. Viscosity is the friction between molecules of a liquid or gas which causes them to adhere to each other (cohesion) and, in water, to a submerged body (adhesion). Water is more viscous than air, and this friction between molecules is what causes resistance to motion. The effects of drag and viscosity naturally promote the slow motion-like movements of tai chi.

Body Positioning

Attention to posture and breathing is important to proper body positioning. The back is straight with the head held erect. Participants should imagine their head is suspended from above to avoid a stiff vertical posture. Vision should be focused straight ahead, but sometimes follow the movements of the hands. Breathing should be deep and relaxed, with the mind alert and focused. Exhale through the mouth and inhale through the nose in a natural fashion. Joints of the arms should be relaxed, with the shoulders sunk and elbows slightly flexed.

Tai chi is rooted in the feet, issued through the legs, controlled by the waist and expressed through the hands. All of the moves originate from the main energy center in the abdomen, which is called the t'an t'ien (pronounced don chien). Participants work from a low center of gravity, softening the knees and using only the amount of energy needed to execute the movements.

Water tai chi is based on the yang style and chi kung, which consist of more than 100 changing postures and require extensive practice. The aquatic adaptations are much simpler and involve more repetition. Some of the water tai chi movements are true to form, while others are creative adaptations. For example, "Wave hands like clouds," a frequent posture in the yang form, repeats three times while moving laterally to the left. The water version incorporates the movement numerous times while traveling in both directions. On land, upper body movements like "box both ears," "raising the chi" and "push hands" are performed with constantly changing leg stances. Interesting upper body movements can accompany a variety of water walking movements like the step and kick front, side step, and step and pivot. Simplification of the complex postures of tai chi enables more students to participate and enjoy.

It helps to use imagery-based commands when leading water tai chi classes. For example, use instructions like "move arms like water flowing from a hose," "coordinate movements of the whole body like a string of pearls," move arms as if they were massaging a ball, sink and pivot," "turn the waist" and "sink and rise like a cat."

Yin and Yang

Another component of tai chi is the concept of yin and yang, two opposing types of energy. Yin is calm and static, while yang is active and dynamic. Chi flows only when these two forces are in balance. For example, the lower body is firmly grounded to the earth while the upper body moves like clouds in the wind. Tai chi is based on the laws of nature. Many of the movements and postures relate to animals, tile sea and the sky. "Parting the Wild Horse's Mane," "Repulse the Monkey" and "White Crane Spreads Wings" are some examples.

The early roots of tai chi are steeped in folklore and imagination. It is believed that an ancient Taoist priest had a dream of a rattlesnake and crane in combat, and thus was inspired to create the first movements of tai chi.

Water Tai Chi Movements

The following are some water tai chi movements to incorporate into your aquatic class:

- Chinese Torso Twist: Face forward and bend your knees slightly, standing with your feet firmly anchored three to four inches beyond your shoulder width. Extend both arms out to the side with your elbows and wrists relaxed. Rotate your upper torso while swinging your arms to the left. Keep your feet anchored, and your back and head erect as you rotate back to the right. Inhale and exhale with the movement while contracting your abdominal muscles. Imagine your arms as water flowing from a hose. Repeat 12 times.

- Side Kicks: Stand with your feet, several inches apart and lift both arms out to your sides at shoulder level. Lift your right knee while lowering your arms and bringing them across your chest. Then kick your leg out to the side while extending your arms, positioning the fingertips up and keeping the elbows soft. Lower your arms and leg, bend your knees slightly and repeat with your left leg. Travel forward and then backward for variety. Always keep one foot anchored. Repeat 15 times, alternating legs.

- Embracing the Moon: Face forward with your feet positioned shoulder width apart. Hold your hands as if you were carrying a basketball—one palm up and the other palm down. Begin rotating the imaginary ball in a figure-eight pattern while gradually increasing your range of motion. Keep your elbows soft and your shoulders down. Move the opposite leg like a pendulum while rotating the ball to the side of your anchored leg. Repeat 15 times.

- Wave Hands Like Clouds: Stand with your feet several inches apart and lift your arms to shoulder level. Step laterally with the right foot, and simultaneously circle both arms under and out of the water. The right arm circles clockwise and the left arm counter-clockwise. Repeat four times and then travel left. Repeat entire sequence three times.

- Tai Chi Expressive Hands: Integrate these moves into water walking or deep water classes:

Alternate Push Hands—With elbows sunk, position hands with fingertips up, one palm facing the chest and the other palm facing forward. Imagine pulling taffy.
Box Both Ears—Make two fists with elbows sunk in front of the body. Rotate the palms up while opening hands, and pull them down and behind the body. Open arms out to the side and reposition with fisted hands.
Cross Hands—Position arms crossed in front of the chest as if you were holding a large ball. Slowly lift the arms up while uncrossing them. Open arms out to the side, scoop under the water and return to crossed position with opposite arm in front.
Raise Hands and Push—Position arms in front of body with palms down and elbows sunk. Slowly lift arms to top of head, lower them to chest and push forward. Keep palms facing down until the arms are at chest level.

—by Carol Argo

Carol Argo is an AFAA certified instructor and trainer for the Aquatic Exercise Association and owner of The Fitness Company, an aquatic and personal training business in Palos Verdes, California. She has studied tai chi for three years and teaches it on land and in water.

Chapter 25

Check Your Smoking I.Q.

An Important Quiz for Older Smokers

If you or someone you know is an older smoker, you may think that there is no point in quitting now. Think again. By quitting smoking now, you will feel more in control and have fewer coughs and colds. On the other hand, with every cigarette you smoke, you increase your chances of having a heart attack, a stroke, or cancer. Need to think about this more? Take this older smokers' I.Q. quiz. Just answer "true" or "false" to each statement below. Be sure to read the correct answers and explanations at the bottom of this test.

True or False?

1. If you have smoked for most of your life, it's not worth stopping now.

2. Older smokers who try to quit are more likely to stay off cigarettes.

3. Smokers get tired and short of breath more easily than non-smokers the same age.

4. Smoking is a major risk factor for heart attack and stroke among adults 60 years of age and older.

National Heart, Lung, and Blood Institute (NHLBI), NIH Pub No. 91-3031, October 1991.

269

5. Quitting smoking can help those who have already had a heart attack.

6. Most older smokers don't want to stop smoking.

7. An older smoker is more likely to smoke more cigarettes than a younger smoker.

8. Someone who has smoked for 30 to 40 years probably won't be able to quit smoking.

9. Very few older adults smoke cigarettes.

10. Lifelong smokers are more likely to die of diseases like emphysema and bronchitis than nonsmokers.

Results of the Smoking Quiz

1. False: Nonsense! You have every reason to quit now and quit for good—even if you've been smoking for years. Stopping smoking will help you live longer and feel better. You will reduce your risk of heart attack, stroke and cancer; improve blood flow and lung function; and help stop diseases like emphysema and bronchitis from getting worse.

2. True: Once they quit, older smokers are far more likely than younger smokers to stay away from cigarettes. Older smokers know more about both the short-and long-term health benefits of quitting.

3. True: Smokers, especially those over 50 years old, are much more likely to get tired, feel short of breath, and cough more often. These symptoms can signal the start of bronchitis or emphysema, both of which are suffered more often by older smokers. Stopping smoking will help reduce these symptoms.

4. True: Smoking is a major risk factor for four of the five leading causes of death including heart disease, stroke, cancer, and lung diseases like emphysema and bronchitis. For adults 60 and over, smoking is a major risk factor for six of the top 14 causes of death. Older male smokers are nearly twice as likely to die from stroke as older men who do not smoke. The odds are nearly as high for older female smokers. Cigarette smokers of any age have a 70 percent greater heart disease death rate than do nonsmokers.

5. True: The good news is that stopping smoking does help people who have suffered a heart attack. In fact, their chances of having another attack are smaller. In some cases, ex-smokers can cut their risk of another heart attack by half or more.

6. False: Most smokers would prefer to quit. In fact, in a recent study, 65 percent of older smokers said that they would like to stop. What keeps them from quitting? They are afraid of being irritable, nervous, and tense. Others are concerned about cravings for cigarettes. Most don't want to gain weight. Many think it's too late to quit—that quitting after so many years of smoking will not help. But this is not true.

7. True: Older smokers usually smoke more cigarettes than younger people. Plus, older smokers are more likely to smoke high nicotine brands.

8. False: You may be surprised to learn that older smokers are actually more likely to succeed at quitting smoking. This is more true if they're already experiencing long-term smoking-related symptoms like shortness of breath, coughing, or chest pain. Older smokers who stop want to avoid further health problems, take control of their life, get rid of the smell of cigarettes, and save money.

9. False: One out of five adults aged 50 or older smokes cigarettes. This is more than 11 million smokers, a fourth of the country's 43 million smokers! About 25 percent of the general U.S. population still smokes.

10. True: Smoking greatly increases the risk of dying from diseases like emphysema and bronchitis. In fact, over 80 percent of all deaths from these two diseases are directly due to smoking. The risk of dying from lung cancer is also a lot higher for smokers than nonsmokers: 22 times higher for males, 12 times higher for females.

For more information on stopping smoking, write:

NHLBI Information Center
P.O. Box 30105
Bethesda, MD 20824-0105

Part Four

Being a Prudent Medical Customer

Chapter 26

Health Quackery

Quacks—people who sell unproven remedies-have been around for years. You may remember the "snake oil" salesman who traveled from town to town making amazing claims about his "fabulous" product. Today's quack is only a little more slick. Sometimes only money is wasted, but it can be a serious problem if quackery prevents you from seeking professional medical care.

Who Are the Victims?

To the quack, people of all ages are fair game, but older people form the largest group of victims. In fact, a Government study found that 60 percent of all victims of health-care fraud are older people.

Most people who are taken in by a quack's worthless and often dangerous treatments are desperate for some offer of hope. Because older people as a group have more chronic illnesses than younger people, they are likely targets for fraud.

What Do Quacks Promise?

- Anti-Aging. The normal processes of aging are a rich territory for medical quackery. In a youth-oriented society, quacks find it easy to promote a wide variety of products. They simply say their products can stop or reverse aging processes or relieve conditions associated with old age. While there are products

National Institute on Aging (NIA) "Age Page," 1995.

that may reduce wrinkles or reverse baldness for some people, these products cannot slow the body's aging process. However, not smoking, eating a healthy diet, and getting regular exercise may help prevent some diseases that occur more often as people age.

- Arthritis Remedies. Arthritis "remedies" are especially easy to fall for because symptoms of arthritis tend to come and go. People with arthritis easily associate the remedy they are using with relief from symptoms. Arthritis sufferers have paid for bottled seawater, "extracts" from New Zealand green-lipped mussels, and Chinese herbal medicines (which have no herbs but may contain drugs that are dangerous).

There is no cure for most forms of arthritis, but treatments that can help reduce pain and enable greater movement are available. These include drugs, heat treatments, a balance of rest and exercise, and in some cases, surgery.

- Cancer Cures. Quacks prey on the older person's fear of cancer by offering "treatments" that have no proven value—for example, a diet dangerously low in protein or drugs such as Laetrile. By using unproven methods, patients may lose valuable time and the chance to receive proven, effective therapy. This can reduce the chance for controlling or curing the disease.

How To Protect Yourself

One way to protect yourself is to question carefully what you see or hear in ads. Although there are exceptions, the editors of newspapers, magazines, radio, and TV do not regularly screen their ads for truth or accuracy.

Find out about a product before you buy it. Check out products sold door-to-door through an agency such as the Better Business Bureau.

The following are common ploys used by dishonest promoters:

- promising a quick or painless cure,

- promoting a product made from a "special" or "secret" formula,

- usually available through the mail and from only one sponsor,

- presenting testimonials or case histories from satisfied patients,

- advertising a product as effective for a wide variety of ailments, or

- claiming to have the cure for a disease (such as arthritis or cancer) that is not yet understood by medical science.

- Remember if it seems too good to be true it probably is.

Resources

If you have questions about a product, talk to your doctor or contact one of the following agencies.

Food and Drug Administration
HFE-88
5600 Fishers Lane
Rockville, MD 20857
The Food and Drug Administration answers questions about medical devices, medicines, and food supplements that are mislabeled, misrepresented, or in some way harmful.

U.S. Postal Service
Office of Criminal Investigation
Washington, DC 20260-2166
U.S. Postal Service monitors quack products purchased by mail.

Council of Better Business Bureaus
4200 Wilson Boulevard
8th Floor
Arlington, VA 22209
The Council of Better Business Bureaus offers publications and advice on products.

Federal Trade Commission
Room 421
6th Street and Pennsylvania Avenue, NW.
Washington, DC 20580
The Federal Trade Commission looks into charges of false advertising in publications or on the radio and TV.

Cancer Information Service (CIS)
800-4-CANCER
The CIS, funded by the National Cancer Institute, can answer questions about a broad range of cancer-related issues, including foods and products.

National Arthritis, Musculoskeletal and Skin Diseases Information Clearinghouse (NIAMS)
Box AMS
9000 Rockville Pike
Bethesda, MD 20892
301-495-4484
The NIAMS Information Clearinghouse answers questions about issues and products related to arthritis.

The National Institute on Aging (NIA)
P.O. Box 8057
Gaithersburg, MD 20898-8057
800-222-2225
800-222-4225 (TTY)
The NIA offers a variety of information on health and aging.

Chapter 27

Unproven Medical Treatments Lure Elderly

Americans spend upwards of $20 billion each year on unproven medical treatments. Sixty percent of those who try untested therapies are over 65 and spend an estimated $10 billion on them, according to a 1984 House Subcommittee on Health and Long-Term Care report, "Quackery: A $10 Billion Scandal."

Approximately 80 percent of older Americans have one or more chronic health problems, according to John Renner, M.D., a Kansas City-based champion of quality health care for the elderly. He says their pain and disability lead to despair, making them excellent targets for deception.

"Despite disappointments with promised cures, they continue to hold out hope that next quick 'cure' will work," says anti-fraud activist Stephen Barrett, M.D.

Frightened of losing a parent or grandparent, family members, too encourage them to try everything, especially unproven remedies, according to Barrie R. Cassileth, Ph.D., writing in *CA—A Cancer Journal for Clinicians.*

And, indeed, sometimes people get better when using unproven treatments. But because these therapies have not passed scientific muster, it is impossible to know if improvement is associated with the treatment, represents spontaneous change, or is due to the "placebo" effect. (A placebo is an inactive substance with no known therapeutic value. The "placebo effect" is the phenomenon of people

Food and Drug Administration (FDA), *FDA Consumer*, December 1994.

getting better while taking an inactive substance they believe to be therapeutic.)

"It's important to remember," says Barrett, "that many conditions get better on their own, or appear to get better if we believe they will."

What's the Danger?

Taking a chance on unproven treatments is not simply useless, it is often dangerous, according to the Food and Drug Administration, which divides such products into two categories: direct health hazards and indirect health hazards.

Direct health hazards are likely to cause serious injuries. For example, muscle stimulators, promoted falsely as muscle toners, carry a risk of severe electric shock.

Indirectly harmful products are those that cause people to delay or reject proven remedies, according to FDA. For example, if cancer patients reject proven therapies in favor of unproven ones, their disease may advance beyond the point where proven therapies can help.

All types of unproven therapies can be economically harmful, often draining precious dollars from older Americans' limited resources.

FDA's Health Fraud Staff, in its Center for Drug Evaluation and Research, investigates any product for which a disease claim is made. Joel Aronson, director of the health Fraud Staff, points out that once a manufacturer claims a product can treat or prevent a disease or condition, "whether that product is bottled water or an herb, it is considered a drug and falls under FDA jurisdiction." A product is also considered a drug if it claims to alter the structure or function of the body.

FDA's Center for Food Safety and Applied Nutrition becomes involved with issues such as health claims for herbs, vitamins, and other dietary supplements (see "Dietary Supplements: Making Sure Hype Doesn't Overwhelm Science" in the November 1993 *FDA Consumer*). For a reprint of this article, contact your local FDA office, or write FDA, HFE-88, 5600 Fishers Lane, Rockville, MD 20857.

FDA's Promotion and Advertising Staff, in its Center for Devices and Radiological Health, investigates health and disease claims made about devices. Byron Tart, acting director, explains that such devices fall into two main categories: devices approved for some medical use but promoted for an unapproved use, and devices not approved for any medical use at all.

Targeting Older Americans

Commonly, unproven products are pushed zealously on the elderly. Promoters often claim their products prevent aging and such conditions as arthritis, Alzheimer's disease, heart disease, and impotence.

According to the National Institute on Aging, however, "while a healthy lifestyle will help delay many of the conditions associated with aging processes, no preparation or device can stop aging." The 1984 House Subcommittee report estimated that people spent at least $2 billion per year on anti-aging remedies. Some anti-aging products are also promoted to either prevent or treat Alzheimer's disease.

According to JoAnn McConnell, Ph.D., of the Alzheimer's Association, "so-called new `cures' for Alzheimer's surface constantly."

But there are no cures, which may cause Alzheimer's patients and their families to be susceptible to products holding out false hope.

There is, however, one approved treatment for Alzheimer's disease: the drug Cognex (tacrine hydrochloride), which was approved in September of 1993 specifically to treat the symptoms of Alzheimer's disease. "It is not a cure for Alzheimer's disease," says FDA Commissioner David A. Kessler, M.D., "but it provides some relief for patients and their families."

Particularly susceptible to deception are the 37 million Americans—many of them over 65—who have arthritis. One reason is that arthritis symptoms come and go, causing people to associate their spontaneous relief with a new "remedy." The Arthritis Foundation says that older Americans spend an estimated $2 billion annually for unproven arthritis remedies.

A Closer Look

Here's a closer look at some unproven therapies promoted for a variety of ills common in older people:

- Cellular therapy promoters claim an extract from animal hearts can strengthen human hearts, eye extracts can cure eye disease, and so on. FDA says there are no scientific studies demonstrating the safety and effectiveness of cellular therapy for any medical purpose and warns of health problems, including severe allergic reactions and death.

- Chaparral is an herb used in teas, capsules and tablets that promoters purport delays aging, cleanses the blood, and treats cancer. In early 1993, FDA warned consumers not to use it because

281

it had caused serious liver and kidney troubles. Most manufacturers voluntarily withheld chaparral- containing products from sale, and consumers are advised not to use remaining products.

- Coenzyme Q-10, a synthetically produced version of a naturally occurring enzyme, is promoted to slow aging by enhancing the immune system. Not only is there no proven benefit, but it may be dangerous for people with poor circulation, according to Edward L Schneider, M.D., of the National Institute on Aging. Overall, there is no evidence that "boosting" the immune system delays aging, nor is there any evidence that it's possible to do so, according to Schneider.

- DHEA (dehydroepiandrosterone) is a naturally occurring chemical. Because levels decline with aging, some scientists speculate it may play some role in aging processes. But there is not proof that DHEA delays aging, according to Schneider.

- DMSO, or dimethyl sulfoxide, is a solvent similar to turpentine promoted for arthritis relief. In a sterile form called Rimso-50, it is approved by FDA for treating a rare bladder condition called interstitial cystitis. For this approved use, it is instilled into the bladder for short times (20 to 30 minutes). This is the only approved human use. There are no controlled studies demonstrating its safety and effectiveness in relieving swollen, inflames arthritis joins, and in an impure form it can harbor bacterial toxins that can enter the bloodstream even when applied topically. It is one of the few compounds rapidly absorbed through the skin. It can be especially dangerous if used as an enema, as recommended by its promoters.

- Electrical stimulators are approved by FDA when prescribed by physicians for various conditions, including after-stroke therapy. However, FDA has not approved them for wrinkle removal and face lifts.

- Geranium, an inorganic, nonessential element sold as a dietary supplement. Promoters claim it prevents and treats Alzheimer's, and advise users to apply bandage wraps with it to treat arthritis and headaches. Not only is geranium ineffective, but is has caused serious irreversible kidney damage and death, according to FDA.

- Gerovital-H3, originating in Romania more than 30 years ago, was brought here illegally and sold as a cure for arthritis, atherosclerosis, angina pectoris, hypertension, deafness, Parkinson's disease, depression, diabetes, and impotence. One of its ingredients is procaine hydrochloride, an anesthetic approved for dental use. No health claims for Gerovital have been substantiated, and FDA considers it an unapproved new drug. It has caused low blood pressure, respiratory difficulties, and convulsions in some users.

- Herbal products are centuries-old, but mostly unproven, "cures" for everything from constipation to anxiety. They are available in various forms, including teas, capsules and tablets. Some are potentially dangerous. Chamomile tea, for example, can cause a severe allergic reaction in people allergic to ragweed. Lobelia can cause vomiting, breathing problems, convulsions, and even coma and death when used in large amounts; people with heart disease are especially susceptible. Comfrey has caused severe and even fatal liver disease. (See "Beware the Unknown Brew: Herbal Teas and Toxicity" in the May 1991 *FDA Consumer*.)

- Lecithin, a naturally occurring component of certain body tissues, is touted for lowering cholesterol and treating Alzheimer's disease. There's no proof that it's effective for either one.

- Low-intensity lasers are promoted to relieve arthritis pain, but FDA has not approved them for this or any other use.

- Magnetism: Pressure dots with tiny magnets affixed to adhesive strips that are worn over the arthritic area are promoted for curing arthritis; a magnet in men's briefs is purported to cure impotence; and a magnet used a suppository is promoted for curing hemorrhoids. There is no scientific basis for any of these claims.

- Retin-A has been approved by FDA as a topical treatment for acne. The agency, however, has not determined whether it is safe and effective as a wrinkle remover.

- RIFE generator promoters claim that they can insert a person's photograph into their device and diagnose medical conditions. FDA has not approved the marketing of this device, nor is there any scientific basis for this claim.

- RNA, or ribonucleic acid, a natural body chemical that carries genetic information, is a common ingredient in anti-aging compounds and is also promoted for Alzheimer's. Promoters claim it rejuvenates old cells, improves memory, and prevents wrinkling. But there have been no controlled scientific studies to back up these claims.

• Superoxide dismutase (SOD) is a normal body chemical that is promoted as being able to slow aging and treat Alzheimer's disease. According to the National Institute on Aging's Schneider, writing in the *New England Journal of Medicine*, some studies have shown higher tissue levels of SOD in longer-living species. A survey of a large number of different animal species revealed, in fact, that the longest-lived species, human beings, had the highest tissue levels of superoxide dismutase. But there is no evidence that SOD works to delay aging or prolong life, nor is there any evidence that taking SOD tablets raises blood or tissue levels of SOD.

Hearing Aids

FDA is taking action to improve the patient care of people who buy hearing aids. Though hearing aids have significantly improved the quality of life for many older Americans, the agency is concerned that some manufacturers are making unsubstantiated claims about their devices and are giving inaccurate portrayals of their devices' risks and benefits.

The agency last November proposed changes to hearing aid regulations to require a hearing assessment in all cases before a person is sold a hearing aid. The regulation will also require that this assessment be done by a qualified health professional licensed by the state. A public hearing on the proposal was held Dec. 6 and 7 near FDA headquarters in Rockville, Md.

Although a 1977 regulation restricts hearing aid sales to people who have had a hearing evaluation by a doctor within six months, FDA Commissioner Kessler pointed out that the "regulation also included a provision allowing fully informed adult patients to waive the medical examination." Kessler said this waiver has been "overused and misrepresented."

Before proposing the regulation changes, FDA reviewed promotional materials for a number of hearing aids and found that several manufacturers were making unsubstantiated and misleading claims that created unrealistic expectations about the performance of the devices. In addition, the materials failed to disclose significant information and did not accurately disclose the device's potential risks and benefits.

At press time, FDA was reviewing public comments on the proposed regulation changes.

Avoiding Fraud

According to FDA, these red flags should make you think twice about remedies not prescribed by your doctor:

- celebrity endorsements

- inadequate labeling (a legitimate non-prescription medication is labeled with indications for use, as well as how to use it and when to seek medical help)

- claims that the product works by a secret formula

- promotion of the treatment only in the back pages of magazines, over the phone, by direct mail, in newspaper ads in the format of new stories, or 30-minute commercials in talk show format.

The Arthritis Foundation says the following claims are also warning signs that a "cure" has but questionable therapeutic value:

- It's effective for a wide range of disorders, such as cancer, arthritis and sexual dysfuntion. ("But, says FDA's Aronson, "don't misinterpret this to believe a product promoted for only one disease is safe and effective.")

- It's all natural.

- It's inexpensive and has no side effects.

- It works immediately and permanently, making a visit to the doctor unnecessary.

Older Americans, along with younger folks, should remember that falling victim to health fraud is "not a matter of being weaker or foolish," says Renner. "It is a matter of being in pain or having more than one chronic illness—or both."

Barrett offers a final word of advise: "When you feel your physician isn't doing enough to help, don't stray from scientific health care in a desperate attempt to find a solution." Instead, ask your physician to provide a more detailed explanation or to refer you to another doctor.

—by Kristine Napier

Kristine Napier is a registered dietitian and writer in Mayfield Village, Ohio.

Chapter 28

Pills, Patches, and Shots: Can Hormones Prevent Aging?

Hormones are powerful chemicals that help keep our bodies working normally. They are made naturally, by the body, and can affect us in far-reaching ways. Levels of some hormones decrease as a normal part of aging. In other cases, the body may fail to make enough of a hormone for other reasons. In either case, the body's hormone levels can be increased by taking hormone supplements—pills, shots, or medicated skin patches.

Certain hormone supplements have received a lot of attention lately, including DHEA (dehydroepiandrosterone), human growth hormone (hGH), melatonin, and testosterone. Unproven claims that taking these supplements can make people feel young again or that they can prevent aging have been appearing in the news. However, when it comes to hormones, more is not necessarily better.

The fact is that no one has yet shown that supplements of these hormones add years to people's lives. And while some supplements provide health benefits for people with genuine deficiencies of certain hormones, they also can cause harmful side effects. The right balance of hormones helps us stay healthy, but the wrong amount might be dangerous.

Another concern is that some hormone supplements are not regulated as drugs by the Food and Drug Administration; they are sold as nutritional supplements, instead. For this reason, the rules controlling how they are produced and sold are not as strict as the rules for drugs. For example, producers of DHEA and melatonin are not

National Institute on Aging (NIA), undated.

required to include important health information on the labels of their bottles. Researchers also have found that the dose listed on the label of some bottles of melatonin may be different from the dose inside the bottle.

The National Institute on Aging (NIA), part of the National Institutes of Health, conducts research to find out how hormone supplements affect people. In the case of most hormone supplements, it is not yet known how much is too much or too little, and for some, whether hormone supplements should be taken at all. This fact sheet provides information about what is known so far and about what researchers are doing to find out more.

Talk to Your Doctor

The NIA does not recommend taking supplements of DHEA, growth hormone, or melatonin, because not enough is known about them. People who have a genuine deficiency of testosterone or human growth hormone (see below) should take them only under a doctor's supervision. The NIA does not recommend taking any supplement as an anti-aging remedy, because no supplement has been proven to serve this purpose. Talk to your doctor to make sure that over-the-counter supplements will not interfere with other medications you are taking and that they will not affect any medical conditions you may have. You might want to show this fact sheet to your doctor, to help explain your concerns.

How Hormones Work

Groups of special cells—glands—make chemicals called hormones and release them into the bloodstream. Hormones taken as supplements also end up in the bloodstream. In either case, the blood then carries hormones to different parts of the body. There, hormones influence the way organs and tissues work.

Hormone supplements may not have exactly the same effects on us that our own naturally produced hormones have, because the body may process them differently. Another difference is that high doses of supplements, whether pills, skin patches, or shots, may result in higher amounts of hormones in the blood than are healthy. When that happens, any negative effects that even the body's own hormones can cause may increase. Tiny amounts of these powerful chemicals, whether made by the body or taken as supplements, can have widespread effects.

DHEA

DHEA is made by the adrenal glands, which sit on top of each kidney. Although it is not known whether DHEA itself causes hormonal effects, the body breaks DHEA down into two hormones that are known to affect us in many ways: estrogen and testosterone (see below). Supplements of DHEA can be bought without a prescription, and also may be found under the name "dehydroepiandrosterone." After people reach the age of about 30, their bodies start to make less DHEA, and the amount of DHEA found in the bloodstream continues to drop as people grow older. Supplements are sold as an anti-aging remedy claimed, by some, to improve energy, strength, and immunity. DHEA is also said to increase muscle and decrease fat.

Right now, there is no reliable evidence that DHEA supplements do any of these things. However, there are early signs that DHEA supplements may lead to liver damage, even when taken briefly.

Some people's bodies make large amounts of estrogen and testosterone from DHEA, while others make smaller amounts. There is no way to predict who will make more and who will make less. Researchers are concerned that DHEA supplements may cause high levels of estrogen or testosterone in some people. The body's own testosterone plays a role in prostate cancer, and high levels of naturally produced estrogen are suspected of increasing breast cancer risk. It is not yet known for certain if supplements of estrogen and testosterone, or supplements of DHEA, also increase the risk of developing these types of cancer. In women, high testosterone levels increase the risk of heart disease and cause growth of facial hair.

Overall, the studies that have been done so far do not provide a clear picture of the risks and benefits of DHEA. For example, some studies show that DHEA helps build muscle, but other studies do not. Researchers are working to find more definite answers about DHEA's effects on aging, muscles, and the immune system. In the meantime, people who are thinking about taking supplements of this hormone should understand that its effects are not fully known. Some of these unknown effects might turn out to be harmful.

Growth Hormone

Human growth hormone (hGH) supplements also are claimed, by some, to reduce the signs of aging—that is, to increase muscle and decrease fat, and to give people a feeling of well-being and energy.

Even though there is no proof that hGH can prevent aging, some people spend a great deal of money on supplements. Shots of the hormone can cost more than $15,000 a year. They are available only by prescription and should be given by a doctor.

Human growth hormone is made by the pituitary gland, just under the brain, and is important for normal development and maintenance of our tissues and organs. It is especially important for normal growth in children. Human growth hormone levels often decrease as people age.

Studies have shown that supplements are helpful to certain people. Sometimes, children are unusually short because their bodies do not make hGH. When they take supplements, their growth improves. Young adults who have no pituitary gland (because of surgery for a pituitary tumor, for example) cannot make the hormone, and they become obese. When they are given supplements, they lose weight.

Researchers are doing studies to find out if hGH can help make older people stronger by building up their muscles and whether it can reduce body fat. They are watching their patients very carefully, because side effects can be serious in older adults. Side effects of hGH treatment can include diabetes and pooling of fluid in the skin and other tissues, which may lead to high blood pressure and heart failure. Joint pain and carpal tunnel syndrome also may occur.

People in search of the "fountain of youth" may have a hard time finding a doctor who will give them shots of hGH. Some people put themselves in danger by trying to get it any way they can. For example, some people went to a clinic in Mexico to get supplements. The clinic was shut down later because side effects were not being carefully monitored by doctors.

Melatonin

The hormone melatonin is made by the pineal gland, in the brain, and decreases with age in some people.

Supplements of melatonin can be bought without a prescription. Some people claim that melatonin is an anti-aging remedy, a sleep remedy, and an antioxidant (antioxidants protect against "free radicals," naturally occurring molecules that cause damage to the body). Early test-tube studies suggest that melatonin may be effective against free radicals, in large doses. However, cells produce antioxidants naturally, and in test-tube experiments, cells reduce the amount they make when they are exposed to additional antioxidants.

Claims that melatonin can slow or reverse aging are very far from proven. Studies of melatonin have been much too limited to support these claims, and have focused on animals, not people.

Research on sleep shows that melatonin does play a role in the sleeping and waking cycle people go through daily, and that supplements can improve sleep in some cases. If melatonin is taken at the wrong time, though, it can disrupt the sleep/wake cycle. The effects of supplements differ from person to person, and more research is needed to find out under what conditions melatonin helps, not disturbs, sleep.

Side effects of melatonin may include confusion, drowsiness, and headache the next morning. Animal studies suggest that melatonin may cause blood vessels to constrict, a condition that could be dangerous for people with high blood pressure or other cardiovascular problems.

The dose of melatonin usually sold in stores—3 milligrams—can result in amounts in the blood up to 40 times higher than normal. It is important to remember that melatonin may be found to have far-reaching effects that are still unknown even at the body's own normal levels, to say nothing of the levels that can be caused by megadoses taken for long periods of time.

Researchers are working to find out more about melatonin's effects.

Testosterone

Testosterone is thought of as a male hormone, but it is found in both men and women. Because men have more testosterone, their voices are deeper, they have more facial hair, and their muscles are larger. Testosterone also plays a role in sex drive and erection.

Testosterone levels may drop as men age, and changes that take place in older men often are wrongly blamed on lower testosterone. For example, the loss of erection some older men experience often is due to unhealthy arteries, not low testosterone levels.

Supplements of testosterone are available, only by prescription, for men whose bodies do not make enough of the hormone. Examples of men who do not make enough testosterone are those whose pituitary glands have been destroyed by infections or tumors, or whose testes have been damaged (the testes are the glands that make testosterone in men, and the pituitary gland helps regulate it).

Supplements provide many benefits for men with a genuine deficiency of testosterone. Men's muscles and bones become smaller and weaker without the hormone, and their sex drive and ability to have erections decrease. Supplements help prevent such problems by restoring normal levels.

But too much testosterone is harmful. Stories about athletes who damaged their health by taking steroids—testosterone supplements— to build up muscle and strength have made headlines. Now, stories about how testosterone can make older men feel young again, and can restore their muscles and their sex drive, have become popular.

The problem is that most of these men already have enough testosterone, and supplements cause them to have more than is normal. The result can be an enlarged prostate gland; harmful cholesterol levels, which may lead to heart disease; psychological problems; infertility; and acne. It is not yet known for certain if testosterone supplements increase the risk of prostate cancer.

Estrogen

Because many women take estrogen supplements for symptoms of menopause, estrogen is included in this fact sheet. Many large, reliable studies have been done on this hormone, and show why it is important to discover both the helpful and harmful effects of a supplement. It is clear that estrogen replacement is helpful to some women after menopause. Women with certain risk factors, however, might decide, along with their doctors, that estrogen supplements are not right for them.

Women have much less estrogen after menopause because the ovaries make dramatically reduced amounts of this reproductive hormone in later life. Studies suggest that reduced estrogen levels are associated with a higher risk of heart disease and osteoporosis—a condition that weakens bones, allowing them to break more easily. These are just two examples of the many areas of the body that can suffer without adequate estrogen.

Research has shown that estrogen supplements prescribed by a doctor can help some women avoid osteoporosis and lower their risk factors for heart disease, the number-one killer of women in the United States. Osteoporosis can lead to severe bone fracture. Patients who are hospitalized for a broken hip have a death rate 12 to 20 percent higher than others in their age group, due to complications. Estrogen helps prevent osteoporosis.

A recent study suggests that estrogen supplements also may delay the onset of Alzheimer's disease, but more research must be done to confirm this early finding.

On the other hand, some studies have raised concerns about a link between estrogen and cancer of the uterus and a possible link between estrogen and breast cancer. It appears that estrogen given to women after menopause also increases the risk of blood clots. Heart attacks, strokes, and other circulation problems may result from blood clots.

Although much is known about estrogen, scientists are learning more. For example, a recent study suggests that older women whose bones are found to be at lower risk of osteoporosis may be at higher risk of breast cancer (doctors can predict a woman's likelihood of developing osteoporosis by measuring bone mineral density). Researchers think this increased breast cancer risk may occur in some women whose bodies have produced high amounts of natural estrogen over their lifetime. More research is needed to tell whether estrogen supplements alone increase the risk of breast cancer.

Researchers have studied estrogen for many years. As a result, doctors are better informed about which women are likely to benefit from supplements and about the right doses to prescribe so that the risk of side effects is reduced. Adding progestin, another female hormone, to estrogen supplements lowers risk of uterine cancer.

The decision whether or not to take estrogen is a personal one. Each woman, along with her doctor, should ask herself: Is there heart disease in my family? Or breast cancer? What are the results of my bone mineral density measurement? Have I had blood clots before, or has my doctor told me that I am prone to blood clots?

There is no right or wrong answer to these questions. Each woman must weigh her answers, based on her health history, with her doctor.

Studies Under Way

The NIA sponsors many research projects that will reveal more about the risks and benefits of hormone supplements. One goal is to discover how DHEA, melatonin, and other supplements affect people over time.

Trophic factors are substances that help control the growth and repair of our tissues and organs throughout our lives. Some trophic factors are considered hormones. Researchers are studying them to find out if decreasing levels of these factors are responsible, at least in part, for the diseases and disabilities seen in aging. Now in its fourth year, a group of 5-year studies of trophic factors is under way. Testosterone, estrogen, and growth hormone are included in the study.

It is important to remember that these studies may not give immediate or final answers, especially in the case of DHEA, melatonin, and human growth hormone, since research on these supplements is fairly new. For example, some of the studies may simply give researchers more information about what kinds of questions they should ask in their next studies. Research is a step-by-step process, and larger studies may be needed to give more definite answers.

Until more is known about DHEA, melatonin, and hGH, consumers should view them with a good deal of caution—and doubt. Despite what advertisements or stories in the media may claim, hormone supplements have not been proven to prevent aging. Some harmful side effects already have been discovered, and further research may uncover others.

More is known about estrogen and testosterone, and people who are concerned about genuine deficiencies of these hormones should consult with their doctors about supplements. Meanwhile, people who choose to take any hormone supplement without a doctor's supervision do so at their own risk.

For more information about free publications from the National Institute on Aging, call 1-800-222-2225 (1-800-222-4225 TTY) or visit our website at http://www.nih.gov/nia.

For more information about Alzheimer's disease, call 1-800-438-4380 or visit our website http://www.alzheimers.org/adear.

Chapter 29

Talking with Your Doctor

Why Does It Matter? Choosing a Doctor You Can Talk To

The first step in good communication is finding a doctor with whom you can talk. Having a main doctor (often called your primary doctor) is one of the best ways to ensure your good health. This doctor knows you and what your health normally is like. He or she can help you make medical decisions that suit your values and daily habits and can keep in touch with other medical specialists and health care providers you may need.

If you don't have a primary doctor or are not at ease with the doctor you currently see, now may be the time to find a new doctor. The suggestions below can help you find a doctor who meets your needs.

1. Decide what you are looking for in a doctor—A good first step is to make a list of qualities that are important to you. Then, go back over the list and decide which are most important and which are nice, but not essential.

2. Identify several possible doctors—After you have a general sense of what you are looking for, ask friends and relatives, medical specialists, and other health professionals for the names of doctors with whom they have had good experiences. A doctor whose name comes up often may be a strong possibility. Rather than just getting a name, ask about the person's

Excerpted from *Talking with Your Doctor: A Guide for Older People*, National Institute on Aging (NIA), NIH Pub. No. 94-3452, December 1994.

experiences. For example, say "What do you like about Dr. Smith?" It may be helpful to come up with a few names to choose from, in case the doctor you select is not currently taking new patients.

3. Consult reference sources—*The Directory of Physicians in the United States* and the *Official American Board of Medical Specialties Directory of Board Certified Medical Specialists* are available at many libraries. These references won't recommend individual doctors, but they will provide a list to choose from. Doctors who are "board certified" have had training after regular medical school and have passed an exam certifying them as specialists in certain fields of medicine. This includes the primary care fields of general internal medicine, family medicine, and geriatrics. Board certification is one way to tell about a doctor's expertise, but it doesn't address the doctor's communication skills.

4. Learn more about the doctors you are considering—once you have selected two or three doctors, call their offices. The office staff can be a good source of information about the doctor's education and qualifications, office policies, and payment procedures. Pay attention to the office staff—you will have to deal with them often! You may want to set up an appointment to talk with a doctor. He or she is likely to charge you for such a visit.

5. Make a choice—After choosing a doctor, make the first appointment. This visit may include a medical history and a physical examination. Be sure to bring your medical records and a list of your current medicines with you. If you haven't interviewed the doctor, take time during this visit to ask any questions you have about the doctor and his or her practice. After the appointment, ask yourself whether this doctor is a person with whom you could work well. If you are not satisfied, schedule a visit with one of your other candidates.

Summary: Choosing a Doctor You Can Talk To:

- Decide what you are looking for in a doctor.

- Identify several possible doctors.

- Consult reference sources, current patients, and colleagues.

- Learn more about the doctors you are considering.

- Make a choice.

Things to Consider When Selecting a Doctor:

- Is the location of the doctor's office important? How far can I travel to see the doctor?

- Is the hospital the doctor admits patients to important to me?

- Is the age, sex, race, or religion of the doctor important?

- Do I prefer a single doctor or a group practice?

- Do I have to choose a doctor who is covered by my insurance plan?

- Does the doctor accept Medicare?

- Is the doctor board-certified? In what field?

What Are the Doctor's Office Policies?

- Is the doctor taking new patients?

- What days/hours does the doctor see patients?

- Does the doctor ever make house calls?

- How far in advance do I have to make appointments?

- What is the length of an average visit?

- In case of an emergency, how fast can I see the doctor?

- Who takes care of patients after hours or when the doctor is away?

Questions to Ask the Doctor:

- Do you have many older patients? What are your views on health and aging?

- How do you feel about involving the patient's family in care decisions?

- Will you honor living wills, durable powers of attorney for health care, and other advance directives ?

- Do you still work with your patients when they move to a nursing home?

What Can I Do? Tips for Good Communication

A basic plan can help you communicate better with your doctor, whether you are starting with a new doctor or continuing with the doctor you've been visiting. The following tips can help you and your doctor build a partnership.

Getting Ready for Your Appointment

1. Be prepared: make a list of your concerns—Before going to the doctor, make a list of what you want to discuss. For example, are you having a new symptom you want to tell the doctor about? Did you want to get a flu shot or pneumonia vaccine? If you have more than a few items to discuss, put them in order so you are sure to ask about the most important ones first. Take along any information the doctor or staff may need such as insurance cards, names of your other doctors, or your medical records. Some doctors suggest you put all your medicines in a bag and bring them with you, others recommend bringing a list of medications you take.

2. Make sure you can see and hear as well as possible—Many older people use glasses or need aids for hearing. Remember to take your eyeglasses to the doctor's visit. If you have a hearing aid, make sure that it is working well, and wear it. Let the doctor and staff know if you have a hard time seeing or hearing. For example, you may want to say, "My hearing makes it hard to understand everything you're saying. It helps a lot when you speak slowly."

3. Consider bringing a family member or friend—Sometimes it is helpful to bring a family member or close friend with you. Let your family member or friend know in advance what you want from your visit. The person can remind you what you planned to discuss with the doctor if you forget, and can help you remember what the doctor said.

4. Plan to update the doctor—Think of any important information you need to share with your doctor about things that have happened since your last visit. If you have been treated in the emergency room, tell the doctor right away. Mention any changes you have noticed in your appetite, weight, sleep, or energy level. Also tell the doctor about any recent changes in the medication you take or the effect it has had on you.

Your doctor may ask you how your life is going. This isn't just polite talk or an attempt to be nosy. Information about what's happening in your life may be useful medically. Let the doctor know about any major changes or stresses in your life, such as a divorce or the death of a loved one. You don't have to go into detail; you may just want to say something like, "I thought it might be helpful for you to know that my sister passed away since my last visit with you," or "I had to sell my home and move in with my daughter."

Summary: Getting Ready for Your Appointment

- Be prepared: make a list of concerns.

- Make sure you can see and hear as well as possible.

- Consider bringing a family member or friend.

- Plan to update the doctor

Sharing Information with Your Doctor

1. Be honest—It is tempting to say what you think the doctor wants to hear; for example, that you smoke less or eat a more balanced diet than you really do. While this is natural, it's not in your best interest. Your doctor can give you the best treatment only if you say what is really going on.

2. Stick to the point—Although your doctor might like to talk with you at length, each patient is given a limited amount of time. To make the best use of your time, stick to the point. Give the doctor a brief description of the symptom, when it started, how often it happens, and if it is getting worse or better.

3. Ask questions—Asking questions is key to getting what you want from the visit. If you don't ask questions, your doctor may think that you understand why he or she is sending you for a test or that you don't want more information. Ask questions when you don't know the meaning of a word (like aneurysm, hypertension, or infarct) or when instructions aren't clear (e.g., does taking medicine with food mean before, during, or after a meal?). You might say, "I want to make sure I understand. Could you explain that a little further?" It may help to repeat what you think the doctor means back in your own words and ask, "Is this correct?" If you are worried about cost, say so.

4. Share your point of view—Your doctor needs to know what's working and what's not. He or she can't read your mind, so it is important for you to share your point of view. Say if you feel rushed, worried, or uncomfortable. Try to voice your feelings in a positive way. For example, "I know you have many patients to see, but I'm really worried about this. I'd feel much better if we could talk about it a little more." If necessary, you can offer to return for a second visit to discuss your concerns.

Summary: Sharing Information With Your Doctor

-   Be honest.

-   Stick to the point.

-   Ask questions.

-   Share your point of view.

Getting Information from Your Doctor and Other Health Professionals

1. Take notes—It can be difficult to remember what the doctor says, so take along a note pad and pencil and write down the main points, or ask the doctor to write them down for you. If you can't write while the doctor is talking to you, make notes in the waiting room after the visit. Or, bring a tape recorder along, and (with the doctor's permission) record what is said. Recording is especially helpful if you want to share the details of the visit with others.

2. Get written or recorded information—Whenever possible, have the doctor or staff provide written advice and instructions. Ask if your doctor has any brochures, cassette tapes, or videotapes about your health conditions or treatments. For example, if your doctor says that your blood pressure is high, he or she may give you brochures explaining what causes high blood pressure and what you can do about it. Some doctors have videocassette recorders for viewing tapes in their offices. Ask the doctor to recommend other sources, such as public libraries, nonprofit organizations, and government agencies, which may have written or recorded materials you can use.

3. Remember that doctors don't know everything—Even the best doctor may be unable to answer some questions. There still is

much we don't know about the human body, the aging process, and disease. Most doctors will tell you when they don't have answers. They also may help you find the information you need or refer you to a specialist. If a doctor regularly brushes off your questions or symptoms as simply part of aging, think about looking for another doctor.

4. Talk to other members of the health care team—Today, health care is a team effort. Other professionals, including nurses, physician assistants, pharmacists, and occupational or physical therapists, play an active role in your health care. These professionals may be able to take more time with you.

Summary: Getting Information From Your Doctor and Other Health Professionals

- Take notes.

- Get written or recorded information.

- Remember that doctors don't know everything.

- Talk to other members of the health care team.

Where Do I Begin? Getting Started with a New Doctor

Your first meeting is the best time to begin communicating positively with your new doctor. When you see the doctor and office staff, introduce yourself and let them know how you like to be addressed. The first few appointments with your new doctor also are the best times to:

1. Learn the basics of the office—Ask the office staff how the office runs. Learn what days are busiest and what times are best to call. Ask what to do if there is an emergency, or when the office is closed.

2. Share your medical history—Tell the doctor about your illnesses or operations, medical conditions that run in your family, and other doctors you see. You may want to ask for a copy of the medical history form before your visit so you have all the time and information you need to complete it. Your new doctor may ask you to sign a medical release form to get copies of your medical records from doctors you have had before. Be prepared to give the new doctor your former doctors' names and addresses, especially if they are in a different city.

3. Give information about your medications—Many people take several medicines. It is possible for medicines to interact, causing unpleasant and sometimes dangerous side effects. Your doctor needs to know about ALL of the medicines you take, including over-the-counter (non-prescription) drugs, so bring everything with you to your first visit, including eye drops, vitamins, and laxatives. Tell the doctor how often you take each and describe any drug allergies or reactions you have had and which medications work best for you. Be sure your doctor has the phone number of your regular drug store.

4. Tell the doctor about your habits—To provide the best care, your doctor must understand you as a person and know what your life is like. The doctor may ask about where you live, what you eat, how you sleep, what you do each day, what activities you enjoy, your sex life, and if you smoke or drink. Be open and honest with your doctor. It will help him or her to understand your medical conditions fully and recommend the best treatment choices for you.

Summary: Getting Started with a New Doctor

- Learn the basics of how the office runs.
- Share your medical history.
- Give information about your medications.
- Tell the doctor about your habits.

Is the Doctor's Office Convenient?

- Where is the doctor's office located?
- Is parking available nearby? What is the cost?
- Is the office on a bus or subway line?
- Does the building have an elevator? Ramps for a wheelchair? Adequate lighting?

What Should I Say? Talking about Your Health

Talking about your health means sharing information about how you feel both physically and emotionally. Knowing how to describe your symptoms, discuss treatments, and talk with specialists will help you become a partner in your health care. Here are some issues that may be important to you when you talk with your doctor.

Preventing Disease and Disability

Until recently, preventing disease in older people received little attention. But things are changing. It's never too late to stop smoking, improve your diet, or start exercising. Getting regular checkups and seeing other health professionals such as dentists and eye specialists help promote good health. Even people who have chronic diseases, like arthritis or diabetes, can prevent further disability and in some cases, control the progress of the disease.

If a certain disease or health condition runs in your family, ask your doctor if there are steps you can take to help prevent it. If you have a chronic condition, ask how you can manage it and if there are things you can do to prevent it from getting worse. If you want to discuss health and disease prevention with your doctor, say so when you make your next appointment. This lets the doctor plan to spend more time with you as well as to prepare for the discussion.

Questions to Ask Your Doctor about Prevention:

- Should I get a flu shot, pneumonia shot, and/or other immunizations?

- How often should I have a breast or prostate examination?

- Would changing my diet or exercise habits help me avoid specific diseases ?

Sharing Any Symptoms

It is very important for you to be clear and concise when describing your symptoms. Your description helps the doctor identify the problem. A physical exam and medical tests provide valuable information, but it is your symptoms that point the doctor in the right direction.

Tell the doctor when your symptoms started, what time of day they happen, how long they last (seconds? days?), how often they occur, if they seem to be getting worse or better, and if they keep you from going out or doing your usual activities. Take the time to make some notes about your symptoms before you call or visit the doctor. Concern about your symptoms is not a sign of weakness. It is not necessarily complaining to be honest about what you are experiencing.

Questions to Ask Yourself about Your Symptoms:

- What exactly are my symptoms?
- Are the symptoms constant? If not, when do I experience them?
- Do the symptoms affect my daily activities? Which ones? How?

Learning More about Medical Tests

Sometimes doctors need to do blood tests, x-rays, or other procedures to find out what is wrong or to learn more about your medical condition. Some tests, such as Pap smears, mammograms, glaucoma tests, and screenings for prostate and colorectal cancer, are done on a regular basis to check for hidden medical problems.

Before having a medical test, ask your doctor to explain why it is important and what it will cost, and, if possible, to give you something to read about it. Ask how long the results of the test will take to come in.

When the results are ready, make sure the doctor tells you what they are and explains what they mean. You may want to ask your doctor for a written copy of the test results. If the test is done by a specialist, ask to have the results sent to your primary doctor.

Questions to Ask Your Doctor about Medical Tests:

- What will we know after the test?
- How will I find out the results? How long will it take to get the results?
- What steps does the test involve? How should I get ready ?
- Are there any dangers or side effects?

Discussing Your Diagnosis and What You Can Expect

If you understand your medical condition, you can help make better decisions about treatment. If you know what to expect, it may be easier for you to deal with the condition.

Ask the doctor to tell you the name of the condition and why he or she thinks you have it. Ask how it may affect your body, and how long it might last. Some medical problems never go away completely. They can't be cured, but they can be treated or managed. You may want to write down what the doctor says to help you remember.

It is not unusual to be surprised or upset by hearing you have a new medical problem. Questions may occur to you later. When they do, make a note of them for your next appointment.

Sometimes the doctor may want you to talk with other health professionals who can help you understand how to manage your condition. If you have the chance to work with other health professionals, take advantage of it. Also, find out how you can reach them if you have questions later.

Questions to Ask Your Doctor about the Diagnosis:

- What may have caused this condition? Will it be permanent?

- How is this condition treated or managed? What will be the long-term effects on my life?

- How can I learn more about it?

Talking about Treatments

Although some medical conditions do not require treatment, most can be helped by medicine, surgery, changes in daily habits, or a combination of these. You will benefit most from treatment when you know what is happening and are involved in making decisions. If your doctor suggests a treatment, be sure you understand what it will and won't do and what it involves. Have the doctor give you directions in writing, and feel free to ask questions.

If your doctor suggests a treatment that makes you uncomfortable, ask if there are other treatments to consider. For example, if the doctor recommends medicine for your blood pressure, you may want to ask if you can try lowering it through diet and exercise first. If cost is a concern, ask the doctor if less expensive choices are available. The doctor can work with you to develop a treatment plan that meets your needs.

Questions to Ask Your Doctor about Treatment:

- How soon should treatment start? How long will it last?
- Are there other treatments available?
- How much will the treatment cost? Will my insurance cover it?
- Are there any risks associated with the treatment?

Making the Most of Medications

Your doctor may prescribe a drug for your condition. Make sure you know the name of the drug and understand why it has been prescribed for you. Ask the doctor to write down how often and how long you should take it. Make notes about any other special instructions such as foods or drinks you should avoid. If you are taking other medications, make sure your doctor knows, so he or she can prevent harmful drug interactions.

Sometimes medicines affect older people differently than younger people. Let the doctor know if your medicine doesn't seem to be working or if it is causing problems. Don't stop taking it on your own. If another doctor (for example, a specialist) prescribes a medication for you, call your primary doctor to let him or her know. Also call to check with your doctor before taking any over-the-counter medications. You may find it helpful to keep a chart of all the medicines you take and when you take them.

The pharmacist also is a good source of information about your medicines. In addition to answering questions, the pharmacist keeps records of all the prescriptions you get filled at that drug store. Because your pharmacist keeps these records, it is helpful to use a regular drug store.

A pharmacist also can help you select over-the-counter medicines that are best for you. At your request, the pharmacist can fill your prescriptions in easy-to-open containers and may be able to provide large print prescription labels.

Questions to Ask Your Doctor and Pharmacist about Medications:

- What are the common side effects? What should I pay attention to?

- What should I do if I miss a dose?

- Are there foods, drugs, or activities I should avoid while taking this medicine?

Changing Your Daily Habits

Doctors and other health professionals may suggest you change your diet, activity level, or other aspects of your life to help you deal with medical conditions. Sometimes the doctor's suggestions may not be acceptable to you. For example, the doctor might recommend a diet that includes foods you cannot eat or do not like. Tell your doctor if you don't feel a plan will work for you and explain why. There may be other choices. Keep talking with your doctor to come up with a plan that works.

Questions to Ask Your Doctor about Changing Your Habits:

- How will this change help me?

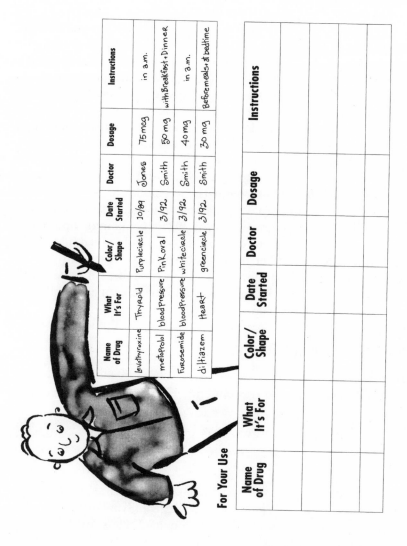

Name of Drug	What It's For	Color/ Shape	Date Started	Doctor	Dosage	Instructions
Levothyroxine	Thyroid	Purple circle	10/89	Jones	75 mcg	in a.m.
metoprolol	blood pressure	Pink oval	3/92	Smith	50 mg	with Breakfast + Dinner
Furosemide	blood pressure	white circle	3/92	Smith	40 mg	in a.m.
diltiazem	Heart	green circle	3/92	Smith	30 mg	Before meals + at bedtime

For Your Use

Name of Drug	What It's For	Color/ Shape	Date Started	Doctor	Dosage	Instructions

Figure 29.1.

- Do you have any reading material or videotapes on this topic?

- Are there support groups or community services that might help me?

Seeing Specialists

Your doctor may send you to a specialist for further evaluation. You also may request to see one yourself, although your insurance company may require that you have a referral from your primary doctor.

When you see a specialist, ask that he or she send information about further diagnosis or treatment to your primary doctor. This allows your primary doctor to keep track of your medical care. You also should let your primary doctor know at your next visit about any treatments or medications the specialist recommended.

A visit to the specialist may be short. Often, the specialist already has seen your medical records or test results and is familiar with your case. If you are unclear about what the specialist tells you, ask him or her questions. For example, if the specialist says that you have a medical condition that you aren't familiar with, you may want to say, "I don't know very much about that condition. Could you explain what it is and how it might affect me?" or, "I've heard it's painful. What can be done to prevent or manage the pain?" You also may ask for written materials to read or call your primary doctor to clarify anything you haven't understood.

Questions to Ask Your Specialist:

- What is your diagnosis?

- What treatment do you recommend? How soon do I need to begin the new treatment?

- Will you discuss my care with my primary doctor?

Surgery

In some cases, surgery may be the best treatment for your condition. If so, your doctor will refer you to a surgeon. Knowing more about the operation will help you make an informed decision. It also will help you get ready for the surgery, which, in turn, makes for a better recovery. Ask the surgeon to explain what will be done during the operation and what reading material or videotapes you can look at before the operation. Find out if you will have to stay overnight in the hospital to have the surgery, or if it can be done on an outpatient basis. Minor surgeries that don't require an overnight stay can sometimes be done at medical centers called "ambulatory surgical centers."

When surgery is recommended, it is common for the patient to seek a second opinion. In fact, your insurance company may require it. Doctors are used to this practice, and most will not be insulted by your request for a second opinion. Your doctor may even be able to suggest other doctors who can review your case. Hearing the views of two different doctors can help you decide what's best for you.

Questions to Ask Your Surgeon about Surgery:

- What is the success rate of the operation? How many of these operations have you done successfully?

- What problems occur with this surgery? What kind of pain and discomfort can I expect?

- Will I have to stay in the hospital overnight? How long is recovery expected to take? What does it involve?

If You Are Hospitalized

If you have to go to the hospital, some extra guidelines may help you. First, most hospitals have a daily schedule. Knowing the hospital routine can make your stay more comfortable. Find out how much choice you have about your daily routine, and express any preferences you have about your schedule. Doctors generally visit patients during specific times each day. Find out when the doctor is likely to visit so you can have your questions ready.

In the hospital, you may meet with your primary doctor and various medical specialists, as well as nurses and other health professionals. If you are in a teaching hospital, doctors-in-training, known as medical students, interns, residents, and fellows, also may examine you. Many of these doctors-in-training already have a lot of knowledge. They may be able to take more time to talk with you than other staff. Nurses also can be an important source of information, especially since you will see them on a regular basis.

Questions to Ask Medical Staff in the Hospital:

- How long can I expect to be in the hospital?

- When will I see my doctor? What other doctors and health professionals will I see?

- What is the daily routine in this part of the hospital?

If You Have to Go to the Emergency Room

A visit to the emergency room is always stressful. If possible, take along the following items: your health insurance card or policy number, a list of your medications, a list of your medical problems, and the names and phone numbers of your doctor and one or two family members or close friends. Some people find it helpful to keep this information on a card in their wallets or purses.

While in the emergency room, ask questions if you don't understand tests or procedures that are being done. Before leaving, make sure you understand what the doctor told you. For example, if you have bandages that need to be changed, be sure you understand how and when it is to be done. Tell your primary doctor as soon as possible about your emergency room care.

Questions to Ask Medical Staff in the Emergency Room:

- Will you talk to my primary doctor about my care?
- Do I need to arrange any further care?
- May I get instructions for further care in writing?

Can I Really Talk about That? Discussing Sensitive Subjects

Much of the communication between doctor and patient is personal. To have a good partnership with your doctor, it is important to talk about sensitive subjects, like sex or memory problems, even if you are embarrassed or uncomfortable. Doctors are used to talking about personal matters and will try to ease your discomfort. Keep in mind that these topics concern many older people. For more information on the topics discussed below, see the resource list at the end of this book.

It is important to understand that problems with memory, depression, sexual function, and incontinence are not normal parts of aging. If your doctor doesn't take your concerns about these topics seriously or brushes them off as being part of normal aging, you may want to consider looking for a new doctor.

1. Sexuality—Most health professionals now understand that sexuality remains important in later life. If you are not satisfied with your sex life, don't automatically assume it's due to

310

your age. In addition to talking about age-related changes, you can ask your doctor about the effects of an illness or a disability on sexual function. Also, ask your doctor what influence medications or surgery may have on your sexual life. If you aren't sure how to bring the topic up, try saying, "I have a personal question I would like to ask you..." or, "I understand that this condition can affect my body in many ways. Will it affect my sex life at all?"

2. Incontinence—About 15 to 30 percent of older people living at home have problems controlling their bladder this is called urinary incontinence. Often, certain exercises or other measures are helpful in correcting or improving the problem. If you have trouble with control of your bladder or bowels, it is important to let the doctor know. In many cases, incontinence is the result of a treatable medical condition. When discussing incontinence with your doctor, you may want to say something like, "Since my last visit there have been several times that I couldn't control my bladder. I'm concerned, because this has never happened to me before."

3. Grief, mourning, and depression—As people grow older, they experience losses of significant people in their lives, including spouses and cherished friends. A doctor who knows about your losses is better able to understand how you are feeling. He or she can make suggestions that may be helpful to you.

   Although it is normal to feel grief and mourning when you have a loss, later life does not have to be a time of ongoing sadness. If you feel down all the time or for more than a few weeks, let your doctor know. Also tell your doctor about symptoms such as lack of energy, poor appetite, trouble sleeping, or lack of interest in life. These could be signs of medical depression. If you feel sad and withdrawn and are having trouble sleeping, give your doctor a call. Depression can be a side effect of medications or a sign of a medical condition that needs attention. It often can be treated successfully—but only if your doctor knows about it.

4. Memory problems—One of the greatest fears of older people is problems with their ability to think and remember. For most older people, thinking and memory remain good throughout the later years. If you seem to have problems remembering recent

events or thinking clearly, let your doctor know. Try to be specific about the changes you have noticed, for example, "I've always been able to balance my checkbook without any problems, but lately I'm finding that I get very confused." The doctor will probably want you to undergo a thorough checkup to see what might be causing your symptoms.

In many cases, these symptoms are caused by a passing, treatable condition such as depression, infection, or a side effect of medication. In other cases, the problem may be Alzheimer's disease or a related condition that causes ongoing loss of skills such as learning, thinking, and remembering. While there currently is no way to determine for sure if a person has Alzheimer's disease, a careful history, physical evaluation, and mental status examination are still important. They help the doctor rule out any other, perhaps treatable, causes of your symptoms and determine the best plan of care for you.

5. Care in the event of a serious illness—You may have some concerns or wishes about your care if you become seriously ill. If you have questions about what choices you have, ask your doctor. You can specify your desires through documents called advance directives such as a living will or durable power of attorney for health care. Advance directives allow you to say what you'd prefer if you were too ill to make your wishes known. In an advance directive you can name a family member or other person to make decisions about your care if you aren't able.

    In general, the best time to talk with your doctor about these issues is when you are still relatively healthy. If you are admitted to the hospital or a nursing home, you will be asked if you have any advance directives. If the doctor doesn't raise the topic, do so yourself. To make sure that your wishes are carried out, write them down. You also should talk with family members so that they understand your wishes.

6. Problems with family—Even strong and loving families can have problems, especially under the stress of illness. Although family problems can be painful to discuss, talking about them can help your doctor help you. Your doctor may be able to suggest steps to improve the situation for you and other family members.

If you feel you are being mistreated in some way, let your doctor know. Some older people are subjected to abuse by family members or others. Abuse can be physical, verbal, psychological, or even financial in nature. Your doctor may be able to provide resources or referrals to other services that can help you if you are being mistreated.

7. Feeling unhappy with your doctor—Misunderstandings can come up in any relationship, including between a patient and his or her doctor. If you feel uncomfortable with something your doctor or the doctor's staff has said or done, be direct. For example, if the doctor does not return your telephone calls, you may want to say something like, "I realize that you care for a lot of patients and are very busy, but I feel frustrated when I have to wait for days for you to return my call. Is there a way we can work together to improve this?" Being honest is much better for your health than avoiding the doctor. If you have a long-standing relationship with your doctor, working out the problem may be more useful than looking for a new doctor.

Summary

If you have questions or worries about a subject that your doctor does not talk about with you, bring them up yourself. Practice with family or friends what you will tell or ask the doctor. If there are brochures or pamphlets about the subject in the doctor's waiting room, use them as a way to begin to talk. Talking with your doctor about sensitive subjects is important. Although talking about these subjects may be awkward for both you and your doctor, don't avoid it. If you feel the doctor doesn't take your concerns seriously, remember that you can always change doctors.

Who Else Will Help? Involving Your Family and Friends

It can be helpful to take a family member or friend with you when you go to the doctor's office. You may feel more confident if someone else is with you. Also, a friend or relative can help you remember what you planned to tell or ask the doctor. He or she also can help you remember what the doctor says. But don't let your companion take too strong a role. The visit is between you and the doctor. You may want some time alone with the doctor to discuss personal matters. For best results, let your companion know in advance how he or she can be most helpful.

If a relative or friend helps with your care at home, having that person along when you visit the doctor may be useful. In addition to the questions you have, your caregiver may have concerns he or she wants to discuss with the doctor. Some things caregivers may find especially helpful to discuss are: what to expect in the future, sources of information and support, community services, and ways they can maintain their own well-being.

Even if a family member or friend can't go with you to your appointment, he or she can still help. For example, the person can serve as your sounding board, helping you to practice what you want to say to the doctor before the visit. And after the visit, talking about what the doctor said can remind you about the important points and help you come up with questions to ask next time.

What's Next? Some Closing Thoughts

Good health care always depends on good communication with your doctor and other health professionals. We hope this book will help you take an active role in your health care.

If you have suggestions to add to future editions of this book or other ideas for making it more helpful, please write to Freddi Karp, Editor, National Institute on Aging, Public Information Office, Building 31, Room 5C27, 31 Center Drive MSC 2292, Bethesda, MD 20892-2292.

Getting More Information

You can make the best use of your time with your doctor by being informed. This often includes drawing on other sources of health information such as home medical guides, books and articles available at libraries, organizations such as the American Heart Association and the Arthritis Foundation, other institutes within the National Institutes of Health, and self-help groups.

The National Institute on Aging (NIA) has information about a variety of issues related to aging, including menopause, incontinence, and pneumonia. Large-print Age Pages are available on topics such as depression, stroke, safe use of medications, and types of doctors you may see.

To order publications or to request a publications list, call the NIA Information Center at 1-800-222-2225; TTY 1-800-2224225. You also may want to encourage your doctor to order these publications for his or her office.

For a fact sheet and other publications about Alzheimer's disease, contact the NIA Alzheimer's Disease Education and Referral (ADEAR) Center at 1-800-438-4380.

Additional Resources

Sexuality

Sexuality Information and Education Council of the United States
Suite 2500, 130 West 42nd Street
New York, NY 10036
212-819-9770

Incontinence

Help for Incontinent People (HIP)
P.O. Box 544
Union, SC 29379
800-BLADDER

The Simon Foundation
P.O. Box 835
Wilmette, IL 60091
800-237-4666

Grief, Mourning, and Depression

NIMH Depression Awareness, Recognition and Treatment Program
Room 10-85, 5600 Fishers Lane
Rockville, MD 20857
800-421-4211

Memory Problems

Alzheimer's Association
Suite 1000, 919 North Michigan Avenue
Chicago, IL 60611
800-272-3900

Alzheimer's Disease Education and Referral (ADEAR) Center
P.O. Box 8250
Silver Spring, MD 20907-8250
800-438-4380

National Stroke Association
Suite 1000, 8480 East Orchard Road
Englewood, CO 80111-5015
800-367-1990

Care in the Event of a Terminal Illness

National Hospice Organization
Suite 901, 1901 North Moore Street
Arlington, VA 22209
800-658-8898

Problems With Family

Children of Aging Parents
Suite 302-A 1609 Woodbourne Road
Levittown, PA 19057-1511
215-945-6900

Eldercare Locator Service
Suite 100, 1112 16th Street NW
Washington, DC 20036
800-677-1116

National Center on Elder Abuse
Suite 500, 810 First Street NE
Washington, DC 20002
202-682-2470

Chapter 30

Preventive Medical Tests, Immunizations, and Counseling

Clinical Preventive Services for Normal-Risk Adults (18 years and older) Recommended by Most U.S. Authorities

Table 30.1. Screening

Ages (1)	Who	Screening	How Often
18-75 years	Men and women	Blood pressure	Periodically
18-75 years	Men and women	Height and weight	Periodically
18-75 years	Men and women	Dental	Periodically
18-75 years	Men and women	Alcohol use	Periodically
18-75 years	Women	Pap smear	Every 1-3 years
35-65 years	Men	Cholesterol	Every 5 years
45-65 years	Women	Cholesterol	Every 5 years
50-70 years(2)	Women	Mammography	Every 1-2 years
50-75 years	Men and women	Sigmoidoscopy	Every 5-10 years
50-75 years	Men and women	Fecal occult blood	Yearly
65-75 years	Men and women	Vision	Periodically
65-75 years	Men and women	Hearing	Periodically

(1) Upper age limits should be determined on a case-by-case basis.
(2) See counseling section for mammography recommendations.

U.S. Department of Health and Human Services, Public Health Service 1997.

Table 30.2. Immunizations

Ages	Who	Immunization	How Often
18-75 years	Men and women	Tetanus-Diphtheria	Every 10 years
18-75 year	Men and women who have not had chicken pox	Varicella (chicken pox)	Once (2 doses)
18-50 years	Nonimmune women of child-bearing age	Measles, mumps, rubella	Once (1 dose)
65-75 years	Men and women	Pneumococcal	Once in a lifetime
65-75 years	Men and women	Influenza (flu)	Yearly

Table 30.3. Counseling. Your health care provider should take time to discuss the following topics with you.

Who	Topic	How Often
Women ages 18-75 years	Calcium intake	Periodically
Women of childbearing age	Folic acid	Periodically
Peri- and postmenopausal women	Hormone replacement	Periodically
Women ages 40-75 years	Mammography	Periodically
Men ages 50-75 years	Prostate cancer	Periodically
Men and women	Tobacco cessation	Periodically
Men and women	Drug and alcohol use	Periodically
Men and women	Sexually transmitted diseases and HIV	Periodically
Men and women	Family planning	Periodically
Men and women	Domestic violence	Periodically
Men and women	Unintentional injuries	Periodically
Men and women	Seat belt use	Periodically
Men and women	Nutrition	Periodically
Men and women	Physical activity	Periodically
Men and women	Polypharmacy	Periodically
Elderly men and women	Fall prevention	Periodically

Chapter 31

Cancer Tests You Should Know About: A Guide For People 65 And Over

Most people don't like to think about cancer. But think about this: The earlier cancer is found, the better the chances of beating it.

Cancer Tests You Should Know About describes simple tests that can help find cancer early, long before any symptoms appear. You may have heard of some of them, such as mammograms or rectal and prostate exams.

Despite what many people think, most people who are tested will not have cancer. But if it turns out you do, this booklet can help you find the best care.

Why Is It Important To Find Cancer Early?

Cancers that are found early may be easier to cure. Early treatment can be simpler, making it easier to go about daily life. All in all, finding cancer early could:

- Save your life.
- Help you live life to the fullest.

Why Should You Think About Cancer?

Anyone can get cancer. But you are more likely to get cancer as you get older—even if no one in your family has had it. It may surprise

National Cancer Institutes (NCI), NIH Pub. No. 93-3256, 1993.

you to learn that more than one-half of all cancers occur in people age 65 and over.

If You Did Have Cancer, Wouldn't You Know It?

Most cancers in their earliest, most treatable stages do not cause any symptoms or pain. That is why it is so important to have regular cancer tests. They can find problems early—long before you would notice anything wrong.

But What If You Do Notice Something Wrong?

Certain changes could be a sign of cancer. For example, a change in bowel habits could mean cancer of the colon or rectum. A breast lump could mean breast cancer. Don't assume these or other changes are just a normal pan of growing older. See your doctor right away.

Who Should You Ask About Cancer Tests?

Perhaps you see one doctor just for your back or another doctor just for your heart. Maybe you see one doctor for checkups, but the subject of cancer has not come up. Why not bring it up yourself? Ask your family doctor, internist, or other trusted health professional about getting tested for cancer. The next section tells you about the tests to detect cancer early.

Cancer Tests

The tests in this booklet are right for most people age 65 and over.* But you and your doctor need to decide what is right for you. You may need certain tests more often if you have had cancer before, have some other medical conditions, or have a family member who has had cancer.

Most of the cancer tests described in this booklet take little time. Some tests may be uncomfortable, but they are not painful. Cancer tests are usually done right in your doctor's office.

Bring this booklet the next time you see your doctor. Together you can schedule your cancer tests. Then, as you get each test, write the date in the space provided.

You may be concerned about the cost of these cancer tests. Ask your doctor if Medicare will help or ask your own insurance company if they cover these tests. Medicare helps pay for some mammograms and Pap smears.

* For guidelines for people under 65, call the Cancer Information Service toll-free at 1-800-4-CANCER (1-800-422-6237).

Breasts

A woman's risk of breast cancer increases with age. Fortunately, women can take three steps to find cancer early:

Mammogram

This x-ray of the breast can reveal problems up to 2 years before a lump can be felt. To find out where to get a mammogram, ask your doctor. Or, call the National Cancer Institute's Cancer Information Service at: 1-800-4-CANCER (1-800-422-6237).
Recommended: Every year.

Breast Exam

Your doctor should check your breasts for problems or changes that could be a sign of breast cancer.
Recommended: Every year, or as part of your regular health checkup.

Breast self-exam

Ask your doctor or nurse for instructions. You also can call the Cancer Information Service at 1-800-4-CANCER (1-800-422-6237) for a free booklet.
Recommended: Every month.

Uterus and Cervix

As women get older they have a higher risk of cancers of the female sex organs—especially cancers of the uterus and cervix. If you stopped seeing your gynecologist after menopause (change of life), it is important to ask your doctor about the following tests:

Pelvic Exam

The doctor feels the internal sex organs, bladder, and rectum for any changes in size or shape.
Recommended: Every year.

Pap smear

A Pap smear, also called a Pap test, is usually done at the same time as the pelvic exam. During this test, the doctor removes a few cells from the cervix with a swab. The cells then are checked under a microscope. After three normal annual Pap tests, your doctor may decide not to do the test for the next 1 to 3 years.

Recommended: Every year.

Colon and Rectum

Cancers of the colon and rectum are more likely to occur as people get older. Three tests can help find these cancers early:

Rectal Exam

In this test, the doctor gently feels for any bumps or irregular areas on the rectum.

Recommended: Every year, or as part of your regular health checkup.

Guaiac Stool Test

The guaiac (pronounced "gwy-ack") stool test is sometimes called a "fecal" or "stool" occult test or "hemoccult" test. This test can find unseen blood in stool samples. Your doctor can give you a simple kit to collect stool samples at home. Or, your doctor can do the test as part of a rectal exam.

Recommended: Every year.

Sigmoidoscopy or "procto"

The doctor looks for cancer in the colon and rectum with a thin, lighted instrument called a sigmoidoscope.

Recommended: Every 3 to 5 years.

Prostate

Prostate cancer is the most common cancer in American men—especially older men. More than 80 percent of prostate cancer cases occur in men age 65 and over.

Rectal Exam

The doctor feels the prostate through the rectum. Hard or lumpy areas may mean cancer is present.

Recommended: Every year.

PSA

The prostate-specific antigen test (PSA) measures the level of a specific protein in a man's blood. The protein seems to increase in cases of prostate cancer and other prostate diseases.

The National Cancer Institute is studying whether screening with the PSA test along with a rectal exam may help decrease deaths from prostate cancer.

TRUS

Transrectal ultrasound (TRUS) detects cancer by using sound waves produced by an instrument inserted into the rectum. The waves bounce off the prostate, and the pattern of the echoes made by the waves is converted to a picture by computer. TRUS is not a routine test. The doctor will use this exam to help diagnose a man's problem.

Colon and Rectum

The three tests suggested for women also are suggested for men.

Rectal exam

Recommended: Every year, or as part of your regular health checkup.

Guaiac stool test

Recommended: Every year.

Sigmoidoscopy or "procto"

Recommended: Every 3 to 5 years.

What If You Find Out You Have Cancer?

Today, there are new and better ways to treat cancer. If you are told you have cancer, take these steps to get the best possible care:

1. Find a doctor who is right for you and the kind of cancer you have. Oncologists are doctors specially trained to treat cancer.

2. Find out what your treatment choices are and which are best for you. If you don't understand something, ask.

3. Get a second opinion from another doctor before treatment begins. Doctors and most insurance companies expect their patients to do this. Many doctors will help you get a second opinion.

4. Talk to your family and friends and ask for their support. Or ask your doctor to help you find other people or groups who can help. No one needs to handle cancer alone.

5. Call the Cancer Information Service at 1-800-4-CANCER (1-800-422-6237) for help with all these steps. Staff members can give you information about treatment and where to get it. They also can direct you to groups that may be able to help with transportation, finances, and dealing with your problems. Spanish-speaking staff members can be reached at this toll-free number.

6. Ask your doctor to check the National Cancer Institute's PDQ system. This computer system has the most up-to-date treatment information in the United States. You or your doctor can call the Cancer Information Service (1-800-4-CANCER) to learn more about PDQ.

Want To Learn More About Cancer?

Call the Cancer Information Service toll-free at 1-800-4-CANCER (1-800-422-6237) for information and booklets about cancer.
Or, write to:

Office of Cancer Communications
National Cancer Institute
Building 31, Room 10A24
Bethesda, MD 20892

For more information on aging, write to:

National Institute on Aging
P.O. Box 8057
Gaithersburg, MD 20898-8057

Why Get Tested for Cancer?

Most cancers in their earliest stages do not cause symptoms or pain. Get checked for cancer when you're feeling well... for good health and a good life.

Chapter 32

Be Informed: Questions to Ask Your Doctor Before You Have Surgery

Are you facing surgery? You are not alone. Millions of Americans have surgery each year. Most operations are not emergencies. This means you have time to ask your surgeon questions about the operation and time to decide whether to have it, and if so, when and where. The information presented here does not apply to emergency surgery.

The most important questions to ask about elective surgery are why the procedure is necessary for you and what alternatives there are to surgery. If you do not need to have the operation, then you can avoid any risks that might result. All surgeries and alternative treatments have risks and benefits. They are only worth doing if the benefits are greater than the risks.

Your primary care doctor, that is, your regular doctor, may be the one who suggests that you have surgery and may recommend a surgeon. You may want to identify another independent surgeon to get a second opinion. Check to see if your health insurance will pay for the operation and the second opinion. If you are eligible for Medicare, it will pay for a second opinion. You should discuss your insurance questions with your health insurance company or your employee benefits office.

Overview

Following are 12 questions to ask your primary care doctor and surgeon before you have surgery, and the reasons for asking them.

Agency for Health Care Policy and Research (AHCPR) Pub. No. 95-0027, January 1995.

The answers to these questions will help you be informed and help you make the best decision. Sources are listed at the end of these questions to help you get more information from other places.

Your doctors should welcome questions. If you do not understand the answers, ask the doctors to explain them clearly. Patients who are well informed about their treatment tend to be more satisfied with the outcome or results of their treatment.

1.   What operation are you recommending?

Ask your surgeon to explain the surgical procedure. For example, if something is going to be repaired or removed, find out why it is necessary to do so. Your surgeon can draw a picture or a diagram and explain to you the steps involved in the procedure.

Are there different ways of doing the operation? One way may require more extensive surgery than another. Ask why your surgeon wants to do the operation one way over another.

2.   Why do I need the operation?

There are many reasons to have surgery. Some operations can relieve or prevent pain. Others can reduce a symptom of a problem or improve some body function. Some surgeries are performed to diagnose a problem. Surgery also can save your life. Your surgeon will tell you the purpose of the procedure. Make sure you understand how the proposed operation fits in with the diagnosis of your medical condition.

3.   Are there alternatives to surgery?

Sometimes, surgery is not the only answer to a medical problem. Medicines or other nonsurgical treatments, such as a change in diet or special exercises, might help you just as well or more. Ask your surgeon or primary care doctor about the benefits and risks of these other choices. You need to know as much as possible about these benefits and risks to make the best decision.

One alternative may be "watchful waiting," in which your doctor and you check to see if your problem gets better or worse. If it gets worse, you may need surgery right away. If it gets better, you may be able to postpone surgery, perhaps indefinitely.

4.   What are the benefits of having the operation?

Ask your surgeon what you will gain by having the operation. For example, a hip replacement may mean that you can walk again with ease.

Ask how long the benefits are likely to last. For some procedures, it is not unusual for the benefits to last for a short time only. There might be a need for a second operation at a later date. For other procedures, the benefits may last a lifetime.

When finding out about the benefits of the operation, be realistic. Sometimes patients expect too much and are disappointed with the outcome, or results. Ask your doctor if there is any published information about the outcomes of the procedure.

5.   What are the risks of having the operation?

All operations carry some risk. This is why you need to weigh the benefits of the operation against the risks of complications or side effects.

Complications can occur around the time of the operation. Complications are unplanned events, such as infection, too much bleeding, reaction to anesthesia, or accidental injury. Some people have an increased risk of complications because of other medical conditions.

In addition, there may be side effects after the operation. For the most part, side effects can be anticipated. For example, your surgeon knows that there will be swelling and some soreness at the site of the operation.

Ask your surgeon about the possible complications and side effects of the operation. There is almost always some pain with surgery. Ask how much there will be and what the doctors and nurses will do to reduce the pain. Controlling the pain will help you be more comfortable while you heal, get well faster, and improve the results of your operation.

6.   What if I don't have this operation?

Based on what you learn about the benefits and risks of the operation, you might decide not to have it. Ask your surgeon what you will gain—or lose—by not having the operation now. Could you be in more pain? Could your condition get worse? Could the problem go away?

7.   Where can I get a second opinion?

Getting a second opinion from another doctor is a very good way to make sure having the operation is the best alternative for you. Many health insurance plans require patients to get a second opinion before they have certain non-emergency operations. If your plan does not require a second opinion, you may still ask to have one. Check with your insurance company to see if it will pay for a second opinion. If you get one, make sure to get your records from the first doctor so that the second one does not have to repeat tests.

8.   What has been your experience in doing the operation?

One way to reduce the risks of surgery is to choose a surgeon who has been thoroughly trained to do the procedure and has plenty of experience doing it. You can ask your surgeon about his or her recent record of successes and complications with this procedure. If it is more comfortable for you, you can discuss the topic of surgeons' qualifications with your regular or primary care doctor.

9.   Where will the operation be done?

Most surgeons practice at one or two local hospitals. Find out where your operation will be performed. Have many of the operations you are thinking about having been done in this hospital? Some operations have higher success rates if they are done in hospitals that do many of those procedures. Ask your doctor about the success rate at this hospital. If the hospital has a low success rate for the operation in question, you should ask to have it at another hospital.

Until recently, most surgery was performed on an inpatient basis and patients stayed in the hospital for one or more days. Today, a lot of surgery is done on an outpatient basis in a doctor's office, a special surgical center, or a day surgery unit of a hospital. Outpatient surgery is less expensive because you do not have to pay for staying in a hospital room.

Ask whether your operation will be done in the hospital or in an outpatient setting. If your doctor recommends inpatient surgery for a procedure that is usually done as outpatient surgery, or just the opposite, recommends outpatient surgery that is usually done as inpatient surgery, ask why. You want to be in the right place for your operation.

10.   What kind of anesthesia will I need?

Anesthesia is used so that surgery can be performed without unnecessary pain. Your surgeon can tell you whether the operation calls for local, regional, or general anesthesia, and why this form of anesthesia is recommended for your procedure.

Local anesthesia numbs only a part of your body for a short period of time, for example, a tooth and the surrounding gum. Not all procedures done with local anesthesia are painless.

Regional anesthesia numbs a larger portion of your body, for example, the lower part of your body for a few hours. In most cases, you will be awake with regional anesthesia.

General anesthesia numbs your entire body for the entire time of the surgery. You will be unconscious if you have general anesthesia.

Anesthesia is quite safe for most patients and is usually administered by a specialized physician (anesthesiologist) or nurse anesthetist. Both are highly skilled and have been specially trained to give anesthesia.

If you decide to have an operation, ask to meet with the person who will give you anesthesia. Find out what his or her qualifications are. Ask what the side effects and risks of having anesthesia are in your case. Be sure to tell him or her what medical problems you have including allergies and any medications you have been taking, since they may affect your response to the anesthesia.

11.   How long will it take me to recover?

Your surgeon can tell you how you might feel and what you will be able to do or not do the first few days, weeks, or months after surgery. Ask how long you will be in the hospital. Find out what kind of supplies, equipment, and any other help you will need when you go home. Knowing what to expect can help you cope better with recovery.

Ask when you can start regular exercise again and go back to work. You do not want to do anything that will slow down the recovery process. Lifting a 10-pound bag of potatoes may not seem to be "too much" a week after your operation, but it could be. You should follow your surgeon's advice to make sure you recover fully as soon as possible.

12.   How much will the operation cost?

Health insurance coverage for surgery can vary, and there may be some costs you will have to pay. Before you have the operation, call your insurance company to find out how much of these costs it will pay and how much you will have to pay yourself.

Ask what your surgeon's fee is and what it covers. Surgical fees often also include several visits after the operation. You also will be billed by the hospital for inpatient or outpatient care and by the anesthesiologist and others providing care related to your operation.

Surgeons' Qualifications

You will want to know that your surgeon is experienced and qualified to perform the operation. Many surgeons have taken special training and passed exams given by a national board of surgeons. Ask if your surgeon is "board certified" in surgery. Some surgeons also have the letters F.A.C.S. after their name. This means they are Fellows of the American College of Surgeons and have passed another review by surgeons of their surgical practices.

For More Information

Surgery

The American College of Surgeons (ACS) has a free series of pamphlets on "When You Need an Operation." For copies, write to the ACS, Office of Public Information, 55 E. Erie Street, Chicago, IL 60611, or call 312-664-4050. Pamphlets in this series range from those providing general information about surgery to those explaining specific surgical procedures.

Second Opinion

For a free brochure on "Medicare Coverage for Second Surgical Opinions: Your Choice Facing Elective Surgery," write to Health Care Financing Administration, Publications, NI-26-27, 7500 Security Blvd., Baltimore, Maryland 21244-1850. Ask for Publication No. HCFA 02173.

To get the name of a specialist in your area who can give you a second opinion, ask your primary doctor or surgeon, the local medical society, or your health insurance company. Medicare beneficiaries may also obtain information from the U.S. Department of Health and Human Services' Medicare hotline: call toll-free 800-638-6833.

Anesthesia

Free booklets on what you should know about anesthesia are available from the American Society of Anesthesiologists (ASA) or the American Association of Nurse Anesthetists (AANA). For copies, write to ASA at 520 North Northwest Highway, Park Ridge, IL 60068, or call 708-825-5586; or AANA at 222 S. Prospect Avenue, Park Ridge, IL 60068-4001, or call 708-692-7050.

Pain Control

"Pain Control After Surgery: A Patient's Guide" is available free from the Agency for Health Care Policy and Research (AHCPR). For a copy of this consumer version of the AHCPR-supported clinical practice guideline and for information on other patient guides, write to the AHCPR Publications Clearinghouse, P.O. Box 8547, Silver Spring, MD 20907, or call toll-free 800-358-9295.

General

For almost every disease, there is a national or local association or society that publishes consumer information. Check your local telephone directory. There are also organized groups of patients with certain illnesses that can often provide information about a condition, alternative treatments, and experience with local doctors and hospitals. Ask your hospital or doctors if they know of any patient groups related to your condition. Also, your local public library has medical reference materials about health care treatments.

Some of these issues are covered in greater detail in a guidebook and video program, "PREPARED(TM) for Health Care: A Consumer's Guide to Better Medical Decisions," by J.C. Gambone, D.O., and R.C. Reiter, M.D., Copyright 1993, Great Performance, Beaverton, Oregon. For information on obtaining copies, write to Great Performance, Inc. at P.O. Box 91400, Portland, OR 97291-0400.

For further information you may also wish to see "The Savvy Patient: How to Be an Active Participant in Your Medical Care," by David R. Stutz, M.D., Bernard Feder, Ph.D., and the Editors of Consumer Reports Books, Copyright 1990, published by Consumers Union of U.S., Inc., Yonkers, NY, 10703.

Reference to these materials does not constitute endorsement by the U.S. Department of Health and Human Services.

Chapter 33

Medication and Older Adults

Mary Parker of Oak Ridge, Tenn., is quick to joke about her health problems. Her vibrant smile and upbeat attitude belie her 78 years. But last year she had a health problem she didn't find amusing. The medication she took for her swollen sinuses left her so weak and dizzy she couldn't get out of bed.

"I felt like I wanted to die," she remembers. "It was awful."

She learned an important lesson from the episode. She thinks twice before taking any medication, questions her doctors and pharmacists, and reviews all her medications regularly with her primary physician.

Parker's attitude is a good one for older adults to have, experts say. As people age, they often develop a number of problems taking medications. Being aware that problems may occur is the first way to minimize them.

"You are a partner in your health care," urges Madeline Feinberg, Pharm.D., a pharmacist and director of the Elder Health program of the University of Maryland School of Pharmacy. "This is a partnership between you, your doctor, and your pharmacist. You need to be assertive and knowledgeable about the medications you take."

The Food and Drug Administration is also working to make drugs safer for older adults, who consume a large share of the nation's medications. Adults over age 65 buy 30 percent of all prescription drugs and 40 percent of all over-the-counter drugs.

U.S. Food and Drug Administration (FDA), *FDA Consumer*, September-October 1997.

"Almost every drug that comes through FDA [for approval] has been examined for effects in the elderly," says Robert Temple, M.D., associate director for medical policy in FDA's Office of Drug Evaluation and Research. "If the manufacturer hasn't done a study in the elderly, we ask for it."

More than 15 years ago, the agency established guidelines for drug manufacturers to include more elderly patients in their studies of new drugs. Upper age limits for drugs were eliminated, and even patients who had other health problems were given the green light to participate if they were able. Also, drugs known to pass primarily through the liver and kidneys must be studied in patients with malfunctions of those organs. This has a direct benefit for older adults, who are more likely to have these conditions.

In several surveys, FDA discovered that drug manufacturers had been using older adults in their drug studies; however, they weren't examining that age group for different reactions to the drugs. Now, they do. Today, every new prescription drug has a section in the labeling about its use in the elderly.

Says Temple, "The FDA has done quite a bit and worked fully with academia and industry to change drug testing so that it does analyze the data from elderly patients. We're quite serious about wanting these analyses."

When More Isn't Necessarily Better

Of all the problems older adults face in taking medication, drug interactions are probably the most dangerous. When two or more drugs are mixed in the body, they may interact with each other and produce uncomfortable or even dangerous side effects. This is especially a problem for older adults because they are much more likely to take more than one drug. Two-thirds of adults over age 65 use one or more drugs each day, and a quarter of them take three drugs each day.

Not all drug combinations are bad. High blood pressure is often treated with several different drugs in low doses. Unless supervised by a doctor, however, taking a mixture of drugs can be dangerous.

For example, a person who takes a blood-thinning medication for high blood pressure should not combine that with aspirin, which will thin the blood even more. And antacids can interfere with certain drugs for Parkinson's disease, high blood pressure, and heart disease. Before prescribing any new drug to an older patient, a doctor should be aware of all the other drugs the patient may be taking.

"Too often, older people get more drugs without a reassessment of their previous medications," says Feinberg. "That can be disastrous."

There is also evidence that older adults tend to be more sensitive to drugs than younger adults are, due to their generally slower metabolisms and organ functions. As people age, they lose muscle tissue and gain fat tissue, and their digestive systems, liver, and kidney functions slow down. All this affects how a drug will be absorbed into the bloodstream, react in the organs, and how quickly it will be eliminated. The old adage "Start low and go slow" applies especially to the elderly.

Older adults who experience dizziness, constipation, upset stomach, sleep changes, diarrhea, incontinence, blurred vision, mood changes, or a rash after taking a drug should call their doctors. The following suggestions may also help:

• Don't take a drug unless absolutely necessary. Try a change in diet or exercise instead. Ask your doctor if there's anything else you can do besides drug therapy for the condition.

• Tell your doctor about all the drugs you take. If you have several doctors, make sure they all know what the others are prescribing, and ask one doctor (such as an internist or general practitioner) to coordinate your drugs.

• Ask for drugs that treat more than one condition. Blood pressure medicine might also be good for heart disease, for example.

• Keep track of side effects. New symptoms may not be from old age but from the drug you're taking. Try another medication if possible until you find one that works for you.

• Learn about your drugs. Find out as much as you can by asking questions and reading the package inserts. Both your doctor and pharmacist should alert you to possible interactions between drugs, how to take any drug properly, and whether there's a less expensive generic drug available.

• Have your doctor review your drugs. If you take a number of drugs, take them all with you on a doctor's visit.

• Ask the doctor, "When can I stop taking this drug?" and, "How do we know this drug is still working?"

• Watch your diet. Some drugs are better absorbed with certain foods, and some drugs shouldn't be taken with certain foods. Ask a pharmacist what foods to take with each drug.

• Follow directions. Read the label every time you take the medication to prevent mistakes, and be sure you understand the timing and dosage prescribed.

- Don't forget. Use a memory aid to help you—a calendar, pill box, or your own system. Whatever works for you is best.

Medicine and Special Needs

Arthritis, poor eyesight, and memory lapses can make it difficult for some older adults to take their medications correctly. Studies have shown that between 40 and 75 percent of older adults don't take their medications at the right time or in the right amount. About a quarter of all nursing home admissions are due at least in part to the inability to take medication correctly.

A number of strategies can make taking medication easier. Patients with arthritis can ask the pharmacist for an oversized, easy-to-open bottle. For easier reading, ask for large-type labels. If those are not available, use a magnifying glass and read the label under bright light.

Invent a system to remember medication. Even younger adults have trouble remembering several medications two or three times a day, with and without food. Devise a plan that fits your daily schedule. Some people use meals or bedtime as cues for remembering drugs. Others use charts, calendars, and special weekly pill boxes.

Mary Sloane, 78, keeps track of five medications a day by sorting her pills each evening into separate dishes. One is for morning pills, the other for the next evening. Then she turns each medicine bottle upside down after taking the pill so she can tell at a glance if she has taken it that day.

"You have to have a system," Sloane says. "Because just as soon as I get started taking my pills, the phone rings, and when I come back to it, I think, 'Now have I taken that?'"

Drug-taking routines should take into account whether the pill works best on an empty or full stomach and whether the doses are spaced properly. To simplify drug-taking, always ask for the easiest dosing schedule possible—just once or twice a day, for example.

Serious memory impairments require assistance from family members or professionals. Adult day-care, supervised living facilities, and home health nurses can provide assistance with drugs.

Active Lives

Not all older adults are in danger of drug interactions and adverse effects. In fact, as more and more people live active lives well into their 80s or beyond, many take few medications at all. Among healthy older adults, medications may have the same physical effects as they do in younger adults. It is primarily when disease interferes that the problems begin.

To guard against potential problems with drugs, however, older adults must be knowledgeable about what they take and how it makes them feel. And they should not hesitate to talk to their doctors or pharmacists about questions and problems they have with a medication.

Says the University of Maryland's Feinberg: "We need to have educated patients to tell us how the drugs are working."

—by Rebecca D. Williams

Rebecca D. Williams is a writer in Oak Ridge, Tenn.

Cutting Costs

The cost of medications is a serious concern for older adults, most of whom must pay for drugs out of pocket. Even those who have insurance to supplement Medicare must often pay a percentage of the cost of their medicines.

For a new prescription, don't buy a whole bottle but ask for just a few pills. You may have side effects to the medication and have to switch. If you buy just a few, you won't be stuck with a costly bottle of medicine you can't take.

For ongoing conditions, medications are often less expensive in quantities of 100. Only buy large quantities of drugs if you know your body tolerates them well. But be sure you can use all of the medication before it passes its expiration date.

Call around for the lowest price. Pharmacy prices can vary greatly. If you find a drug cheaper elsewhere, ask your regular pharmacist if he or she can match the price.

Other ways to make your prescription dollars go further include:

- Ask for a senior citizens discount.

- Ask for a generic equivalent.

- Get drug samples free. Pharmaceutical companies often give samples of drugs to physicians. Tell your doctor you'd be happy to have them. This is especially convenient for trying out a new prescription.

- Buy store-brand or discount brand over-the-counter products. Ask the pharmacist for recommendations.

- Call your local chapter of the American Association for Retired Persons (AARP) and your local disease-related organizations (for diabetes, arthritis, etc.) They may have drugs available at discount prices.

- Try mail order. Mail-order pharmacies can provide bulk medications at discount prices. Use this service only for long-term drug therapy because it takes a few weeks to be delivered. Compare prices before ordering anything.

—by R.D.W.

What to Ask the Doctor

Before you leave your doctor's office with a new prescription, make sure you fully understand how to take the drug correctly. Your pharmacist can also provide valuable information about how to take your medicines and how to cope with side effects. Ask the following questions:

- What is the name of this drug, and what is it designed to do? Is this a generic or a name brand product?

- What is the dosing schedule and how do I take it?

- What should I do if I forget a dose?

- What side effects should I expect?

- How long will I be on this drug?

- How should I store this drug?

- Should I take this on an empty stomach or with food? Is it safe to drink alcohol with this drug?

—by R.D.W.

Chapter 34

Over-the-Counter Drugs: Safe If Used Wisely

Market surveys show that older Americans spend less money on over-the-counter drugs (OTCs) than they do on prescriptions. Even so, the elderly use between 40 and 50 percent of all OTCs consumed to relieve complaints such as arthritis pain, insomnia, constipation, indigestion, and headaches.

As any shopper knows, the variety of OTCs to choose from can be overwhelming; about 300,000 types of over-the-counter drugs (OTCs) are sold in the United States today. These products contain more than 700 different active ingredients. Annual sales of OTCs amount to billions of dollars, indicating a strong consumer demand for medications that can be used to self-treat uncomplicated health problems.

When presented with so many options, how much do you know about what you buy? How safe are these preparations? And, how safe is your use of them? Some consumers think of OTCs as benign "home remedies"; they are not. Others avoid OTCs because of unwarranted concerns about their safety or effectiveness.

Using OTCs appropriately can be beneficial; uninformed use carries risks. Where should the balance be struck? Many over-the-counter medications have active ingredients that can cause problems under some circumstances. At the same time, surveys show that the vast majority of consumers are satisfied with the results they obtain from the OTCs they use.

Reprinted with permission from the *National Policy and Resource Center on Women and Aging Letter*, Volume 2 Number 6, March 1998.

This chapter offers information about the benefits of OTCs and ways to avoid their hazards. Before reading further, however, you may wish to test your knowledge with the quiz at the end of the chapter.

"Safe and Effective"

At the beginning of the 20th century, patent medicines were widely advertised, often with extravagant claims about their effectiveness. Their safety was addressed less often. But in 1937 the market underwent a significant change. Following the deaths of more than 100 persons from an antibiotic containing ethylene glycol (antifreeze), the political climate was ripe for consumer protection laws; and Congress passed the first drug safety act. Since then, consumers have welcomed new OTCs while continuing to need assurance of safety. In response, through amendments to the original law, Congress has sought to maintain a balance between drug innovation and safety regulations.

With a vast number of products coming onto the market, the U.S. Food and Drug Administration (FDA) has had to develop methods to respond to standards set by Congress. Medications that had been on the market for many years were "grandfathered" into compliance if they had not demonstrated any significant safety problems.

Newer OTCs presented a more difficult challenge. By 1972, the FDA found itself unable to review the thousands of new OTCs individually and asked its scientific advisory committees to review the safety and effectiveness of their active ingredients. At the completion of the process—one that lasted 22 years—the agency had assessed 1,454 active ingredients for specific uses in 90 therapeutic categories.

Mark Novitch, a former FDA Deputy Commissioner, describes the more than two-decade review as the single largest undertaking ever. Hundreds of OTC products could not be demonstrated to be effective; lesser numbers were found to be potentially unsafe and were removed from the market immediately.

New OTCs continue to enter the market. Many of them were previously available only by prescription. The federal government has actively encouraged the development of these so-called "switch" products. Prescription drug coverage is costly for medical insurers; consumers pay for OTCs directly. Switch drugs are more readily regulated than other OTCs because they already have received approval for use at prescription level doses. Their manufacturers have only to demonstrate that the lower doses in the OTC versions are effective and that consumers who may have misdiagnosed their symptoms will not be harmed by the drug.

The Risk of Misuse

The drug regulatory process in the United States is one of the most demanding in the world. Congress requires the FDA, in addition to approving active ingredients, to determine the clarity of labels so that consumers can understand a drug's use, potential adverse effects, and drug interactions.

So how safe are over-the-counter drugs? Very safe—if they are used properly. The most difficult safety issues arise when the drugs reach our medicine cabinets. Experts disagree about how well consumers can self-medicate. A trade organization, Non-Prescription Drug Manufacturers' Association (NDMA), believes that "consumers readily understand what a drug is for, its limits, who should use the product, and what other drugs should not be taken in combination."

Others disagree. For example, Elaine Brody of the Philadelphia Geriatric Center did research in the 1980s on how the elderly use OTCs. Her conclusion? Misuse is a serious problem.

Older persons experience two to three times more adverse drug reactions than do younger adults, most often from OTCs. One reason for this is that older persons use more medications. They also consult more physicians, increasing the likelihood of duplications and drug interactions.

Despite this risk, older individuals are much less likely to receive counseling or directions regarding drug use. Not surprisingly, surveys show that elderly consumers cannot identify from one-quarter to one-third of the OTCs they are using.

When to Watch Out

Inappropriate use of OTCs takes many people to the hospital. A three-year study reported in the *Journal of the American Medical Association* in 1974 attributed 18 percent of admissions to OTC misuse. Most problems arise from analgesics (aspirin), antiarthritics (nonsteroidal anti-inflammatory drugs), and antacids.

Non-steroidal anti-inflammatory drugs (NSAIDs) include such familiar brands as Advil, Motrin, and Nuprin as well as newer switch products such as Actron, Orudis-KT, and Aleve. Consumers are less familiar with the effects of NSAIDs than with those of aspirin.

One New Hampshire pharmacist, responsible for tracking drug-related hospital admissions, has seen many cases of excessive bleeding among older persons who are taking blood-thinning agents (i.e., warfarin) and who then use NSAIDs and develop stomach ulcers.

Not all adverse events stem from taking prescription drugs and OTCs together; alcohol consumption also can affect the body's reaction to medications. In fact, a family physician interviewed for this article believes that drinking alcohol while using certain OTCs contributes to many of the adverse reactions to OTCs.

This can be the case with sleep aids and cough medicines that contain diphenhydramine (Benadryl). Used in combination with alcohol or other drugs, the mild drowsiness and confusion associated with diphenhydramine alone may increase to dangerous levels.

Pain relievers and alcohol do not mix either. The FDA recently asked the makers of pain relievers to add warnings to their labels against the use of these products by persons consuming three or more alcoholic beverages a day. While few people experience ill effects from mixing alcohol and pain pills, those who do are often severely affected—by liver damage in the case of acetaminophen (Tylenol and others) and by stomach bleeding in the case of aspirin and NSAIDs.

Other safety issues arise from the way our bodies handle drugs as we age. Elderly persons typically need lower doses of medications than younger persons to achieve the same effects, either beneficial or harmful. For example, many older persons are particularly susceptible to kidney damage from excessive use of NSAIDs. Use of these drugs by people with pre-existing kidney problems can precipitate kidney failure.

Similarly, aging diminishes our ability to adapt to adverse effects from drugs. For example, the dizziness and confusion often associated with the use of some OTCs have a greater impact on older people who have a tendency to fall or whose mental agility is diminished.

Misdiagnosis

Consumers at any age can misdiagnose the ailment for which they are using OTCs. Most consumers do not consult a medical practitioner before using OTCs to treat medical problems. Regulation standards are written to avoid the hazards of misdiagnosis, but they cannot ensure that consumers will make appropriate decisions.

Misdiagnosis can be serious if unrecognized. Heart attacks, ulcers, and esophageal cancer have been mistakenly treated as heartburn. Although not life-threatening, antifungal preparations often are used inappropriately to treat bacterial infections. Not only do such treatments fail to resolve the infection, but drug-resistant yeast organisms may be encouraged.

Before Taking OTCs

Using OTCs carries virtually no risk if you use them wisely. What can you do individually to lower your chances of experiencing adverse effects?

Self-education is the prescription for safety. Learn to treat OTCs as drugs and remember: Each drug affects different people differently.

Consumers and health care providers need to share more information with one another. Many people do not tell their health care providers or pharmacists about the OTCs that they use—nor how much and how often. And providers usually do not ask—although that is changing.

Many consumers learn about OTCs from brand-name advertisements that can lead consumers to expect quick and safe "fixes" from the use of these products. These ads neither inform consumers about less costly generic preparations nor do they typically suggest ways to relieve symptoms without medication.

Take the problem of insomnia. Sleep aids are advertised regularly on television and purchased disproportionately by older people. Regular exercise, bedtime routines, substituting music for television and warm milk for alcohol and caffeine, and having the bedroom at a comfortable temperature may be as effective as medications.

Here are some specific suggestions to help you stay on the safe side of OTCs:

- Ask your pharmacist. No other health professionals have as much training in prescription and OTC drugs as pharmacists. Also, because nearly all pharmacies are computerized, your pharmacist is most likely to know all the medications you are taking.

- Keep a list of all drugs you use. Do this for both prescription and over-the-counter medications. Your medical records, as well as your pharmacy's record, should also list this information. In the interest of your safety, make certain that all such records are complete. Obtaining all your medications from the same pharmacy will help prevent oversights. To get you started, "Elder Health"—a program of the University of Maryland School of Pharmacy—offers booklets in which to record personal medical information and responses to medications (see Resources, below).

- Seek out and investigate non-drug solutions to health problems. When you have a health problem, ask your health care provider whether an OTC is the best remedy and what alternatives there might be. Pharmacies often make this kind of information available as well. For example, Searle (a large manufacturer of OTCs) has placed information on ways to alleviate insomnia in pharmacies around the country.

- Read the label carefully once you decide to use an OTC. The FDA requires that OTC drug manufacturers provide legible and readily understood information on product ingredients, safe dosages, and warnings on potential side effects and interactions. After reading the label, if you have any questions about the safety of the drug for your circumstances, consult an accessible and knowledgeable resource—your pharmacist.

- Seek medical attention if the condition for which you are using OTCs does not resolve or if you are experiencing the condition for the first time and are "just guessing" about what it is.

- Report adverse reactions to your health care provider, pharmacist, and the FDA hotline (see Resources, below).

Resources

AARP Health Newsletter: "Ask Your Pharmacist" answers questions about OTCs. Published by the AARP Pharmacy. PO Box 883, Libertyville, IL 60048. Tel: 800-456-2277.

Complete Drug Reference: Published by Consumer Reports Books. Tel: 800-500-9760. Cost: $39.95.

Elder Health: This center produces pamphlets on a variety of health issues, including personal pharmaceutical records. Elder Health, University of Maryland School of Pharmacy, 20 North Pine St., Baltimore, Maryland 21201.

FDA Hotline: Keeps track of adverse reactions to OTCs in ongoing reassessments of drug regulations. 800-FDA-4010. Their web site is at www.fda.gov.

Healthtouch Online: Provides information on over 7,000 prescription and OTC drugs. Web site: www.healthtouch.com.

Medical Drug Reference: An easy to use CD-ROM offering consumer information on OTC and prescription drugs. Parsons Technology, One Parsons Drive, PO Box 100, Hiawatha, Iowa 52233-0100. Tel: 800-223-6925. Cost: $29.

National Council on Patient Information and Education. Helps consumers and providers understand drug treatments. Tel: 202-347-6711.

"Pharmacist On Call": Senior members of American Express can use pharmacists on call 7 days a week (8 am-1 pm) for confidential answers to questions on OTCs, prescription, and generic medications. Tel: 800-633-2639.

The Physician's Desk Reference (PDR) for Nonprescription Drugs and the *American Pharmaceutical Association's Handbook of Nonprescription Drugs*. Clinicians and pharmacists keep published references such as these on hand. Ask health professionals for information that is not available elsewhere.

Test Your Over-the-Counter Knowledge

Circle T (true) or F (false) after the following statements; then check your answers below.

1. Unlike prescription drugs, over-the-counter medications are not regulated by the government. True or false?

2. Older persons are more at risk than others for side-effects from OTC drugs. True or false?

3. If you have three or more drinks of alcohol every day, you should not take OTC pain relievers. True or false?

4. Some OTCs should not be taken with certain other OTCs or certain prescription medications. True or false?

5. Non-steroidal anti-inflammatory drugs (antiarthritics) can cause kidney failure if taken by persons with pre-existing kidney problems. True or false?

6. The production and sale of hormones such as "anti-aging" DHEA and melatonin are classified as "food additives" by the FDA and therefore are not regulated as strictly as are prescription medications and OTCs. True or false?

Answers: 1. F 2. T 3. T 4. T 5. T 6. T

by Dr. Ann T. Schulz

Dr. Ann T. Schulz is a nurse practitioner who specializes in women's health.

The *Women & Aging Letter* is a project of Brandeis University, in co-operation with the American Society on Aging, the National Black Women's Health Project, and the Coalition of Labor Union Women. The Center is located at the Heller School, Brandeis University, Waltham, MA 02254-9110, tel: 800-929-1995. For information about subscribing to the *Women and Aging Letter*, contact the Center as noted above.

Chapter 35

Polypharmacy

Many elderly persons are taking multiple drugs for several health problems. When this is the case it is important to assess the medication regimen. This includes the reason for the medication, the number of drugs being taken and how and where they are obtained. Some health problems may be chronic, for example congestive heart failure or diabetes. Others, may be acute conditions such as a urinary tract infection (UTI) or pneumonia. The individual may also be taking vitamins, sleeping, and pain medicines, laxatives, or cold remedies bought over the counter (OTC). Some medications may be from different pharmacies, various health care professionals, or even borrowed from neighbors. When assessing medications, it is important to know which of the medications are temporary and which are for long-term use.

What Is Polypharmacy?

Polypharmacy is the consistent use of multiple drugs on a regular basis. Remember this can be both prescribed and OTC medications.

Medicine is a drug or remedy and the term medication is used when talking about a particular drug or remedy. Medications may be prescribed by a licensed professional or bought without a prescription, called over the counter. The use of multiple medications is not always dangerous and undesirable. Many elderly patients require a complex regime to relieve symptoms of a wide range of diseases. However, the older person can be at risk from three problems:

- Medication error: the more medication an individual takes the more likely a mistake will be made in the time and/or amount taken. There is also the possibility with confusion of drug names.

- Adverse side effects: medications may cause dizziness, loss of appetite, depression, incontinence, weakness, and skin rashes among other symptoms.

- Adverse interactions: some medication may increase or block the action of other drugs.

Elderly persons do not process drugs as efficiently as younger ones do. The physical changes in the liver and kidneys slow down the rate of chemical breakdown and the excretion of many substances. These substances remain in the body for abnormally long periods of time. Certain chronic diseases may also slow down this process. It is also believed that the elderly may be more sensitive to drugs affecting the cardiovascular system and central nervous system. In other words, less of the drug may be needed to have the same effect as with a younger person. Functional impairments, such as vision or memory loss and limited mobility may make it difficult for the elderly to take medication as prescribed, resulting in errors. Aunt Jane may find it easier to take all her medication at one time—and she can honestly say she takes her medicine every day! Poor nutrition and dehydration may lead to changes in the way drugs are used by the body. Medications are very expensive and may be hoarded, borrowed, or outdated when money is tight. Cultural differences may influence issues of independence and willingness to follow a prescribed treatment plan.

Who Is Susceptible?

Persons who are already ill with diseases and who have trouble following a complicated medication schedule are at risk. Individuals who are anxious or in pain may overmedicate themselves to relieve symptoms. All the elderly must be careful of medication interaction and side effects due to the increased effect of medications on the aging body systems. These include those individuals:

- With multiple chronic diseases
- Who take many medications

- Who have many health care professionals
- With disabilities, particularly diminished cognitive functioning
- Who live alone
- Who use multiple pharmacy sources

Is It Preventable?

The prevention of adverse effects from polypharmacy requires careful monitoring of the medication regimen by health care professionals and the patient (or patient's family). The patient and family members should:

- Know the side effects of medications

- Know possible interactions of prescribed and OTC medicine

- Discard outdated medicines on a routine basis, this includes reviewing the drug dosage being taken with what had been ordered

- Bring all medications being taken when visiting the health care professional

- Express concerns to the health care professional

- Seek another opinion if concerns are ignored

- Encourage use of one pharmacy or supplier

- Discourage the borrowing or lending of medications

What Is the Active Approach?

Practice Prevention!

- Obtain a list of all the medications being taken.

- Observe your family member for signs of confusion, memory loss, fatigue, inability to function normally, changes in eating, complaints of diarrhea, stomach upset, double vision, headaches, or skin rashes.

- Notify the health care professional of the symptoms and concerns that may be caused by medications. Remember that the HCP may not be aware of all the drugs being taken. Many elderly persons have multiple providers or may still be taking medicines prescribed years ago.

- Develop a method for proper medication administration. This should be a schedule of when and how to take the medication and what food, drink, or activity to avoid.

- Assess whether someone needs to monitor or assist in the taking of medication.

On A Positive Note

By careful monitoring the serious risks of medication errors and interactions can be avoided. This allows persons with multiple diseases to truly benefit from their treatment. Today, many people remain healthy, active, and alert due to several factors, among which include healthier life styles, planning for the future, and advancing medical knowledge.

Part Five

Safety Concerns

Chapter 36

Crime and Older People

Older people and their families worry about crime, and with good reason. Though the elderly are less likely to be victims of crime than teenagers and young adults, the number of crimes against older people is hard to ignore. Each year, about two million older people become crime victims.

The elderly are targets for robbery, personal and car theft, and burglary. Older people are more likely than younger victims to face attackers who are strangers. They are more often attacked at or near their homes. Chances are that an older victim may be more seriously hurt than a younger person.

It isn't only strangers who hurt older people. Sometimes, family members, friends, or caretakers may physically, mentally, or financially abuse older people through neglect, violence, or by stealing money or property.

Even though there are risks, do not let a fear of crime stop you from enjoying life. There are things you can do to be safer. Be careful and be aware of what goes on around you.

Fighting Crime

You can fight crime. The best thing you can do at home is to lock your doors and windows. You can also protect yourself at home in other ways:

- Always try to see who's there before opening your door. Look through a peephole or a safe window. Ask any stranger to tell

National Institute on Aging, "Age Page," 1996.

you his or her name and to show proof that he or she is from the identified company or group. Remember, it is okay to keep the door locked if you are uneasy.

- Make sure that locks, doors, and windows are strong and cannot be broken easily. A good alarm system can help. Many police departments will send an officer to your home to suggest changes that could improve your security.

- Mark valuable property by engraving an identification number on it, such as your driver's license number. Make a list of expensive items such as jewelry or silver. Take a picture of the valuable items and store the details in a safe place like a bank safety deposit box.

On the street, stay alert at all times, even in your own neighborhood and at your own door. Walk with a friend. Try to stay away from places where crimes happen, such as dark parking lots or alleys. You can also:

- Have monthly pension or Social Security checks sent direct-deposit, right to the bank. If you visit the bank often, vary the time of day you go.

- Don't carry a lot of cash. Try not to carry a purse. Put your money, credit cards, or wallet in an inside pocket. If you are stopped by a robber, hand over any cash you have.

- Don't dress in a flashy way. Leave good jewelry, furs, and other valuables in a safe place to avoid tempting would-be robbers.

Money and property crimes come in many forms and are a big problem. Older people may be victims of consumer fraud such as con games or insurance scams. Even family members or friends can sometimes steal an older person's money or property. Trust what you feel. Protect yourself:

- Don't take money from your bank account if a stranger tells you to. In one common scam a thief may pretend to be a bank employee and ask you to take out money to "test" a bank teller. Banks do not check out their employees this way.

- Stay away from deals that are "too good to be true." Beware of deals that ask for a lot of money up front and promise you sure success. Check with your local Better Business Bureau.

- Don't give your credit card or bank account number over the phone to people who have called you to sell a product or ask for a contribution.

- Don't be taken in by quick fixes or miracle cures for health problems. People who are not trained or licensed may try to sell you miracle "cures" for cancer, baldness, arthritis, or other problems. Ask your doctor before you buy. Be sure to go to licensed professionals.

Neglect or mistreatment of older people is called elder abuse. It can happen anywhere, at home by family or friends, or in a nursing home by other caregivers. Physical, financial, or emotional abuse by family or friends is very hard to deal with. There is help for people who are being abused. Most states and many local governments have Adult Protective Services programs. Check the phone book or call directory assistance. You can also talk to your clergy, a lawyer, or doctor. Your local Area Agency on Aging may help. The Eldercare Locator (1-800-677-1116) can direct you to a local agency.

Reporting Crime

You can help your friends and neighbors by reporting crime when it happens. Police say that more than half of all crimes go unreported. If you don't report a crime, because of embarrassment or fear, the criminals stay on the streets.

If you are the victim of a crime, there is help. Contact the National Organization for Victim Assistance (NOVA), 1757 Park Rd., NW, Washington, D.C. 20010. NOVA's 24 hour hotline is 1-800-TRY-NOVA.

Other Resources

American Association of Retired Persons (AARP)
Criminal Justice Services
601 E Street, NW
Washington, D.C. 20049
202-434-2222

Council of Better Business Bureaus
4200 Wilson Boulevard, Suite 800
Arlington, VA 22209
703-525-0100
Ask for the pamphlet called "Tips on Elderly Consumer Problems" and other publications.

United Seniors Health Cooperative (USHC)
1331 H Street, NW, Suite 500
Washington, D.C. 20045-4706
Publications are available on a variety of health-related consumer issues.

For a list of free publications from the National Institute on Aging (NIA), contact:
NIA Information Center
P.O. Box 8057
Gaithersburg, MD 20898-8057
800-222-2225
800-222-4225 (TTY)
E-mail: niainfo@access.digex.net

Chapter 37

Preventing Falls and Fractures

An injury from falling can limit a person's ability to lead an active, independent life. This is especially true for older people. Each year thousands of older men and women are disabled, sometimes permanently, by falls that result in broken bones. Yet many of these injuries could be prevented by making simple changes in the home.

As people age, changes in their vision, hearing, muscle strength, coordination, and reflexes may make them more likely to fall. Older persons also are more likely to have treatable disorders that may affect their balance—such as diabetes or conditions of the heart, nervous system, and thyroid. In addition, compared with younger people, older persons often take more medications that may cause dizziness or lightheadedness.

Preventing falls is especially important for people who have osteoporosis, a condition in which bone mass decreases so that bones are more fragile and break easily. Osteoporosis is a major cause of bone fractures in women after menopause and older people in general. For people with severe osteoporosis, even a minor fall may cause one or more bones to break.

Steps to Take

Falls and accidents seldom "just happen," and many can be prevented. Each of us can take steps to make our homes safer and reduce

National Institute on Aging, "Age Page," updated August 1998.

the likelihood of falling. Here are some guidelines to help prevent falls and fractures.

- Have your vision and hearing tested regularly and properly corrected.

- Talk to your doctor or pharmacist about the side effects of the medicines you are taking and whether they affect your coordination or balance. Ask for suggestions to reduce the possibility of falling.

- Limit your intake of alcohol. Even a small amount of alcohol can disturb already impaired balance and reflexes.

- Use caution in getting up too quickly after eating, lying down, or resting. Low blood pressure may cause dizziness at these times.

- Make sure that the nighttime temperature in your home is at least 65F degrees. Prolonged exposure to cold temperatures may cause a drop in body temperature, which in turn may lead to dizziness and falling. Many older people cannot tolerate cold as well as younger people can.

- Use a cane, walking stick, or walker to help maintain balance on uneven or unfamiliar ground or if you sometimes feel dizzy. Use special caution in walking outdoors on wet and icy pavement.

- Wear supportive rubber-soled or low-heeled shoes. Avoid wearing smooth-soled slippers or only socks on stairs and waxed floors. They make it very easy to slip.

- Maintain a regular program of exercise to improve strength and muscle tone, and keep your joints, tendons, and ligaments more flexible. Many older people enjoy walking and swimming. Mild weight-bearing activities, such as walking or climbing stairs, may even reduce the loss of bone due to osteoporosis. Check with your doctor or physical therapist to plan a suitable exercise program.

Make Your Home Safe

Many older people fall because of hazardous conditions at home. Use this checklist to help you safeguard against some likely hazards.

Stairways, hallways, and pathways should have:

- good lighting and be free of clutter,

- firmly attached carpet, rough texture, or abrasive strips to secure footing,

- tightly fastened handrails running the whole length and along both sides of all stairs, with light switches at the top and bottom.

Bathrooms should have:

- grab bars located in and out of tubs and showers and near toilets,

- nonskid mats, abrasive strips, or carpet on all surfaces that may get wet,

- nightlights.

Bedrooms should have:

- nightlights or light switches within reach of bed(s),

- telephones (easy to reach), near the bed(s).

Living areas should have:

- electrical cords and telephone wires placed away from walking paths,

- rugs well secured to the floor,

- furniture (especially low coffee tables) and other objects arranged so they are not in the way,

- couches and chairs at proper height to get into and out of easily.

For More Information

For more complete information on simple, relatively inexpensive repairs and safety recommendations for your home, write to the U.S. Consumer Product Safety Commission, Washington, DC 20207; or call (800) 638-2772. The Commission also can send you a free copy of the booklet *Home Safety Checklist for Older Consumers*.

Chapter 38

Older Consumer Home Safety Checklist

Each year, many older Americans are injured in and around their homes. The U.S. Consumer Product Safety Commission (CPSC) estimates that in 1981, over 622,000 people over age 65 were treated in hospital emergency rooms for injuries associated with products they live with and use everyday.

CPSC believes that many of these injuries result from hazards that are easy to overlook, but also easy to fix. By spotting these hazards and taking some simple steps to correct them, many injuries might be prevented.

Use this checklist to spot possible safety problems which may be present in your home. Answer yes or no to each question. Then go back over the list and take action to correct those items which may need attention.

Keep this checklist as a reminder of safe practices, and use it periodically to re-check your home.

This checklist is organized by areas in the home. However, there are some potential hazards that need to be checked in more than just one area of your home. These are highlighted at the beginning of the checklist and short reminders are included in each other section of the checklist.

All Areas Of The Home

In all areas of your home, check all electrical and telephone cords; rugs, runners and mats; telephone areas; smoke detectors; electrical

U.S. Consumer Product Safety Commission, Washington, DC 20207, CPSC Document No. 4701.

outlets and switches; light bulbs; space heaters; woodburning stoves; and your emergency exit plan.

Check All Cords

Question: Are lamp, extension, and telephone cords placed out of the flow of traffic?

Recommendation: Cords stretched across walkways may cause someone to trip.

- Arrange furniture so that outlets are available for lamps and appliances without the use of extension cords.
- If you must use an extension cord, place it on the floor against a wall where people can not trip over it.
- Move the phone so that telephone cords will not lie where people walk.

Question: Are cords out from beneath furniture and rugs or carpeting?

Recommendation: Furniture resting on cords can damage them, creating fire and shock hazards. Electric cords which run under carpeting may cause a fire.

- Remove cords from under furniture or carpeting.
- Replace damaged or frayed cords.

Question: Are cords attached to the walls, baseboards, etc., with nails or staples?

Nails or staples can damage cords, presenting fire and shock hazards.

- Remove nails, staples, etc.
- Check wiring for damage.
- Use tape to attach cords to walls or floors.

Question: Are electrical cords in good condition, not frayed or cracked?

Damaged cords may cause a shock or fire.

- Replace frayed or cracked cords.

Question: Do extension cords carry more than their proper load, as indicated by the ratings labeled on the cord and the appliance?

Overloaded extension cords may cause fires. Standard 18 gauge extension cords can carry 1250 watts.

- If the rating on the cord is exceeded because of the power requirements of one or more appliances being used on the cord, change the cord to a higher rated one or unplug some appliances.

- If an extension cord is needed, use one having a sufficient amp or wattage rating.

Check All Rugs, Runners, and Mats

Question: Are all small rugs and runners slip-resistant?

CPSC estimates that in 1982, over 2,500 people 65 and over were treated in hospital emergency rooms for injuries that resulted from tripping over rugs and runners. Falls are also the most common cause of fatal injury for older people.

- Remove rugs and runners that tend to slide.
- Apply double-faced adhesive carpet tape or rubber matting to the backs of rugs and runners.
- Purchase rugs with slip-resistant backing.
- Check rugs and mats periodically to see if backing needs to be replaced.
- Place rubber matting under rugs. (Rubber matting that can be cut to size is available.)
- Purchase new rugs with slip-resistant backing.

Note: Over time, adhesive on tape can wear away. Rugs with slip-resistant backing also become less effective as they are washed. Periodically, check rugs and mats to see if new tape or backing is needed.

Question: Are emergency numbers posted on or near the telephone?

Recommendation: In case of emergency, telephone numbers for the Police, Fire Department, and local Poison Control Center, along with a neighbor's number, should be readily available.

- Write the numbers in large print and tape them to the phone, or place them near the phone where they can be seen easily.

Question: Do you have access to a telephone if you fall (or experience some other emergency which prevents you from standing and reaching a wall phone)?

- Have at least one telephone located where it would be accessible in the event of an accident which leaves you unable to stand.

Check Smoke Detectors

Question: Are smoke detectors properly located?

Recommendation: At least one smoke detector should be placed on every floor of your home.

- Read the instructions that come with the smoke detector for advice on the best place to install it.
- Make sure detectors are placed near bedrooms, either on the ceiling or 6-12 inches below the ceiling on the wall.
- Locate smoke detectors away from air vents.

Question: Do you have properly working smoke detectors?

Recommendation: Many home fire injuries and deaths are caused by smoke and toxic gases, rather than the fire itself. Smoke detectors provide an early warning and can wake you in the event of a fire.

- Purchase a smoke detector if you do not have one.
- Check and replace batteries and bulbs according to the manufacturer's instructions.
- Vacuum the grillwork of your smoke detector.
- Replace any smoke detectors which can not be repaired.

Note: Some fire departments or local governments will provide assistance in acquiring or installing smoke detectors.

Check Electrical Outlets and Switches

Question: Are any outlets and switches unusually warm or hot to the touch?

Unusually warm or hot outlets or switches may indicate that an unsafe wiring condition exists.

- Unplug cords from outlets and do not use the switches.
- Have an electrician check the wiring as soon as possible.

Question: Do all outlets and switches have cover plates, so that no wiring is exposed?

Recommendation: Exposed wiring presents a shock hazard.

- Add a cover plate.

Question: Are light bulbs the appropriate size and type for the lamp or fixture?

Recommendation: A bulb of too high wattage or the wrong type may lead to fire through overheating. Ceiling fixtures, recessed lights, and "hooded" lamps will trap heat.

- Replace with a bulb of the correct type and wattage. (If you do not know the correct wattage, use a bulb no larger than 60 watts.)

Check Space Heaters

Question: Are heaters which come with a 3-prong plug being used in a 3-hole outlet or with a properly attached adapter?

Recommendation: The grounding feature provided by a 3-hole receptacle or an adapter for a 2-hole receptacle is a safety feature designed to lessen the risk of shock.

- Never defeat the grounding feature.
- If you do not have a 3-hole outlet, use an adapter to connect the heater's 3-prong plug. Make sure the adapter ground wire or tab is attached to the outlet.

Question: Are small stoves and heaters placed where they can not be knocked over, and away from furnishings and flammable materials, such as curtains or rugs?

Recommendation: Heaters can cause fires or serious burns if they cause you to trip or if they are knocked over.

- Relocate heaters away from passageways and flammable materials such as curtains, rugs, furniture, etc.

Question: If your home has space heating equipment, such as a kerosene heater, a gas heater or an LP gas heater, do you understand the installation and operating instructions thoroughly?

Recommendation: Unvented heaters should be used with room doors open or window slightly open to provide ventilation. The correct fuel, as recommended by the manufacturer, should always be used. Vented heaters should have proper venting, and the venting system should be checked frequently. Improper venting is the most frequent cause of carbon monoxide poisoning, and older consumers are at special risk.

- Review the installation and operating instructions.
- Call your local fire department if you have additional questions.

Check Woodburning Heating Equipment

Question: Is woodburning equipment installed properly?

Recommendation: Woodburning stoves should be installed by a qualified person according to local building codes.

- Local building code officials or fire marshals can provide requirements and recommendations for installation.

Note: Some insurance companies will not cover fire losses if wood stoves are not installed according to local codes.

Check the Emergency Exit Plan

Question: Do you have an emergency exit plan and an alternate emergency exit plan in case of a fire?

Recommendation: Once a fire starts, it spreads rapidly. Since you may not have much time to get out and there may be a lot of confusion, it is important that everyone knows what to do.

- Develop an emergency exit plan.
- Choose a meeting place outside your home so you can be sure that everyone is capable of escape quickly and safely.
- Practice the plan from time to time to make sure everyone is capable of escape quickly and safely.

Remember periodically to re-check your home.

Kitchen

In the kitchen, check the range area, all electrical cords, lighting, the stool, all throw rugs and mats, and the telephone area.

Check the Range Area

Question: Are towels, curtains, and other things that might catch fire located away from the range?

Recommendation: Placing or storing non-cooking equipment like potholders, dish towels, or plastic utensils on or near the range man result in fires or burns.

- Store flammable and combustible items away from range and oven.
- Remove any towels hanging on oven handles. If towels hang close to a burner, change the location of the towel rack.
- If necessary, shorten or remove curtains which could brush against heat sources.

Question: Do you wear clothing with short or close-fitting sleeves while you are cooking?

Recommendation: CPSC estimates that 70% of all people who die from clothing fires are over 65 years of age. Long sleeves are more likely to catch fire than are short sleeves. Long sleeves are also more apt to catch on pot handles, overturning pots and pans and causing scalds.

- Roll back long, loose sleeves or fasten them with pins or elastic bands while you are cooking.

Question: Are kitchen ventilation systems or range exhausts functioning properly and are they in use while you are cooking?

Recommendation: Indoor air pollutants may accumulate to unhealthful levels in a kitchen where gas or kerosene-fire appliances are in use.

- Use ventilation systems or open windows to clear air of vapors and smoke.

Question: Are all extension cords and appliance cords located away from the sink or range areas?

Recommendation: Electrical appliances and power cords can cause shock or electrocution if they come in contact with water. Cords can also be damaged by excess heat.

- Move cords and appliances away from sink areas and hot surfaces.
- Move appliances closer to wall outlets or to different outlets so you won't need extension cords.
- If extension cords must be used, install wiring guides so that cords will not hang near sink, range, or working areas.
- Consider adding new outlets for convenience and safety; ask your electrician to install outlets equipped with ground fault circuit interrupters (GFCIs) to protect against electric shock. A GFCI is a shock-protection device that will detect electrical fault and shut off electricity before serious injury or death occurs.

Question: Does good, even lighting exist over the stove, sink, and countertop work areas, especially where food is sliced or cut?

Recommendation: Low lighting and glare can contribute to burns or cuts. Improve lighting by:

- Opening curtains and blinds (unless this causes to much glare).
- Using the maximum wattage bulb allowed by the fixture. (If you do not know the correct wattage for the fixture, use a bulb no larger than 60 watts.)
- Reducing glare by using frosted bulbs, indirect lighting, shades or globes on light fixtures, or partially closing the blinds or curtains.
- Installing additional light fixtures, e.g. under cabinet/over countertop lighting. (Make sure that the bulbs you use are the right type and wattage for the light fixture.)

Question: Do you have a step stool which is stable and in good repair?

Recommendation: Standing on chairs, boxes, or other makeshift items to reach high shelves can result in falls. CPSC estimates that in 1982, 1500 people over 65 were treated in hospital emergency rooms when they fell from chairs on which they were standing.

- If you don't have a step stool, consider buying one. Choose one with a handrail that you can hold onto while standing on the top step.
- Before climbing on any step stool, make sure it is fully opened and stable.
- Tighten screws and braces on the step stool.
- Discard step stools with broken parts.

Remember: Check all of the product areas mentioned at the beginning of the checklist.

Living Room/Family Room

In the living room/family room, check all rugs and runners, electrical and telephone cords, lighting, the fireplace and chimney, the telephone area, and all passageways.

Question: Are chimneys clear from accumulations of leaves, and other debris that can clog them?

Recommendation: A clogged chimney can cause a poorly-burning fire to result in poisonous fumes and smoke coming back into the house.

- Do not use the chimney until the blockage has been removed.
- Have the chimney checked and cleaned by a registered or licensed professional.

Question: Has the chimney been cleaned within the past year?

Recommendation: Burning wood can cause a build up of a tarry substance (creosote) inside the chimney. This material can ignite and result in a serious chimney fire.

- Have the chimney checked and cleaned by a registered or licensed professional.

Check the Telephone Area

For information on the telephone area, refer to the beginning of the checklist.

Check Passageways

Question: Are hallways, passageways between rooms, and other heavy traffic areas well lit?

Recommendation: Shadowed or dark areas can hide tripping hazards.

- Use the maximum wattage bulb allowed by the fixture. (If you do not know the correct wattage, use a bulb no larger than 60 watts.)
- Install night lights.
- Reduce glare by using frosted bulbs, indirect lighting, shades or globes on light fixtures, or partially closing blinds or curtains.
- Consider using additional lamps or light fixtures. Make sure that the bulbs you use are the right type and wattage for the light fixture.

Question: Are exits and passageways kept clear?

Furniture, boxes, or other items could be an obstruction or tripping hazard, especially in the event of an emergency or fire.

- Rearrange furniture to open passageways and walkways.
- Remove boxes and clutter.

Remember: Check all of the product areas mentioned at the beginning of the checklist.

Bathroom

In the bathroom, check bathtub and shower areas, water temperature, rugs and mats, lighting, small electrical appliances, and storage areas for medications.

Check Bathtub and Shower Areas

Question: Are bathtubs and showers equipped with non-skid mats, abrasive strips, or surfaces that are not slippery?

Recommendation: Wet soapy tile or porcelain surfaces are especially slippery and may contribute to falls.

- Apply textured strips or appliques on the floors of tubs and showers.
- Use non-skid mats in the tub and shower, and on the bathroom floor.

Question: Do bathtubs and showers have at least one (preferably two) grab bars?

Recommendation: Grab bars can help you get into and out of your tub or shower, and can help prevent falls.

- Check existing bars for strength and stability, and repair if necessary.
- Attach grab bars, through the tile, to structural supports in the wall, or install bars specifically designed to attach to the sides of the bathtub. If you are not sure how it is done, get someone who is qualified to assist you.

Question: Is the temperature 120 degrees or lower?

Water temperature above 120 degrees can cause tap water scalds.

- Lower the setting on your hot water heater to "Low" or 120 degrees. If you are unfamiliar with the controls of your water heater, ask a qualified person to adjust it for you.
- If your hot water system is controlled by the landlord, ask the landlord to consider lowering the setting.

Note: If the water heater does not have a temperature setting, you can use a thermometer to check the temperature of the water at the tap.

- Always check water temperature by hand before entering bath or shower.
- Taking baths, rather than showers, reduces the risk of a scald from suddenly changing water temperatures.

Check Lighting

Question: Is a light switch located near the entrance to the bathroom?

Recommendations: A light switch near the door will prevent you from walking through a dark area.

- Install a night light. Inexpensive lights that plug into outlets are available.
- Consider replacing the existing switch with a "glow switch" that can be seen in the dark.

Check Small Electrical Appliances

Question: Are small electrical appliances such as hair dryers, shavers, curling irons, etc., unplugged when not in use?

Recommendation: Even an appliance that is not turned on, such as a hairdryer, can be potentially hazardous if it is left plugged in. If it falls into water in a sink or bathtub while plugged in, it could cause a lethal shock.

- Unplug all small appliances when not in use.
- Never reach into water to retrieve an appliance that has fallen in without being sure the appliance is unplugged.
- Install a ground fault circuit interrupter (GFCI) in your bathroom outlet to protect against electric shock.

Check Medications

Question: Are all medicines stored in the containers that they came in and are they clearly marked?

Recommendation: Medications that are not clearly and accurately labeled can be easily mixed up. Taking the wrong medicine or missing a dosage of medicine you need can be dangerous.

- Be sure that all containers are clearly marked with the contents, doctor's instructions, expiration date, and patient's name.
- Dispose of outdated medicines properly.
- Request non-child-resistant closures from your pharmacist only when you cannot use child-resistant closures.

Note: Poisonings occur when children visiting grandparents go through the medicine cabinet or grandmother's purse. In homes where grandchildren or other youngsters are frequent visitors, medicines should be purchased in containers with child-resistant caps, and the caps properly closed after each use. Store medicines beyond the reach of children.

Remember: Check all of the product areas mentioned at the beginning of the checklist.

Bedrooms

In the bedroom, check all rugs and runners, electrical and telephone cords, and areas around beds.

Check Areas Around Beds

Question: Are lamps or light switches within reach of each bed?

Recommendation: Lamps or switches located close to each bed will enable people getting up at night to see where they are going.

- Rearrange furniture closer to switches or move lamps closer to beds.
- Install night lights.

Question: Are ash trays, smoking materials, or other fire sources (heaters, hot plates, teapots, etc.) located away from beds or bedding?

Recommendation: Burns are a leading cause of accidental death among seniors. Smoking in bed is a major contributor to this problem. Among mattress and bedding fire related deaths in a recent year, 42% were to persons 65 or older.

- Remove sources of heat or flame from areas around beds.
- Don't smoke in bed.

Question: Is anything covering your electric blanket when in use?

Recommendation: "Tucking in" electric blankets, or placing additional coverings on top of them can cause excessive heat buildup which can start a fire.

Question: Do you avoid "tucking in" the sides or ends of your electric blanket?

Recommendation:

- Use electric blankets according to the manufacturer's instructions.
- Don't allow anything on top of the blanket while it is in use. (This includes other blankets or comforters, even pets sleeping on top of the blanket.)
- Don't set electric blankets so high that they could burn someone who falls asleep while they are on.

Question: Do you ever go to sleep with a heating pad which is turned on?

Recommendation: Never go to sleep with a heating pad if it is turned on because it can cause serious burns even at relatively low settings.

Question: Is there a telephone close to your bed?

Recommendation: In case of an emergency, it is important to be able to reach the telephone without getting out of bed.

Remember: Check all of the product areas mentioned at the beginning of the checklist.

Basement/Garage/Workshop/Storage Areas

In the basement, garage, workshop, and storage areas, check lighting, fuse boxes or circuit breakers, appliances and power tools, electrical cords, and flammable liquids.

Check Lighting

Question: Are work areas, especially areas where power tools are used, well lit?

Recommendation: Power tools were involved in over 5,200 injuries treated in hospital emergency rooms to people 65 and over in 1982. Three fourths of these were finger injuries. Good lighting can reduce the chance that you will accidentally cut your finger.

- Either install additional light, or avoid working with power tools in the area.

Question: Can you turn on the lights without first having to walk through a dark area?

Recommendation: Basement, garages, and storage areas can contain many tripping hazards and sharp or pointed tools that can make a fall even more hazardous.

- Keep an operating flashlight handy.
- Have an electrician install switches at each entrance to a dark area.

Check the Fuse Box or Circuit Breakers

Question: If fuses are used, are they the correct size for the circuit?

Recommendation: Replacing a correct size fuse with a larger size fuse can present a serious fire hazard. If the fuse in the box is rated higher than that intended for the circuit, excessive current will be allowed to flow and possibly overload the outlet and house wiring to the point that a fire can begin.

- Be certain that correct-size fuses are used. (If you do not know the correct sizes, consider having an electrician identify and label the sizes to be used.)

Note: If all, or nearly all, fuses used are 30-amp fuses, there is a chance that some of the fuses are rated too high for the circuit.

Check Appliances and Power Tools

Question: Are power tools equipped with a 3-prong plug or marked to show that they are double insulated?

Recommendation: These safety features reduce the risk of an electric shock.

- Use a properly connected 3-prong adapter for connecting a 3-prong plug to a 2-hole receptacle.
- Consider replacing old tools that have neither a 3-prong plug nor are double insulated.

Question: Are power tools guards in place?

Recommendation: Power tools used with guards removed pose a serious risk of injury from sharp edges or moving parts.

- Replace guards that have been removed from power tools.

Question: Has the grounding feature on any 3-prong plug been defeated by removal of the grounding pin or by improperly using an adapter?

Recommendation: Improperly grounded appliances can lead to electric shock.

- Check with your service person or an electrician if you are in doubt.

Check Flammable and Volatile Liquids

Question: Are containers of volatile liquids tightly capped?

Recommendation: If not tightly closed, vapors may escape that may be toxic when inhaled.

• Check containers periodically to make sure they are tightly closed.

Note: CPSC has reports of several cases in which gasoline, stored as much as 10 feet from a gas water heater, exploded. Many people are unaware that gas fumes can travel that far.

Question: Are gasoline, paints, solvents, or other products that give off vapors or fumes stored away from ignition sources?

Recommendation: Gasoline, kerosene, and other flammable liquids should be stored out of living areas in properly labeled, non-glass safety containers.

• Remove these products from the areas near heat or flame such as heaters, furnaces, water heaters, ranges, and other gas appliances.

Stairs

For all stairways, check lighting, handrails, and the condition of the steps and coverings.

Check Lighting

Question: Are stairs well lighted?

Recommendation: Stairs should be lighted so that each step, particularly the step edges, can be clearly seen while going up and down stairs. The lighting should not produce glare or shadows along the stairway.

• Use the maximum wattage bulb allowed by the light fixture. (If you do not know the correct wattage, use a bulb no larger than 60 watts.)

• Reduce glare by using frosted bulbs, indirect lighting, shades or globes on light fixtures, or partially closing blinds and curtains.

• Have a qualified person add additional light fixtures. Make sure that the bulbs you use are the right type and wattage for the light fixture.

Question: Are light switches located at both the top and bottom of the stairs.

Recommendation: Even if you are very familiar with the stairs, lighting is an important factor in preventing falls. You should be able to turn on the lights before you use the stairway from either end.

- If no other light is available, keep an operating flashlight in a convenient location at the top and bottom of the stairs.
- Install night lights at nearby outlets.
- Consider installing switches at the top and bottom of the stairs.

Question: Do the steps allow secure footing?

Recommendation: Worn treads or worn or loose carpeting can lead to insecure footing, resulting in slips or falls.

- Try to avoid wearing only socks or smooth-soled shoes or slippers when using stairs.

- Make certain the carpet is firmly attached to the steps all along the stairs.

- Consider refinishing or replacing worn treads, or replacing worn carpeting.

- Paint outside steps with paint that has a rough texture, or use abrasive strips.

Question: Are steps even and of the same size and height?

Recommendation: Even a small difference in step surfaces or riser heights can lead to falls.

- Mark any steps which are especially narrow or have risers that are higher or lower than the others. Be especially careful of these steps when using the stairs.

Question: Are the coverings on the steps in good condition?

Recommendation: Worn or torn coverings or nails sticking out from coverings could snag your foot or cause you to trip.

- Repair coverings.
- Remove coverings.
- Replace coverings.

Question: Can you clearly see the edges of the steps?

Recommendation: Falls may occur if the edges of the steps are blurred or hard to see.

- Paint edges of outdoor steps white to see them better at night.
- Add extra lighting.
- If you plan to carpet your stairs, avoid deep pile carpeting or patterned or dark colored carpeting that can make it difficult to see the edges of the steps clearly.

Question: Is anything stored on the stairway, even temporarily?

Recommendation: People can trip over objects left on stairs, particularly in the event of an emergency or fire.

- Remove all objects from the stairway.

Remember Periodically To Re-Check Your Home.

For further information, write:

U.S. Consumer Product Safety Commission, Washington, D.C. 20207. To report a product hazard or a product-related injury, write to the U.S. Consumer Product Safety Commission, Washington, D.C., 20207, or call the toll-free hotline: 800-638-CPSC. A tele-typewriter for the deaf is available on the following numbers: National 800-638-8270, Maryland only 800-492-8104.

Chapter 39

New Test Predicts Crash Risk of Older Drivers

A new vision test may ultimately help the elderly, their families, and physicians decide when it's okay for an older person to continue driving or when it may be time to hang up the car keys. Using a novel "useful field of view" test to measure how drivers process visual information, researchers at the University of Alabama at Birmingham (UAB) found that poor performance on the test was linked to an increased risk of car crashes. Drivers who showed a 40 percent or greater impairment in their useful field of view were more than twice as likely to be involved in a crash within 3 years of testing.

The research, by Cynthia Owsley, Ph.D., Karlene Ball, Ph.D., and colleagues from UAB and Western Kentucky University in Bowling Green, is reported in the April 8, 1998, issue of the *Journal of the American Medical Association (JAMA)*. The study was funded by the National Institute on Aging (NIA).

It is well known that older drivers are at greater risk of crashes or injury when compared to most other age groups. But there are large differences in their skills and abilities. The useful field of view test— and maintaining or improving driving skills through visual attention training programs—may be one way to address those differences and stay away from age-based restrictions on driving, the scientists say. "By measuring the skills directly related to driving, we can identify specific drivers who are at greatest risk," says Owsley. "Setting an arbitrary age limit for driving unjustifiably restricts the mobility and independence of older people. We're trying to help avoid that."

NIH Press Release, Tuesday, April 7, 1998 http://www.nih.gov/nia.

The study marks the first time that scientists have attempted to find out whether or not a visual processing test can predict the likelihood of future crashes for individual older adults. The test differs substantially from standard eye exams, which measure acuity or visual function, or the ability to see an object at a given distance. To assess their visual processing abilities, participants in this study looked at a computer screen with figures of cars, trucks, and other objects. The drivers were asked to identify a particular object amid different kinds of visual distractions on the screen. The useful field of view was defined as the area in which all of this rapidly presented visual information can be used. People who had measured difficulty with the task were considered to have an impaired useful field of view.

Some 294 drivers ranging in age from 55 to 87 participated in the study. In addition to being tested for visual function, information was collected on the participants' general health, mental status, and how often they drove so that the researchers could determine the factors involved in crashes over the 3-year follow-up period from 1990 to 1993. Crash reports involving the participants were collected from a state agency, and researchers compared the useful field of view scores and results from the other types of vision tests with the crash information. During the 3-year follow-up, 56 of the study's drivers were involved in at least one crash.

Performance on the useful field of view test was found to be directly related to involvement in a crash. People with a 40 percent or greater impairment in their useful field of view were more than twice as likely to be involved in a crash. For every 10 points of reduction in a driver's useful field of view measure, his or her crash risk rose by 16 percent, regardless of age. Other vision tests did not predict the risk of future crashes.

This study is very important for older people, their families, and their neighbors, says Jared B. Jobe, Ph.D., chief of the NIA's adult psychological development branch. Older drivers are involved in more crashes and fatalities per mile driven than most other age groups and are more likely to become disabled or die as a result of collisions than younger adults.

"This research shows there may be a way to protect older drivers and the community in a very reasonable way," Jobe states. More research is needed to make this type of testing practical and proven enough for doctors' offices and state licensing agencies. This study, however, goes a long way in demonstrating what may work, he says. Jobe noted that the NIA is funding additional work by Ball, Owsley and their colleagues to see if elements of the useful field of view test may be incorporated into training programs for older people to help those with a reduction in their useful field of view improve their driving skills.

Owsley's research is part of the NIA-sponsored Edward R. Roybal Centers for Research on Applied Gerontology, which were established to help move promising research findings out of the laboratory and into programs that can directly improve the lives of older people and their families. NIA, part of the National Institutes of Health, leads the national effort in research on aging, supporting and conducting basic, clinical, epidemiological, and behavioral and social research.

Note: Two co-authors of the JAMA article, Karlene Ball, Ph.D., and Daniel L. Roenker, Ph.D., own stock in Visual Resources, Inc., the company that holds the patent to the useful field of view visual attention analyzer used in this study.

Chapter 40

Telecommunications Technology for Safety, Independence, and Social Interaction for Old People with Disabilities

Advanced telecommunications technology like the Internet offers exciting immediate and future applications for older people with disabilities. Yet the overwhelming majority of frail elderly people still rely primarily on their telephone for telecommunications. There are many phone features available, and add-on assistive products, that can assist older people with various types of impairments. This chapter takes a look at some of these special phone features, including personal emergency response systems.

The telephone has been available to us for a relatively short time—about 100 years—and today is an essential component of almost every business and home. For older people with disabilities, many of whom live alone and infrequently leave their home, the phone provides a device for social contacts. For elders who have difficulty getting to places outside their home, the phone can be used for banking and shopping. The phone can also be used to call for help, in the event of a fall, an illness, or some other problem such as an unwanted intrusion.

A recent article from the University at Buffalo's Rehabilitation Engineering Research Center on Aging (Mann et al., 1996) suggests that a significant proportion, about 10 percent, of frail elders have problems with the use of the phone they own. The types of problems they are having most typically relate directly to their impairments.

Reprinted with permission from *Generations*, Fall 1997 v21 n3 p28(2). © 1997 American Society on Aging.

People with vision impairment have difficulty reading the numbers and letters on the phone. Those who have difficulty ambulating and getting up or down from a seated position often have difficulty getting up to answer the phone before the calling party hangs up. People with fine motor impairment from conditions like arthritis have difficulty with small buttons, rotary dials, and holding the receiver. People with hearing impairment may have difficulty hearing the phone ring or hearing the person at the other end of the line. People with cognitive impairment may have difficulty remembering important numbers. For each of these impairments, and related problems, there are potential interventions, many of which rely on products readily available.

Features To Address Impairments

A recently published book, *Communications Technologies for the Elderly* (Lubinski and Higginbotham, 1997) describes a number of telephone features to address specific impairments faced by older people.

Many of these features are commonly found in any home—an answering machine, for example, to help a person with mobility problems who has trouble getting to the phone. Other solutions are not so common, but can be obtained. Examples are a voice-activated phone with a speaker feature that can be answered from across the room, or a cordless phone.

Vision impairment in the elderly can of course be addressed with the usual large numbers, letters, symbols, and buttons with good color contrast between the background and the symbols. More high-tech solutions include cordless phones with pager buttons on base units that make it easy to find the headset and also devices that can be added to a home phone so that it "speaks" the number dialed, making it possible for the user to detect mistakes made while dialing.

People with hand impairment can use phones with voice activation. People with hearing impairment have available many features including add-on devices that provide amplification for the receiver, available in portable models for travel and when amplification is required on several phones, and telecommunication devices for the deaf that include a keypad for typing out messages and a display for reading messages from the person on the other end of the line. Phone features to address memory impairment include picture telephones that display a picture of the person or place to be called (for example, the fire department) next to the memory button.

Personal Emergency Response Systems

Personal emergency response systems (PERS) (also referred to as medical emergency response systems) use telephone lines to signal for help in an emergency situation. They can be purchased, leased, or rented. The PERS user carries or wears a device with a radio transmitter and a button that activates a communicator connected to the person's home phone system. The device can be worn as a pendant, on a wrist band, or on a belt or can be carried in a pocket. The emergency signal goes out to a twenty-four-hour monitoring center, which sends appropriate help: ambulance or police, or relative or neighbor. With most systems, even if the line is in use or the phone is off the hook when the device is activated, the PERS will "seize the line" and send out the signal. Some systems include a speaker phone so that the person monitoring the system can speak with the user and determine the type of emergency and the most appropriate response. Other systems include a smoke alarm feature so that fire departments can be quickly alerted in the event of a fire.

Personal emergency response systems typically provide a feeling of security for both the user and family caregivers and friends. However, not all people who might benefit from a PERS have one, for both economic and psychosocial reasons. Cost is sometimes cited as a factor, although in states with waiver programs, Medicaid now covers the cost for many eligible people. Some people feel they do not need the system, denying the impact of the impairments they face. Care providers must be sensitive to the sense of imposition, invasion of privacy, or stigma that a PERS can raise in some people. While the benefits of a PERS are obvious, the negative feelings that might be associated with use of such a device must be recognized and addressed, with both the potential user and significant family members.

Many companies offer the equipment and services for a PERS, and prices vary significantly. (See AARP's 1992 evaluation of personal emergency response systems.) Factors to consider are the following:

- Who will monitor the calls—a healthcare organization, certified professionals?
- Will the monitor stay on the line until help arrives?
- Will the company test the system with the user, before it is fully released to the user?
- Is the user able to change the batteries?
- Are the batteries long-lasting?

- Is the user alerted when the batteries become low?

- Is the button easy for the user to operate, and is the transmitting device waterproof, lightweight, and truly portable?

- Has the company offering the service established a successful record of consumer satisfaction?

- Will the company quote prices over the phone, or will it only give prices in a home visit (during which time high-pressure sales tactics might more easily be employed)?

The personal emergency response system is an example of ways in which older people are successfully using existing telecommunications technology to circumvent functional limitations.

References

American Association of Retired Persons. 1992. Product Report: PERS. Long Beach, Calif.

Lubinski, R., and Higginbotham, D. J. 1997. *Communication Technologies for the Elderly: Vision, Hearing and Speech* San Diego, Calif.: Singular Publishing Group.

Mann, W., et al. 1996. "The Use of Phones by Elders with Disabilities: Problems, Interventions, Costs." *Assistive Technology* 8(1): 23-33.

— by William C. Mann, OTR, Ph.D.

William C. Mann, OTR, PH.D. is professor and director, Rehabilitation Engineering Research Center on Aging, University at Buffalo, New York.

Part Six

Preparing for Final Decisions

Chapter 41

Home Health Care

What Is Home Health Care?

Home health care is skilled care provided in your home when you are confined there due to illness or injury. This care is ordered and supervised by your doctor. A plan of care is developed by you, your doctor, and the home care staff. The plan gives everyone involved in your care direction as to your rehabilitation. Any changes must be approved by your doctor.

What Services Are Offered in the Home?

Home health care agencies provide the services of skilled professionals, such as nurses, medical social workers, and therapists (physical, occupational, speech, and respiratory). They also provide home health aides for personal care.

Nurses do assessments of your condition; dressing changes and other treatments, including intravenous therapy; family counseling; and health care teaching, such as how to handle equipment and give shots. They also supervise the aides.

Therapists work with you to improve your strength and ability to do everyday tasks, such as bathing and dressing. Therapists also look at your home to suggest easier ways to do things and recommend assistive devices that may be helpful.

Reprinted with permission. *Senior Health Advisor* © 1998 Clinical Reference Systems, Ltd.

Aides help you with personal care and do light housekeeping.

Some home care agencies provide other services. They may rent durable medical equipment such as wheelchairs, walkers, portable commodes, and oxygen. Some agencies have private-pay divisions for services not covered by insurance. Through them nurses, aides, or homemakers (workers who do light housekeeping and some personal care) can be hired by the hour or day.

How Do I Choose a Home Care Agency?

Hospital-sponsored home health care agencies are accredited by the Joint Commission for the Accreditation of Health Care Organizations, if the sponsoring hospital is accredited. Independent home health care agencies can choose to be accredited. All Medicare-certified agencies are reviewed by the state health department each year. They must meet federal and state guidelines. As a beginning benchmark, choose an agency that is accredited or Medicare-certified.

Choose an agency that can provide all the services you need or works closely with other providers. Interview the primary nurse that will be involved in your care. Since the staff of the agency comes into your home, there must be a good fit between you and the staff.

You have the right to choose which home health care agency you want to provide your care. There may be many agencies in your town. A hospital or doctor can not dictate which agency you choose.

Does Insurance Pay for Home Care?

Many health care plans cover home health services. Each plan is different, so check with your plan representative. Insurance does not cover nurses, aides, or therapists whose services are not medically needed. Insurance does not cover those services when they are needed for custodial care.

Medicare pays for home health care when these four conditions are met:

- You require intermittent (not 24-hour) skilled nursing care, physical therapy, or speech therapy.
- You are confined to your home.
- Your doctor determines that you need home health care and sets up a plan for you to receive care at home.
- The home care agency you are using participates in Medicare.

A prior stay in the hospital is not required to receive home care benefits under Medicare. There is no deductible for home care services.

Medicare Part A (or Part B if you do not have Part A) pays for covered services for as long as they are medically necessary and reasonable. Medicare pays for the services of skilled nurses, home health aides, medical social workers, and therapists (physical, occupational, speech, and respiratory). These services cannot be provided full time. The home health care benefit also covers the full cost of some medical supplies and 80% of the approved amount for durable medical equipment such as wheelchairs, walkers, hospital beds, and oxygen supplies.

For further information on the home health care agencies in your community, contact your hospital discharge planner or social worker or see the Yellow Pages under nursing.

The information on Medicare coverage of home health care was taken from *Your Medicare Handbook* (publication #HCFA- 10050). To order a free copy, write:

- U.S. Department of Health and Human Services Health Care Financing Administration 7500 Security Boulevard Baltimore, Maryland 21244-1850

— by Carolyn Norrgard, RN-C, BA, MEd.
and Carol Matheis-Kraft, Ph.D., RN-C, NHA

Chapter 42

Housing Highlights: Assisted Living

What Are Assisted Living Residences?

Assisted living residences are:

1. Housing environments which provide individualized health and personal care assistance in a home-like setting. The level of care available is between that provided in congregate housing (housing with meal service) and a skilled nursing facility. In these settings:

   - residents are semi-independent physically or mentally, or frail persons who need frequent assistance;

   - services offered include, personal care assistance, health care monitoring, limited health care services and/or the dispensing of medications;

   - state licensing and regulation by state social welfare agencies is required.

2. Important because they promote independence by meeting residents' supportive needs while preventing inappropriate institutionalization.

Excerpted from *Housing Highlights: Assisted Living,* National Resource and Policy Center on Housing and Long Term Care, USC, Andrus Gerontology Center, Los Angeles, CA 90089-0191.

3. Known by various other names. The most common are: personal care homes, sheltered housing, residential care, homes for adults, managed care, catered living, board and care, and domiciliary care.

Who Resides in Assisted Living Residences?

Assisted living housing is often deemed necessary when you have difficulty performing daily tasks and have no one to help you. Some indicators are:

- needing help preparing meals, bathing, dressing, toileting, or taking medication—needing assistance with housekeeping chores or laundry
- requiring some health care assistance or monitoring
- needing transportation to doctors, shopping, and personal business
- feeling frequently confused or experiencing memory problems

How to Begin

Use this check list to evaluate characteristics you should look for in an assisted living residence:

- Does the residence have a home-like atmosphere?
- Does the residence appear small in size and not feel overwhelming?
- Does the residence offer personalized health care services?
- Does the staff encourage performing tasks yourself with assistance?
- Do units have a full bathroom and kitchenette?
- Is there an emergency call system?
- Are friends and family close enough to visit and are they encouraged to do so?
- What kind of health and personal care support is available?

The Cost and Financial Assistance

Currently most assisted living facilities are privately operated. This means that the costs of care are not usually covered by publicly financed programs. The average fee, which includes meals and personal care assistance, ranges from $1,200 to $2,000 a month. Costs are often keyed to your level of impairment and service need.

In some states, rent or service subsidies are available. However, the typical reimbursement rate provided by Supplemental Security Income (SSI) is often too low to assist those with higher levels of impairment and service needs. Your local social security office and Medicaid Office can determine this.

Where to Get Help

There are several ways to locate an assisted living facility in your area. Contact these organizations to find out if there are facilities in your area:

Eldercare Locator Service
Directs you to the nearest agency on aging. No charge.
(800) 677-1116

Assisted Living Facilities Association of America
9401 Lee Highway, Suite 402
Fairfax, Virginia 22031
(703) 691-8100

An Eye to the Future:

Four factors are affecting the emergence of assisted living as an important long term care alternative for the mentally and physically frail:

1. major increases in long term care costs projected into the next century are staggering;

2. demographically, the number of people over the age of 85 is expected to double in the next 20 years, followed by a doubling again in the next thirty years;

3. most older people are seeking more appealing alternatives to live out the last years of their life; and

4. government agencies are recognizing these trends and are likely to introduce entitlement programs that allow older people to choose an assisted living setting instead of a nursing home.

Chapter 43

Assisted Living Consumer Checklist

The following is a consumer checklist of important services, amenities and accommodations in Assisted Living communities. We recommend making several visits, at various times, to each residence you are considering. As you compare Assisted Living residences, we hope this checklist will assure you that the residence you choose will be one of the highest quality and meets your needs.

Consider the following as you assess an Assisted Living residence:

Atmosphere

- As you arrive at the residence, do you like its location and outward appearance?

- As you enter the lobby and tour the residence, is the decor attractive and homelike?

- Did you receive a warm greeting from staff welcoming you to the residence?

- Does the administrator/staff call residents by name and interact warmly with them as you tour the residence?

- Do residents socialize with each other and appear happy and comfortable?

- Are you able to talk with residents about how they like the residence and staff?

- Do the residents seem to be appropriate housemates for you or your loved one?

- Are staff appropriately dressed, personable and outgoing?

- Do the staff members treat each other in a professional manner?

- Are the staff members that you pass during your tour friendly to you?

- Are visits with the resident welcome at any time?

Physical Features

- Is the community well-designed for resident's needs?

- Is the floor plan easy to follow?

- Are doorways, hallways and rooms accommodating to wheelchairs and walkers?

- Are elevators available for those unable to use stairways?

- Are hand rails available to aid in walking?

- Are cupboards and shelves easy to reach?

- Are floors of a non-skid material and carpets firm to ease walking?

- Does the residence have good natural and artificial lighting?

- Is the residence clean, free of odors and appropriately heated/cooled?

- Does the residence meet local and/or state licensing requirements?

Needs Assessments, Contracts, Costs & Finances

- Is there a written plan for the care of each resident?

- Does the residence have a process for assessing a potential resident's need for services and are those needs addressed periodically?

- Does this process include the resident, their family and facility staff along with the potential resident's physician?

- When may a contract be terminated and what are refund policies?

- Are there any government, private or corporate programs available to help cover the cost of services to the resident?

- Is a contractual agreement available to include accommodations, personal care, health care and supportive services?

- Are additional services available if the resident's needs change?

- Is there a procedure to pay for additional services like nursing care when the services are needed on a temporary basis?

- Are there different costs for various levels or categories of services?

- Do billing, payment and credit policies seem fair and reasonable?

- May a resident handle their own finances with staff assistance if able or should a family member or outside party be designated to do so?

- Are residents required to purchase renters' insurance for personal property in their units?

- Is staff available to meet scheduled and unscheduled needs?

Medication & Health Care

- Does the residence have specific policies regarding storage of medication, assistance with medications, training and supervision of staff and record keeping?

- Is self-administration of medication allowed?

- Is there a staff person to coordinate home care visits from a nurse, physical therapist, occupational therapist, etc. if needed?

- Are staff available to assist residents who experience memory, orientation, or judgment losses?

- Does a physician or nurse visit the resident regularly to provide medical checkups?

- Does the residence have a clearly stated procedure for responding to a resident's medical emergency?

Services

- Can the residence provide a list of services available?

- Is staff available to provide 24-hour assistance with activities of daily living (ADLs) if needed? ADLs include: Dressing; Eating; Mobility; Hygiene and grooming; Bathing, toileting and incontinence; Using the telephone; Shopping; and Laundry.

- Does the residence provide housekeeping services in residents' units?

- Does the residence provide transportation to doctors' offices, the hairdresser, shopping and other activities desired by residents?

- Can residents arrange for transportation on fairly short notice?

- Are pharmacy, barber/beautician and/or physical therapy services offered on-site?

Individual Unit Features

- Do dining room menus vary from day to day and meal to meal?

- Are different sized and types of units available?

- Are units for single and double occupancy available?

- Do residents have their own lockable doors?

- Is a 24-hour emergency response system accessible from the unit?

- Are bathrooms private with handicapped accommodations to accommodate wheelchairs and walkers?

- Are residents able to bring their own furnishings for their unit and what may they bring?

- Do all units have a telephone and cable TV and how is billing handled?

- Is a kitchen area/unit provided with a refrigerator, sink and cooking element?

- May residents keep food in their units?

- May residents smoke in their units? In public spaces?

Social & Recreational Activities

- Is there evidence of an organized activities program, such as a posted daily schedule, events in progress, reading materials, visitors, etc.?

- Do residents participate in activities outside of the residence in the neighboring community?

- Do volunteers, including family members, come into the residence to help with or conduct programs?

- Does the residence create a sense of community by requiring residents to participate in certain activities or perform simple chores for the group as a whole?

- Are residents' pets allowed in the residence? Who is responsible for their care?

- Does the residence have its own pets?

Food Service

- Does the residence provide three nutritionally balanced meals a day, seven days a week?

- Are snacks available?

- May a resident request special foods?

- Are common dining areas available?

- May residents eat meals in their units?

- May meals be provided at a time a resident would like or are there set times for meals?

ALFA's Philosophy of Assisted Living Care

In addition to this checklist, we encourage you to look for a general philosophy of care based on 10 principles—principles that make Assisted Living residents the top priority.

1. Offering cost effective quality care personalized for the individual's needs

2. Fostering independence for each resident

3. Treating each resident with dignity and respect

4. Promoting the individuality of each resident

5. Allowing each resident choice of care and lifestyle

6. Protecting each resident's right to privacy

7. Nurturing the spirit of each resident

8. Involving family and friends in care planning and implementation

9. Providing a safe, residential environment

10. Making the Assisted Living residence a valuable community asset

Chapter 44

Finding a Nursing Home

Introduction

Selecting a nursing home is one of the most important and difficult decisions that you may be asked to make. Though it may be difficult to admit, you may spend several years in a nursing home. So it is important that you make the best decision possible, and base your decision on the most complete and timely information available.

The Health Care Financing Administration (HCFA) wants you to make a good choice when choosing a nursing home. This chapter is designed to help you choose a nursing home. It provides you with a step-by-step process that will assist you. It also provides you with some key resources that will help you conduct a wise search for the nursing home or long-term care facility that best fits your needs.

Step 1: Building a Network

Before you begin searching for a nursing home, it is a good idea to put together a network of people who can help you make the right choice. This team should include the family and friends who are important to you. It should also include the doctors and health professionals who understand your needs. Clergy and social workers may also be valuable network members.

U.S. Department of Health and Human Services, Health Care Financing Administration—Medicare and Medicaid, December 1996.

Consult with your network. Family and friends may be willing to share responsibilities and should be treated as partners. Remember that two heads are better than one, and many heads are better than two.

If you are helping to select a nursing home for a relative, make every effort to involve your relative in the selection process. If your relative is mentally alert, it is essential that his or her wishes be respected. People who are involved in the selection process are better prepared when the time comes to move into a nursing home.

Finding a nursing home that provides the right services for you in a pleasant, comfortable environment atmosphere often requires research. Ideally, you will have ample time to plan ahead, examine several nursing homes, and make the appropriate financial plans. By planning ahead, you will have more control over the selection process, more time to gather good information, and more time to make certain that everyone in your network is comfortable with the ultimate choice. Planning ahead is the best way to ease the stress that accompanies choosing a nursing home, and helps assure that you will make a good choice.

Unfortunately, a great many people must select a nursing home with little notice—frequently during a family crisis or right after a serious illness or operation. If you are in this situation, this chapter should still be helpful. Though you may not be able to follow all of the steps in the upcoming pages, by reading this chapter you will gain valuable information about nursing homes, learn about the people who might be able to help you, and pick up some tips about what to look for in a nursing home.

Step 2: Long-Term Care Options

Until recently, few alternatives to nursing homes existed for people who could no longer take care of themselves. Even today, some people are placed in nursing homes simply because neither they nor their family know about the alternatives to nursing homes. Today, people who cannot live completely independently may choose from a variety of living arrangements that offer different levels of care. For many, these alternatives are preferable to nursing homes.

Home and Community Care. Most people want to remain at home as long as possible. A person who is ill or disabled and needs help may be able to get a variety of home services that might make moving into a nursing home unnecessary. Home services include meals

404

on wheels programs, friendly visiting and shopper services, and adult day care. In addition, there are a variety of programs that help care for people in their homes. Some nursing homes offer respite care— when they admit a person for a short period of time to give the home caregivers a break. Depending on the case, Medicare, private insurance, and Medicaid may pay some home care costs.

Subsidized Senior Housing. There are Federal and State programs that subsidize housing for older people with low to moderate incomes. A number of these facilities offer assistance to residents who need help with certain tasks, such as shopping and laundry, but residents generally live independently in an apartment within the senior housing complex. In this way, subsidized senior housing serves as a lower cost alternative to assisted living—though assisted living communities are frequently newer and more luxurious.

Assisted Living (Non-Medical Senior Housing). Some people need help with only a small number of tasks, such as cooking and laundry. Some may only need to be reminded to take their medications. For those people who need only a small amount of help, assisted living facilities may be worth considering. Assisted living is a general term for living arrangements in which some services are available to residents (meals, laundry, medication reminders), but residents still live independently within the assisted living complex. In most cases, assisted living residents pay a regular monthly rent, and then pay additional fees for the services that they require.

Board and Care Homes. These are group living arrangements (sometimes called group or domiciliary homes) that are designed to meet the needs of people who cannot live independently, but do not require nursing home services. These homes offer a wider range of services than independent living options. Most provide help with some of the activities of daily living, including eating, walking, bathing, and toileting. In some cases, private long-term care insurance and medical assistance programs will help pay for this type of living.

Continuing Care Retirement Communities (CCRCs). CCRCs are housing communities that provide different levels of care based on the needs of their residents—from independent living apartments to skilled nursing in an affiliated nursing home. Residents move from one setting to another based on their needs, but continue to remain a part of their CCRC's community. Many CCRCs require a large payment

405

prior to admission, then charge monthly fees above that. For this reason, many CCRCs are too expensive for older people with modest incomes.

Nursing Homes. A nursing home is a residence that provides room, meals, recreational activities, help with daily living, and protective supervision to residents. Generally, nursing home residents have physical or mental impairments which keep them from living independently. Nursing homes are certified to provide different levels of care, from custodial to skilled nursing (services that can only be administered by a trained professional).

Before deciding which care setting is most appropriate for you or your relative, talk to your doctor or a social worker and get a realistic assessment of care needs. If you are considering home care, be sure you understand all the work that comes with caring for a chronically ill person. If you are considering independent living, consider the risks associated with an unsupervised environment.

Be sure to discuss long-term care options with family members who will be the main home care givers and/or visitors to your new home. Consider how you will pay for your own long-term care.

Remember that caring for someone who is very sick requires a lot of work. Nursing homes are designed to meet the needs of the acutely or chronically ill. The options discussed above may work for people who require less than skilled care, or who require skilled care for only brief periods of time, but many people with long-term skilled care needs require a level and amount of care that cannot be easily handled outside of a nursing home.

Step 3: Gathering Information

Once you have decided that a nursing home is the right choice for you, it is time to gather information about the nursing homes in your area. A good first step in this process is finding out exactly how many nursing homes there are in your area (because nursing homes are frequently located in out of the way areas, there might be more than you think).

There are a number of ways that you can learn about the nursing homes in your area. The easiest ways to find out about local nursing homes begin with the phone book. Your yellow pages list many of the nursing homes in your area. In addition, your local Office on Aging (in the Blue Pages of your Phone Book) should have a listing of nursing homes in your area and will be able to refer you to your local Long-Term Care Ombudsman.

You can get information on the nursing homes in your area from a variety of sources. Word of mouth can be a good source of information. Ask your friends and neighbors if they know people who have stayed in local nursing homes. Learn all you can from these different sources.

Some Facts About Nursing Homes

On any given day, nursing homes are caring for about one in twenty Americans over the age of 65. Almost half of all Americans turning 65 this year will be admitted into a nursing home at least once. One fifth of those people admitted into nursing homes stay at least one year—one tenth stay three years or more.

The Long-Term Care Ombudsman

One of the best sources of information is your local long-term care ombudsman. Nationwide, there are more than 500 local ombudsman programs. Ombudsman visit nursing homes on a regular basis—their job is to investigate complaints, advocate for residents, and mediate disputes. Ombudsman often have very good knowledge about the quality of life and care inside each nursing home in their area.

Ombudsman are not allowed to recommend one nursing home over another. But when asked about specific nursing homes they can provide information on these important subjects:

- the results of the latest survey,
- the number of outstanding complaints,
- the number and nature of complaints lodged in the last year,
- the results and conclusions of recent complaint investigations.

In addition, the ombudsman may provide general advice on what to look for when visiting the various area nursing homes. The phone number of your State Long-Term Care Ombudsman is provided under the "Phone Lists" section.

Other Community Resources

In addition to the Long-Term Care Ombudsman, there are many other resources that you should consult before selecting a nursing home. Some other people who might be helpful are:

- hospital discharge planners or social workers,
- physicians who serve the elderly,
- clergy and religious organizations,
- volunteer groups that work with the elderly and chronically ill,
- nursing home professional associations.

By using these resources, you will tap into a community of people who understand nursing homes and have a good deal of knowledge about the homes in your area. You should now be able to make a list of the homes in your area which have good reputations.

Other Information You Will Need

There are also some types of basic information that should help you narrow your list of nursing homes. Consider some of these factors—a quick phone call to the nursing home should answer these concerns:

1. Religious and Cultural Preferences: If you have religious or cultural preferences, contact the nursing homes on your list and see if they offer the type of environment which you would prefer.

2. Medicare and Medicaid Participation: If you will be using Medicare or Medicaid, make certain that the nursing homes on your list accept Medicare or Medicaid payment. Often, only a portion of the home is certified for Medicare or Medicaid, so make sure that the home has Medicare or Medicaid "beds" available.

3. HMO Contracts: If you belong to a managed care plan that contracts with a particular nursing home or homes in your area, make sure the homes you are considering have contracts with your HMO.

4. Availability: Make certain that the nursing homes on your list will have space available at the time you might need to be admitted.

5. Special Care Needs: If you require care for special medical conditions or dementia, make sure that the nursing homes on your list are capable of meeting these special circumstances.

6. Location: If you have a large number of nursing home choices, it is usually a good idea to consider nursing homes that your family and friends can visit easily. In most cases, it is a mistake

to select a nursing home that is difficult to visit on a regular basis. Frequent visits are the best way to make sure that you or your relative does well in the nursing home. Visitors are important advocates for chronically ill residents. Frequent visits often make the transition to the nursing home easier for new residents and their families.

You will now be able to figure out which homes in your area may or may not be worth visiting. You will also now be better informed when you begin visiting your area's nursing homes.

Paying for Nursing Home Care

Nursing home care is expensive (a skilled nursing home will cost about $200 a day in many parts of the country). For most people, finding ways to finance nursing home care is a major concern. there are several ways that nursing home care is financed:

Personal Resources. About half of all nursing home residents pay nursing home costs out of personal resources. When most people enter nursing homes, they usually pay out of their own savings. As personal resources are spent, many people who stay in nursing homes for long periods eventually become eligible for Medicaid.

Long-Term Care Insurance. Long-Term Care Insurance is private insurance designed to cover long-term care costs. Plans vary widely, and you would be wise to do some research before purchasing any long-term care policy. Generally, only relatively healthy people may purchase long-term care insurance. For further information on this type of insurance, contact the National Association of Insurance Commissioners and ask for their free booklet, *The Shopper's Guide to Long-Term Care Insurance.* Call (816) 374-7259 for your copy.

Medicaid. Medicaid is a State and Federal program that will pay most nursing home costs for people with limited income and assets. Eligibility varies by state, and you should check into your state's eligibility requirements before assuming that you are either eligible or ineligible. Medicaid will only pay for nursing home care provided in Medicaid-certified facilities.

Medicare. Under certain limited conditions, Medicare will pay some nursing home costs for Medicare beneficiaries who require skilled nursing or rehabilitation services. To be covered, you must (after a qualifying hospital stay) receive the services from a Medicare-certified skilled nursing home. HCFA's book, *Your Medicare Handbook*, discusses the conditions under which Medicare will help pay for nursing home costs in a Medicare-certified nursing home. To obtain a free copy of Your Medicare Handbook, call (800) 638-6833.

Medicare Supplemental Insurance. This is private insurance (often called Medigap) that pays Medicare's deductibles and co-insurances, and may cover services not covered by Medicare. Most Medigap plans will help pay for skilled nursing care, but only when that care is covered by Medicare.

In addition, some people have nursing home costs covered, or partially covered, by managed care plans or employer benefit packages.

If you have any questions about how you will pay for nursing home care, what coverage you may already have, or whether there are any government programs that will help with your expenses, there are people who can help. Your State's Insurance Counseling and Assistance (ICA) program has counselors ready to help you figure out how you can finance your long-term care.

Visiting Nursing Homes

The nursing home visit is probably the most important step in selecting the right nursing home. A visit provides you with an opportunity to talk to nursing home staff and, more importantly, with the people who live and receive care at the nursing home.

When you visit the nursing home, you will probably be given a formal tour. while this may be a very useful introduction to the home, it is important that you are not overly influenced by a guided tour. When the tour is over, return to some of the places where staff are caring for residents. Be ready to ask the staff members who are caring for residents questions about their jobs and how they feel about caring for people with so many different needs.

Near the beginning of your visit, spend some time examining the nursing home's most recent survey report. By law, this report must be posted in the nursing home in an area that is accessible to visitors and residents. Surveyors compile a survey report that lists areas in which the nursing home is cited for deficient practices. Keep these deficiencies in mind as you visit the nursing home, and see whether the home has corrected the deficient practices listed on the survey report.

Over the last decade, different laws and regulations have been enacted to raise the standards of nursing home care, particularly with respect to quality of life. The law now requires that residents receive the necessary care and services that will enable them to reach and maintain their highest practicable level of physical, mental and social well-being. In addition, civil rights law ensures equal access in all nursing homes regardless of race, color or national origin.

Ask residents questions about the nursing home. Learn what they like and what their complaints are. Ask visitors or volunteers similar questions.

What is a Survey?

All nursing homes that are certified to participate in the Medicare or Medicaid programs are visited by a team of trained State surveyors approximately once a year. These surveyors (like inspectors) examine the home over several days and inspect the performance of the nursing home in numerous areas—including quality of life and quality of care. At the conclusion of the survey, the team reports its findings. Nursing homes with deficiencies are subject to fines and other penalties if they are not corrected.

Quality of Life

When visiting nursing homes, pay special attention to quality of life issues. People who are admitted into nursing homes do not leave their personalities at the door. Nor do they lose their basic human needs for respect, encouragement, and friendliness. All individuals need to retain as much control over the events in their daily lives as possible.

Nursing home residents should have the freedom and privacy to attend their personal needs—from managing their own finances (if mentally able) to decorating their rooms with favorite items. They should also be able to participate in their care planning and retain the right to examine their medical records. Residents may only be restrained when medically necessary. Most importantly, staff must always respect the dignity of each individual resident.

To check to see if the nursing home respects the dignity of each individual, look into these questions:

- Are staff members courteous to residents and is the home's management responsive to concerns raised by residents?

411

- Does the nursing home provide a variety of activities and allow residents to choose the activities they want to attend?

- Does the nursing home provide menu choices or prepare special meals at the request of residents? (Sample the food if possible.)

- Are family members encouraged to visit, and are they allowed to visit in privacy when requested?

Quality of Care

Unless you have a medical or social work background, it might be difficult to assess how well the nursing home provides high quality health care to its residents. However, there are still a number of actions you can take to evaluate whether the home is providing high quality health care.

- Check the survey report and see if the home was cited for deficient practices in any quality of care areas.

- Ask about the home's staffing, and ask residents if the staff are available when needed. Make sure that you are comfortable with the number of residents assigned to each nurse and nurse aide. Be aware that there might be less staff at night or on the weekends.

- If you have any special care needs (e.g., dementia, ventilator dependency), it is generally a good idea to make sure that the home has experience in working with people who have had the same condition.

- Even if you have a trusted doctor, ask about the nursing home's physician and how often he or she visits the home. Since the home's doctor may be called in case of emergencies, you should be confident that the home's doctor can take care of resident needs.

By law, nursing homes must complete a comprehensive assessment for every new resident within two weeks of admission. The home also must complete a care plan that is designed to help each resident reach or maintain his or her highest level of well-being. Ask the home about its care planning process and make sure you agree with the home's philosophy. Remember that residents who have meaningful activities and are as independent as possible are generally better able to maintain their health.

Step 5: Follow-up Analysis

Now that you have narrowed your search down to a short list of nursing homes, it is time to re-visit some of the earlier steps. Contact the people in your network (from step 1) and make sure they are comfortable with your short list. See if they have any additional information to offer about the homes on your short list.

Follow-up Visits

You should visit the nursing homes on your short list at least one more time (or as many additional times as you think necessary). Make sure that you see the home at least once in the evening and/or on a weekend because staffing is frequently different at these times. Also, your follow-up visit should include attending a meeting of the nursing home's resident council and/or family council. These meetings will give you a unique look at the concerns of the residents and/or their families. If the nursing home does not have resident or family councils, that might tell you something about the philosophy of the home's management.

Follow-up visits should be conducted at different times of the day than your first visit. Be sure at least one of your visits was during the late morning or midday, so you can observe residents when they are out of bed, eating, and attending activities. continue to ask questions, and take special note of the differences between the nursing homes left on your short list.

After your follow-up visits, you should be able to narrow your short list down to a few nursing homes. At this point it still may be difficult to pick one. A final call to the ombudsman and the other people who provided you with information in the past might help. If you have any additional questions, do not hesitate to contact or visit the nursing home again.

You should now be ready to select the nursing home that is best able to meet your needs. The final decision may still be difficult, and it is possible that more than one nursing home will be a good choice for you. However, you should now have enough information to be confident that you are making the wisest possible choice.

Step 6: After Admission

Even if you made a well-reasoned choice and selected a nursing home only after following the steps discussed in this booklet, it is possible that you may not be entirely satisfied with your choice. New nursing home residents may go through a difficult adjustment period, even if the nursing home is doing all that it can.

Be aware that the law gives you and your relatives specific rights in the nursing home. You should be ready to hold the nursing home accountable if it is not honoring the rights of residents and family members. A summary of these rights is detailed below.

Resident Rights in a Nursing Home

Some people think that nursing home residents surrender the right to make medical decisions, manage funds, and control their activities when they enter a nursing home. This is not true. As a nursing home resident, you have the same rights as anyone else, and certain special protections under the law. The nursing home must post and provide new residents with a statement that details each resident's rights. New residents also have these specific rights.

Respect. You have the right to be treated with dignity and respect. You have the right to make your own schedule, bed-time, and select the activities you would like to attend (as long as it fits your plan of care.) A nursing home is prohibited from using physical and chemical restraints except when necessary to treat medical symptoms.

Services and Fees. The nursing home must inform you, in writing, about its services and fees before you enter the home. Most facilities charge a basic rate that covers room, meals, housekeeping, linen, general nursing care, recreation, and some personal care services. there may be extra charges for personal services, such as haircuts, flowers, and telephone.

Managing Money. You have the right to manage your own money or to designate someone you trust to do so. If you allow the nursing home to manage your personal funds, you must sign a written statement that authorizes the nursing home to manage your finances, and the nursing home must allow you access to your funds. Federal law requires that the home protect your funds from any loss by having a bond or similar arrangement.

Privacy, Property, and Living Arrangements. You have the right to privacy. In addition, you have the right to keep and use your personal property, as long as it does not interfere with the rights, health, or safety of others. Your mail can never be opened by the home unless you allow it. the nursing home must have a system in place to keep you safe from neglect and abuse, and to protect your property from theft. If you and your spouse live in the same home, you are entitled to share a room (if you both agree to do so).

Guardianship and Advanced Directives. As a nursing home resident, you are responsible for making your own decisions (unless you are mentally unable). If you wish, you may designate someone else to make health care decisions for you. You may also draw up advance directives. A Durable Power of Attorney will become your legal guardian if you ever become incapable of making your own decisions. You may also make your end of life wishes known in a living will. Depending upon your State's laws, you may need a lawyer to draw up a Durable Power of Attorney orders or a living will. Check with your local Office on Aging to find out if your state has any legal assistance services that help with preparing these documents. You will find the phone number for your local Office on Aging in the Blue Pages of your phone directory.

Visitors. You have the right to spend private time with the visitors of your choice at any reasonable hour. You have the right to make and receive telephone calls in privacy. The nursing home must permit your family to visit you at any time. Any person who provides you with health or legal services may see you at any reasonable times. Of course, you do not have to see anyone you do not wish to see.

Medical Care. You have the right to be informed about your medical condition, medications, and to participate in your plan of care. You have the right to refuse medications or treatments, and to see your own doctor.

Social Services. The nursing home must provide each resident with social services, including counseling, mediation of disputes with other residents, assistance in contacting legal and financial professionals, and discharge planning.

Moving Out. Living in a nursing home is voluntary. You are free to move to another place. However, nursing home admission policies usually require that you give proper notice that you are leaving. If you do not give proper notice, you may owe the nursing home money based on the home's proper notice rules. Residents whose nursing home services are covered by Medicare and Medicaid do not have to give the nursing home proper notice before moving out.

Discharge. The nursing home may not discharge or transfer you unless:

- it is necessary for the welfare, health, or safety of others,

- your health has declined to the point that the nursing home cannot meet your care needs,

- your health has improved to the extent that nursing home care is no longer necessary,

- the nursing home has not received payment for services delivered,

- the nursing home ceases operation.

If you have any concerns about the nursing home in which you live, call your local long-term care ombudsman or your State's survey agency.

Your Rights as a Relative

Relatives and friends have rights too. Family members and legal guardians have the right to privacy when visiting the nursing home (but only when requested by the resident.) They also have the right to meet with the families of other residents. If the nursing home has a family council, you have the right to join or address this group.

By law, nursing homes must develop a plan of care for every resident. Family members are allowed to assist in preparing the development of this care plan, with the resident's permission. In addition, relatives who have legal guardianship of nursing home residents have the right to examine all medical records concerning their loved one. If you are a resident's legal guardian, Federal law gives you the right to make important decisions on behalf of your relative.

It is important to remember that relatives play a major role in making sure that residents are receiving good care. You can make sure your loved one is receiving good care by visiting often, expressing your concerns whenever they arise, and being active in the nursing home's family council (or helping to start a family council if the nursing home does not have one.)

Remember that if your concerns are not being addressed by the nursing home or if you have a complaint, there are people who can help. Contact your state long-term care ombudsman or state survey agency.

Chapter 45

Hospice

The term hospice was used in medieval times to refer to a lodging for travelers where they could be refreshed and looked after on their journeys. Today hospice refers to a concept of compassionate care for people in the final phase of an incurable illness.

If you have a life expectancy of 6 months or less, hospice or home health care may be a better alternative for care than a hospital. Also, if your family or friends can no longer look after you at home, you might want to consider hospice. You would usually be referred to hospice by your primary physician. Referrals can also be made by family members, friends, clergy, or other health professionals.

Hospice seeks neither to hasten nor postpone death. The emphasis is on quality of life and dignity. Hospice recognizes not only your physical needs by controlling pain but also your social, emotional, and spiritual needs. Hospice hopes to prepare you for a peaceful death at home or in a homelike setting.

Treating the Whole Person

Hospice considers your entire family and you, not yourself alone, the unit of care. You and your family are directly involved in making decisions. Whenever possible, you would be encouraged to make decisions about your treatment, your relationships, personal business, and preferences about burial and memorial services. Grief counseling is provided for your family.

Reprinted with permission. *Senior Health Advisor* © 1997 Clinical Reference Systems, Ltd.

417

Providing a Team Approach

The team approach is essential to the hospice philosophy. Services are provided by an interdisciplinary team of trained professionals: physicians, nurses, clergy, social workers, therapists, aides, and volunteers. The team members address your medical, emotional, psychological, and spiritual needs.

Controlling Pain

Even in some of the most painful forms of cancer, 95% of the time you can be given pain-relieving drugs that allow you to feel almost no pain. Usually the dosage can be kept at a level that also allows you to remain alert. Hospice staff is trained in the best methods of pain control and symptom management to ensure that you are as comfortable as possible.

Types of Hospices

Hospice offers intermittent help and support 24 hours a day, 7 days a week. Most often care is offered at home. In some communities there are independent inpatient hospices with no ties to a medical institution. Some hospitals and nursing homes have wings designated for hospice care. If home and an inpatient facility are available, you may spend time in both places.

Cost of Hospice

Studies have shown hospice care often to be less expensive than conventional care during the last six months of life. Usually less high-cost technology is used, and family, friends, and volunteers may provide much of your daily care.

Hospice care is a covered benefit under most private insurance plans. In addition, hospice is a covered Medicare benefit. In some states it is a covered Medicaid benefit.

For More Information

For more information about hospice or to locate a hospice in your area, write or call:

- National Hospice Organization, Suite 901, 1901 North Moore Street, Arlington, Virginia 22209
- Hospice Helpline: 1-800-658-8898

Chapter 46

What You Should Know about Living Wills

It is not easy to think about a time when an elderly relative no longer will be with you. Certainly, death of a loved one is not something anyone likes to talk about. But sometimes these discussions are necessary so that your relatives can know that their wishes will be carried out, even after they no longer are able to speak for themselves.

These wishes may include decisions about specific types of medical care or life sustaining measures that they feel strongly about. In the event that an illness or accident leaves them unable to make decisions about their care, you, your family members and your doctor all may be required to make decisions about their care. A living will is a document that allows people to make these choices before the need arises.

Living wills can relieve others of the legal and emotional burden of making decisions for someone who can't. Signing a living will can help put older people's minds at ease. Knowing that their wishes will be carried out even if they are unable to express them is likely to be a great comfort to them.

You should know that some doctors consider it unethical not to use life prolonging measures. Be sure to discuss the living will with your relative's physician, as well as other involved family members. It also might be helpful to include your lawyer, or to have a clergy member present.

Reprinted with permission from *The Brown University Long-Term Care Quality Letter*, March 13, 1995 v7 n5 p1S(2). © 1995 Manisses Communications Group Inc.

Your relative also can appoint a health care proxy. If he or she decides to do this, it's a good idea to have the document notarized. Some states require notarization for all living wills. Find out your state's mandates on this.

Once the living will has been written, distribute copies to family members, close friends, clergy, or anyone who may be called upon to make decisions if your relative is unable. Ask the doctor to keep a copy in your relative's medical file.

If your relative is considering drawing up a living will, here are some other things that everyone involved should know:

* In the event of a terminal illness or disease, refusing life support measures is not considered suicide.

* Your relative should redate and initial the living will periodically to ensure that his/her wishes have not changed.

* If your relative decides to revoke a living will be or she can sign a witnessed and notarized statement to that effect. Or, simply destroy all copies of the original document.

—by Dallas M. High, Ph.D.

Elderly People Do Not Take Advantage of Living Wills

Elderly people tend not to make use of advance directives—more commonly known as living wills—even after they have been educated about them, according to an article published in the *Journal of Aging and Health*.

"Overall, the study suggests that elderly people are putting off completing living wills to another time or deferring to others when care decisions must be made for them. Also, a very large segment of the elderly population is refusing to become involved in living will discussions at all," says the author, Dallas M. High, Ph.D. The reason, Dr. High suggests, is that the elderly "are confident that they can rely on others." Simply put, they see living wills as unnecessary.

Dr. High suggests that the government should establish a hierarchy of family member health care surrogates that would step in automatically if an elderly person were unable to make a medical decision for him/herself. Then, living wills would be needed only by "those who do not wish for family members to act as surrogates for health care decisions or wish to express treatment preferences and refusals."

If your relative has not considered drawing up a living will or designating a health care proxy, bring up the topic with him or It is important to inform elders of their options, and encourage them to make choices for the future.

For more information about living wills and current legislation in your state, contact an attorney. For copies of a model will, write to Choice in Dying, 250 W. 57th Street, Room 831, New York, NY 10107 or call (212) 366-5540.

Chapter 47

Dying Well: The Unspoken Dimension of Aging Well

"I have observed, as a matter of fact, that it is only people who exceed the age of ninety who attain euthanasia — who die, that is to say, of no disease, apoplexy or convulsion, and pass away without agony of any sort; nay, who sometimes even show no pallor, but expire generally in a sitting attitude, and often after a meal — or, I may say, simply cease to live rather than die. To come to one's end before the age of ninety, means to die of disease, in other words, prematurely."
—Zygmunt Bauman (1992, p. 19, n 6)

Although death is the defining event of old age, there is a curious silence in gerontological circles about death's bearing on the aging experience. Even such pro-aged groups as the American Gerontology Society and the American Association of Retired Persons (AARP) rarely acknowledge the connection. The magazine of the AARP, *Modern Maturity*, for instance, does not allow even the advertising of wheelchairs or any product portraying old age unhealthily, let alone discussion of coping with fatal illnesses. This void exists in professional circles as well. One analysis of more than 2,600 articles published in the *Gerontologist* and the *Journal of Gerontology* found that less than 2% dealt with any aspect of death (Kearl, 1989, p. 125). An analogous content analysis of articles in the *British Ageing and Society* between 1981 and 1991 found less than 4% (Walter, 1993).

Excerpted and reprinted with permission from *American Behavioral Scientist*, Jan 1996 v39 n3 p336(25), © 1996 Sage Publications Inc.

Nevertheless, over the past 3 decades, as the parameters of "successful" aging were being developed, there were concurrent changes in the highly publicized images of death. No longer were the depictions solely about those dying prematurely because of war, disease, poverty, or some natural calamity. Rather, increasing were the images of those desiring death or of those seeking to end the unwanted existences of loved ones, raising basic questions and moral dilemmas about the nature of good death:

- Considerable publicity was given to Betty Rollin's controversial *Last Wish* (1985), wherein described was how she and her husband assisted her terminally ill mother to commit suicide.(1)

- In 1988, New York's highest court ruled that an elderly woman, the victim of a series of debilitating strokes, must be kept alive through artificial feeding even though her daughters insist that she would prefer to die.

- During the 1980s, stories of suicide pacts between older spouses proliferated in the mass media.(2)

- Also increasing were stories of the ethical dilemmas posed by those existing in irreversible vegetative states, such as the 1991 case of 87-year-old Helga Wanglie. Mrs. Wanglie's life had been artificially maintained at the Hennepin Company Medical Center in Minneapolis. She was unaware and unresponsive to her surroundings. After 8 months, the hospital went to court seeking permission to turn off her life support system over the objections of her religious family, who claimed that she would prefer this existence to death.

- The euthanasia/physician-assisted suicide referendums of the Pacific coast states during the 1990s, culminating in Oregon voters passing Ballot Measure 16 ("Shall law allow terminally ill adult Oregon patients voluntary informed choice to obtain physician's subscription for drugs to end life?") in 1994.

- Derek Humphry's how-to suicide manual, *Final Exit: The Practicalities of Self-Deliverance* and *Assisted Suicide for the Dying*, became a New York Times' best seller in 1991.(3)

- The lives ended by the suicide machines of a retired Michigan pathologist, whose business card reads "Jack Kevorkian, M.D. Bioethics and Obituary. Special Death Counseling."

- And, most recently, the 1994 deaths of Jacqueline Kennedy Onassis and Richard Nixon, both of whom rejected medical treatment that could have prolonged their lives.

Such images say a lot about a culture. Indeed, indexes of death rates have become international political "box scores," with such measures as standardized rates of infant mortality, suicide, homicide, lethal diseases, and accidental deaths (in addition to these rates broken down by social class, race, ethnicity, religion, and sex), along with numbers of executions and life expectancies, used as measures of cultural and social development (Kearl, 1989, 1995). This revelatory power of death occurs on a personal level as well, crystallizing the central beliefs, values, and troths of both the dying and the survivors-to-be (Becker, 1973; see Rosenblatt, Greenberg, Solomon, Pyszczynski, & Lyon, 1989 for experimental demonstration). In its revelations of core outlooks, however, death can also highlight fundamental cultural contradictions. Why are we witnessing the emergence of the right-to-die and death-with-dignity movements at a time when social resources are being heavily invested in modern science's battle against death? Why the huge expenditures for extending the lives of the dying when one in five of the young go to bed hungry?

At issue here is the extent to which the absence of connections drawn between the quality of old age and death derives from the framing of the aging experience. Whose perspective is to be taken: society's? physicians'? gerontologists'? that of healthy and productive older persons? Indeed, old age is the phase of the life cycle when individualism triumphs and when there is the greatest heterogeneity among similarly aged persons. It is for these reasons that the present chapter is predicated on the person-centered standards of aging well, which sensitize us to individuals' positive responses to the various challenges (physiological, psychological, social, and cultural) posed by advanced age. And, although there is a general avoidance of discussions involving growing old and dying in our ageist and death-denying culture, it may well be the case that aging well is conditioned by individuals' perceived abilities to die well.

Aging and Dying in America

The essence of old age in America cannot be decontextualized and reduced to sheer biological terms. Its meaning is shaped by the meanings of the other life stages, which, in turn, are determined at the sociocultural order. As Simone de Beauvoir (1972) observed:

It is the meaning that men attribute to their life, it is their entire system of values that define the meaning and value of old age. The reverse applies: by the way in which a society behaves toward its old people it uncovers the naked, and often carefully hidden, truth about its real principles and aims. (p. 87)

As the notion of "childhood" evolved with industrialization, so "old age" is currently evolving with postindustrialization. And as the traditional nonperson status of children owed in large part to their high rates of mortality (as remains the case in the underdeveloped nations of the world, where the vast proportion of deaths occur in this age group (see Aries, 1962), so now the status of older persons is determined by death's general confinement to their stage of the life cycle—a point to which we will return—and by the new meanings of death.

Over the course of the twentieth century throughout much of the West, as death was increasingly hidden from everyday life (Feifel, 1959, p. xii), it was replacing sex as a core cultural taboo (Gorer, 1965). Death was transformed from being something natural and respected into something unnatural and shameful. Instead of signifying a culminating goal of life, death in American society has come to mean but an unwanted interruption of existence.

In the United States, this taboo status of death derives in part from the cultural happiness ethic. To spare the dying person's feelings, those close to him often conceal his condition in a game of information control (Glaser & Strauss, 1965).(4) The patient, on the other hand, is responsible for the management of his stigma of terminal illness, playing the game that others' efforts to ease matters are seen as effective and appreciated (Goffman, 1963). These interpersonal dynamics were to be culturally amplified: Death became denied in order to dampen "the disturbance and the overly strong and unbearable emotion caused by the ugliness of dying and by the very presence of death in the midst of a happy life" (Aries, 1974, p. 87). Such masquerades and information games have frequently diminished the ability of dying persons to control their own deaths. As illustrated by the reluctance of families and physicians to employ the most powerful painkillers for the terminally ill (often out of fears of narcotic addiction), the standards for dying well are increasingly those of survivors and paid attendants, not the dying individual.

The taboo also derives from the individualism and absence of shared fundamental values in postmodern materialistic cultures. The extreme materialism of the United States—so succinctly captured in the bumper-sticker maxim "He who dies with the most toys wins"—fails to provide the spiritual succor of earlier times for personal extinction. Similar is the case of extreme individualism, as Roy Baumeister (1991) observed:

This "value gap" . . . is the single biggest problem for the modern Western individual in making life meaningful. A major part of the modern response to this value gap is to elevate selfhood and the cultivation of identity into basic, compelling values. But if we rely on the quest for identity and self-knowledge to give life meaning, we make ourselves vulnerable to death in an almost unprecedented way. The self comes to an end in death, and it ceases to give value. Thus, death takes away not only our life but also what gave it value. In contrast, our ancestors typically drew comfort from values that would outlive them. (p. 6)

Finally, also contributing to death's tabooed status was a fundamental cultural contradiction in the social identities of those who die: As individualism (and its related narcissism) increased, the social significance of the self was diminishing—particularly in old age. As recently as the early twentieth century, throughout much of the Western world, a single individual's death could still profoundly affect the life of a community (Aries, 1981, p. 559). However, there were to occur changes to both selves and societies that were to thoroughly dampen death's disruptive potential. Instead of being a unique, inner-directed self that others recognized as a biographical accomplishment, the new self increasingly is viewed to be but an other-directed social actor whose performances are largely programmed by mass education, mass communication, mass production, and mass marketing. Instead of being a whole person having intrinsic worth, this new self is no more than the occupant of producer and consumer roles, interchangeable and replaceable. With it no longer self-evident exactly who the public self is or what the precise nature of its social contributions are, its demise became a forbidden topic.

In the case of the elderly—particularly those who have outlived their friends, have been disengaged from work and much of community life, and are often geographically distant from their families—these crises of identity and insignificance can be particularly poignant. In fact, among their central fears is to die with no one noticing or caring.(5) Such social invisibility and insignificance run contrary to our basic needs for attention and esteem. Aging (and dying) well involve not only individuals' own strategies for well-being but also the social recognition of their attempts. This, in turn, requires new cultural standards for assessment and new social arenas for their accomplishments to be recognized.(6)

The medicalization of old age and death. With the rise of scientific rationalism, medicine inherited from religion and law the social responsibility for defining and managing social problems (Freidson, 1970). In no case is this more evident than for the sociocultural "problems" of old age and death. If current generations of older persons are "trailblazers" of a new stage of the life-cycle (to use a metaphor of the AARP's *Modern Maturity*), then it is the physician who has served as trail guide (Kearl, 1985, 1993).

As Tanya Fusco Johnson (1995) developed earlier, physicians have significantly contributed to the cultural framing of age-related problems in biological rather than in psychosocial terms, reflecting the continuing mechanistic legacy of Cartesian-Newtonian science in modern medicine (Dossey, 1982). As a result, the average physician tends to have a limited view of the factors necessary for aging well and of the forces responsible for death, leading to Weisman (1972) observing that "it is our scientism that excludes human and personal elements and decides that only lesions matter in determining death. . . . Medicine forgets that man is more than a simple organism struggling to survive" (p. 163). Nevertheless, as the cultural high priests responsible for addressing the problem of death, physicians have shifted cultural death fears from concerns over postmortem judgments of the moral worthiness of lives lived to concerns over that which kill us and to the dying process.

Several authors (e.g., Butler, 1975; Platt, 1980) have applied the Greek Tithonius myth to the contemporary aging story. In this immortality parable, a beautiful young man asks Aurora, the goddess of morning, to make him immortal. She does. He ages continuously. Finally, pitying his never-ending dissolution, she makes him into a grasshopper. Instead of making the oldest of the old into grasshoppers, the medical establishment has produced a population requiring ever greater services with advanced age—including the million or more nursing home residents so disabled that 24-hour care is required, and the 10,000 individuals existing in irreversible vegetative states. National estimates reveal approximately one quarter of the aged to be in need of some type of long-term care (U.S. House Select Committee On Aging, 1987).

Illich (1976) argued that the medical community has turned death from a religious and cultural phenomenon into a money-(7) and class-based technological one. Over the course of the twentieth century, "death prevention" increasingly became the primary goal of medicine and a primary value in our culture. The prolongation of both living and dying is a big business: The health care industry comprises one seventh of the economy and employs more than 11 million Americans. And, given capitalism's tendency to produce numerous "losers" along with its "winners," access to this life-extending business is unequal. Owing to class differences in ability to afford medical care, life expectancies are highly correlated with individuals' positions within status hierarchies. As of 1992, for instance, White male life expectancy at birth exceeded that of Black males by 8.2 years (Kochanek & Hudson, 1995). Thus we have Illich's (1976) chilling conclusion about the essence of good deaths from the perspective of the American political economy:

Socially approved death happens when man has become useless not only as a producer but also as a consumer. It is the point at which a consumer, trained at great expense, must finally be written off as a total loss. Dying has become the ultimate form of consumer resistance. (pp. 206-207)

In sum, in capitalist economies, one is "alive" as long as one can consume, which, for many, requires one's ability to produce.(8) With the commodification of death and the medicalization of the dying ritual, many industrialized Westerners are robbed of the personalized relationship that their ancestors had with dying and of the control they had over their own deaths. As a result, there is a growing demand for dying to once again be a natural and dignified experience—if one has to die.

The drive to be immortal. How death typically punctuates life has profound personal, social, and cultural consequences. Where death normally cut individuals down prematurely (e.g., before old age), suddenly and unexpectedly, where the notion that "life exists in the midst of death" was an everyday fact instead of a metaphor (Riley, 1983), death often is viewed as something externally caused, often leading to a fatalistic ethos. Where death is basically confined to older populations (and that which is premature being largely man-made—e.g., owing to homicide, accidents, suicide, unsafe sex, or pollution—and hence avoidable) who die on the outskirts of everyday life, coupled with the demonstrated ability to put people on the moon, to map the human chromosome and engage in genetic engineering, and to unleash the power of the atom in nuclear weapons and power plants, the resultant ethos features an anything-is-possible mind-set. And what could be a greater demonstration of sociocultural power than the death of death?

In fact, because most premature death is nowadays man-made, there is a shared sense that such deaths are avoidable and therefore controllable. Judging from the plethora of laws requiring warning labels on 5-gallon buckets (so children will not fall in them and drown), step-ladders (metal extension ladders are now required to carry 37 warning labels, and 30% of the price goes to cover potential liabilities [Fairlie, 1989]), and even balloons, ours is becoming a risk-free culture. Instead of generating moral doubt or dissatisfactions with society's protective umbrella, premature death is now perceived to be caused either by failure to heed warnings, inadequate lifestyle—such as smoking, poor exercise habits, being poor, or, in the case of AIDS, one's sexual preferences—or by the "underconsumption of clinical care." In other words, the individual is generally to be blamed.

Nowhere is this cultural battle against death clearer than in the medical establishment, where practitioners often view death as their own failure. So extensive have Americans' faith in medicine's ability to conquer most forms of untimely death become—reinforced by the highly publicized breakthroughs in the battles against polio and small pox, and stories of the feats of the Christian Baarnards and Robert Salks—that they believe that medical science will provide a cure for anything that ails us, including old age and death. Emerging is an immortalist ethos (Harrington, 1977; Kearl, in press), fueled by such stories as one appearing in a 1992 issue of Life magazine (Darrach, 1992), wherein one researcher claimed that some of those now living may yet be alive in 400 years.(9)

What are the affects of this cultural immortalism on attitudes toward and experiences of aging well? Perhaps it is death's stigma on old age that underlies the cultural obsession with youth: If you don't grow old then you will not die. Built on this cultural logic is the multibillion dollar-a-year antiaging drug and cosmetic industries, producing products to obscure our aging (and hence our mortality). And preserving the myth for the nonold in everyday life is the historical trend toward increasing social segregations of both the old and the dying from everyday life.

Changing death fears: From premature to postmature demises. With modernization, the dreaded liminality between the worlds of the living and the dead has shifted from the period proceeding death to the period preceding it. When fears of death were associated with unanticipated and premature demises, the cultural consolations of preindustrial societies were based on envisionments of individuals' postmortem fates. Dying well meant assurances that one would, for instance, go to heaven or be reincarnated into some better state. In modern cultures, fears are more associated with aging/living well until one dies. For many older persons, the great nightmare is not no longer existing but, rather, being a superannuated Tithonius: totally dependent on others, exhausting family financial and emotional resources, and being without control and dignity in some total institution. Epitomizing this feared state of being are the victims of advanced Alzheimer's: those socially dead and yet biologically alive.(10) Here dying well involves being able to control when and how one dies.

Changing loci of control over the final passage. Also contributing to contemporary fears of dying are the anxieties of dying within institutional settings, particularly nursing homes, where life is often structured for the convenience of staff and where residents suffer the physical and psychological pains of depersonalization.

As developed, such institutionalization of those living life's final chapter reflects the medicalization of death, which has restricted individuals' traditional control over their own deaths. With medicine framing the end of life, one's final rite of passage features technological rituals addressing the biological processes of dying instead of its spiritual aspects. One would suspect, then, that medicalized death would feature pain control as a key service (and legitimator of medical control). However, according to a large 1993 survey of more than 1,400 physicians and nurses from five major hospitals in different parts of the country, such is not the case. Nearly half the attending physicians and nurses and 70% of resident physicians reported acting against their conscience in overtreating the terminally ill, often ignoring patients' requests to withhold life support. The study also revealed a failure to provide adequate pain relief for those experiencing life's end, with 81% of the respondents agreeing that "the most common form of narcotic abuse in caring for dying patients is undertreatment of pain" (Solomon et al., 1993).

This emergent cultural ritual for managing death has clearly not worked for many. Try as we might during the twentieth century to ignore and to sanitize death, its sting continues to fester—perhaps even more so as we have largely forgotten the time-tested traditional rituals that assisted past generations to cope with the inevitable and normal transition from life to death. During the Middle Ages, for instance, with the rise of individualism, death was recognized as the natural force one had to master: "A man insisted upon participating in his own death because he saw in it an exceptional moment—a moment which gave his individuality its definitive form" (Aries, 1975, p. 11). To assist in this mastery, an instructional manual on the art of dying, entitled *Ars Moriendi*, was to be a best seller for 2 centuries (Illich, 1975, pp. 30-31).

Dissatisfactions over medicalized death rituals have led to the emergence of our own Ars Moriendi. Addressing the desires for greater personal control over how, when, where, and with whom one dies has been the rise of the "right-to-die" and "death-with-dignity" movements, the success of Derek Humphry's *Final Exit* (1991), and hospice. Hospice is a philosophy and a method of care for dying well. An alternative to medicalized death, its goal is to neither hasten nor postpone inevitable death but to transcend suffering and to enhance patient autonomy in determining the manner and style of their dying. Between 1983—when federal laws went into effect allowing Medicare reimbursement for home hospice care—and 1992, the number of hospice patients more than doubled nationwide to 207,000 (Belkin, 1992).(11)

Death as a Province of the Elderly and the Rise of Cultural Gerontophobia

One of the great accomplishments of modernization has been the general confinement of death to those who have lived full, complete lives. Following the two-thirds improvement in our species' life expectancy over the course of the twentieth century, now roughly three out of four deaths in the United States occur among those 65 and older (Rothenberg, Lentzner, & Parker, 1991). More than one in five deaths are Americans 85 years of age or older. The assumption that modern citizens will live to see their old age is reflected in a new statistic of the federal government: YPLL, "years of potential life lost" when people die before the age of 65. Interestingly, although the near-guarantee of three quarters of a century of existence should be the occasion for celebration, the status of older persons has become culturally and sociologically problematic.

Social and cultural recipes for navigating this newly guaranteed stage of the lifespan have failed to keep pace with demographic change, hence the precarious ("roleless role") status of old age. Sociologically, there is the problem of the elderly no longer automatically "fitting in" with the rest of society, along with the political debates surrounding mandatory retirement, the entitlement status of Social

Security and its intergenerational distributive justice, Medicare, and Medicaid.

Culturally, old age's problem entails its meaningfulness and desirability as a life stage. Over the course of the past century, an additional contradiction has arisen: As life expectancies have increased, the perceived prime years of the life cycle have declined. Nineteenth century depictions of the stages of a man's/woman's life (see Achenbaum & Kusnerz, 1978, pp. 2-3) reveal the pinnacle occurring during one's 50s.(12) However, in the 1974 "Myth and Reality of Aging in America" (Harris, 1975) survey of Americans (N = 4,254), nearly one half of all Americans viewed the "best years of a person's life" occurring during teens or 20s, with everything "downhill" from the 30s on.

In this vacuum has arisen the retirement ethos, the cultural consolation ideology for those who must die, a life-cycle stage when one supposedly has the earned right to withdraw from social responsibilities. In a highly individualistic and materialistic culture that values happiness, what this can mean is solipsistic self-indulgence—and hence the appearance of the contemporary "greedy geezer" stereotype in American society (Fairlie, 1988). This, in turn, is raising the specter of meaninglessness to the latter years and the worthlessness of those within them. In 1984, then-Colorado governor Richard Lamm argued that older persons have "a duty to die and get out of the way." Three years later, ethicist Daniel Callahan (1987) wrote in *Setting Limits*:

There can be no community at all, much less community among the generations, without some sacrifice of an unlimited quest for individualistic pleasure on the part of the old. Why should the young respect, much less help and support, old people who mean to live for their own pleasure? . . . If the old are to have meaning in their own lives and significance in the larger social world, they cannot claim a right to self-absorption or an exemption from civic duties. (pp. 30, 49)

On the other hand, is it the case that Lamm and Callahan are simply blaming the victims of social disregard and dismissal? I suggest that this dilemma over the status and roles of older persons in contemporary American society is thoroughly interwoven with the problem of death. Because the traditional cultural practice has been to make lesser persons out of those most likely to die,(13) the parameters for aging well are undoubtedly being shaped by the cultural meanings of and social responses to the dying and the dead.

433

On Cultural "Good Deaths" and "Bad"

As life expectancies approach biological limits, as death comes increasingly to those who have lived full lives and who perhaps are more ready to die (perhaps even preferring death to continued existence) than were earlier generations, and as the timing of an increasing proportion of deaths can be controlled, life's conclusion is increasingly a matter of design. And like all human designs—whether they be musical resolutions, the denouements of literature and drama, the final 2 minutes of a football or basketball game, or the conclusions of human biographies—"bad endings" can destroy otherwise good social performances and "good endings" can potentially save otherwise mediocre ones. In other words, the quality and meaningfulness of all life stages can ultimately depend on how the final one is concluded.

There can be little question that some deaths are better than others. Although the notion of "good death" sounds oxymoronic to many contemporary Americans (Shneidman, 1980, pp. xvii-xviii), people cross-culturally make invidious distinctions between good deaths and bad. Compare, for instance, crooner Bing Crosby's sudden death following 18 rounds of his beloved golf with the slow motion expiration of an 80-year-old diabetic. Bedridden following the amputation of his leg, the old man eventually began slipping in and out of consciousness. This continued over a period of years, exhausting the emotional and financial resources of his family. Worn out, his wife, too, fell seriously ill.

As revealed in this comparison, there are a number of perspectives to be taken when considering the essence of good deaths. Deaths become good when they serve not only the needs of the dying but also those of their survivors and of the broader social orders as well.

First, there is the perspective of the dying individual. Is one dying in the way one prefers? The answer to this question undoubtedly varies by individuals' personality type, age, sex, race and ethnicity, social class, and, of course, culture.(14) For those whose deaths are not easy, a good death may involve being allowed to die in character, at their own pace, in their own style (Dempsey, 1977, p. 231), and with a minimization of degradation. In defining an "appropriate death," Avery Weisman (1978) observed:

Someone who dies an appropriate death must be helped in the following ways: He should be relatively pain-free, his suffering reduced, and emotional and social impoverishments kept to a minimum. Within the limits of disability, he should operate on as high a level as possible, even though only tokens of former fulfillments can be offered. He should also recognize and resolve residual conflicts, and satisfy whatever remaining wishes are consistent with his present plight and his own ego ideal. Finally, among his choices, he should be able to yield control to others in whom he has confidence. He also has the option of seeking or relinquishing significant key people. (p. 193)

To this inventory of attributes of good deaths, we should add the conditions of one's death being meaningful, such as dying for a cause; anticipated, so that one has time to put one's affairs in order and to give one's farewells; occurring upon the completion of a major enterprise, as when Thomas Bensen died the day after his completion of a mural for the Missouri state capitol; death being wished-for; and dying assured that one has left some form of symbolic immortality, such as being remembered for some accomplishment, having biological descendants or intellectual heirs, or leaving a legacy.

Second, there is the perspective of the significant others of the dying/deceased. Thanatologists have long stressed death's dualistic nature, involving not only the individual dying but also the survivors-to-be. Here a good death is one that minimizes the sociological and psychological damage wrought by death to those socially connected with the deceased. Deaths are good, for instance, if the quality of life or social status of survivors is enhanced and if their grief work is minimal.

Finally, there is the perspective of the broader society. For societies, deaths are good when they enhance social solidarities or in other ways contribute to the well-being of the living. Death is the great check against excessive populations. It provides upward mobility for the living and the possibility for sociocultural change (as when elderly bigots die). From this viewpoint, aging well involves dying well: dying at the "right time" and in the "right way," "properly" moving from life's stage so that younger generations can take their turn. There are reasons for these qualified descriptors: Notions of the appropriate timing and style of death, and the proper movement from the world of the living to the world of the dead are highly relative.

Owing to dramatic changes of both selves and society during the twentieth century, we currently find ourselves without a cultural consensus about how and when death is ideally to be met. Just as there is a general paucity of cultural role models for aging well, there is also the general absence of models for dying well.(15) One reason is because of the profound changes in who dies and how.

How the Old Die

With death increasingly coming to those of advanced age with chronic disabilities within institutionalized settings, and owing to the increasing number of age-graded roles from which older individuals are typically excluded (or exclude themselves), few Americans die heroically with their proverbial boots on. Instead, the old now die a series of symbolic minideaths—gradually surrendering or losing their roles of worker, civic member, driver, friend, and spouse—before biologically expiring. If not voluntary or desirable (i.e., retiring as opposed to being mandatorily retired), such disengagements can be socially stigmatizing and personally demeaning.

So how do the old actually die? The euthanasia described by Zygmunt Bauman at the beginning of this article is certainly not the norm. Instead, the old nowadays often die slow-motion deaths from chronic ailments, often dying socially before expiring biologically. More than 7 out of 10 older Americans die within institutions—51% in hospital inpatient settings and 21% in nursing homes (McMillan, Mentnech, Lubitz, McBean, & Russell, 1990). Herein, even the timetable of death is decreasingly natural. In 1991, the American Hospital Association estimated that 70% of hospital deaths are preceded by decisions to stop some form of care (Belkin, 1991). Such decisions, however, appear not to be based on older persons' advance directives, such as living wills, proxy appointments, and durable powers of attorney for health care. A study of medical records made between 1991 and 1993 of 114 older persons (average age 83) who had executed advance directives revealed that in three quarters of their 180 hospitalizations, physicians had not consulted their living wills or designated proxies (Morrison, Olson, Mertz, & Meier, 1995).

Based on interviews with relatives of 5,582 elderly Americans who died in 1986, Lentzner, Pamuk, Rhodenhiser, Rothenberg, and Powell-Griner (1992) found that only 14% were fully functional in their last year of life. Ten percent of the deceased had spent their last year living severely restricted lives with physical and mental disabilities. Another study—based on interviews with family members and close friends of 1,227 elderly people who died in Fairfield County, Connecticut—found that on the day before their death, 51% knew family members, 61% experienced no pain, 90% had no diarrhea, 87% no nausea, and 52% could breathe freely (Brock, Holmes, Foley, & Holmes, 1992).

Such "natural" death statistics are not comforting. And there is evidence that at least some segments of the older population would rather expedite the dying process so as to maintain some personal dignity and to minimize the burden placed on the survivors-to-be.

The specter of hastened death. In early 1990, psychoanalyst Bruno Bettelheim swallowed some pills, placed a plastic bag over his head, and quietly laid until he died. This survivor of Buchenwald knew well the need for meaning, having spent a sizable portion of his career working to restore meaning to the lives of autistic children. In his old age, meaning evaporated for Bettelheim. His wife of 43 years had died 6 years earlier and his loss was compounded by a crippling stroke. Six weeks before his death, Bettelheim had moved into a retirement home.

Although the origin of suicidal proclivities has long been debated, the self-destructive activities of older individuals are perhaps most easily understood: The senses of meaninglessness and helplessness, the loss of roles and significant others, and depression are potent dampeners of the will to live. Although composing about one quarter of the population, Americans age 60 and older commit nearly 4 out of 10 suicides in the United States. And their attempts are more lethal: According to McIntosh (1985), whereas the ratio of suicide attempts to completions is 200 to 1 among the young, among the old it is 4 to 1.

According to a 1992 Gallup survey, an estimated 620,000 elderly Americans may have contemplated suicide that year. Common among those with such thoughts were feelings of loneliness, hopelessness, impotence, and worthlessness ("Nationline," 1992). Following a 50-year period of decline between 1981 and 1986, the suicide rate of Americans 65 and older increased some 25%, whereas the rates of all other age groups declined. The suicide rates for women decline with age, whereas those of males, particularly White males, increase. In fact, the ratio of male to female suicides increases from 4 to 1 in the 65 to 69 age range to a 12 to 1 ratio by the age of 85.

Such differences in suicide rates by sex and race (i.e., the more than threefold difference in the rates of White and Black males aged 75 to 84) in this country and their differences cross-culturally (in Japan, for instance, during the mid-1980s, males aged 75 and older were less than 40% more likely to take their own lives than similarly aged females, compared with their tenfold greater likelihood in the United States) suggest differential opportunities or abilities for aging well. The relatively high rates of White males may indicate the absence of anticipatory socializations for later life and overdependency on the social connections and meanings derived from work roles. Perhaps they are too successfully socialized into capitalism's work ethic and require a more potent rite of passage ritual into the retirement years to be able to age well.

437

Older Persons' Attitudes Toward Suicide and Euthanasia

Given their rising suicide rates and increasingly timed deaths, amid abundant media reportings of Jack Kevorkian's suicide machine, and the ethical plights of those in limbo between the worlds of the living and the dead, how have the attitudes of the elderly, our culture's "shock-absorbers of death" (Hochschild, 1973, p. 85), changed between the 1970s and 1990s? Have older persons' desire for control and their abhorrence of dependency made them receptive to the right-to-die/ death with dignity movements?

To analyze (and compare with younger age groups) older Americans' attitudes toward suicide and euthanasia, the results of 12 years (from 1977 to 1994) of the National Opinion Research Center's (NORC) General Social Surveys were analyzed (N = 16,455). Each of these surveys is an independently drawn, full probability sampling of noninstitutionalized, English-speaking individuals 18 years of age or older who live within the continental United States (Davis & Smith, 1994).

To gauge individuals' attitudes toward euthanasia, responses to the following question (EUTHANASIA) were considered:

- When a person has a disease that cannot be cured, do you think doctors should be allowed by law to end the patient's life by some painless means if the patient and his family request it? Recoded 1 = allow, 2 = don't allow/don't know.

Attitudes toward the moral right of the terminally ill to commit suicide were measured by the following question (SUICIDE.ILL):

- Do you think a person has the right to end his or her own life if this person has an incurable disease? Recoded 1 = yes, 2 = no/ don't know.

Between 1977 and 1994, the percentage of American adults agreeing with SUICIDE.ILL increased from 38% to 61% and with EUTHANASIA from 60% to 68%. There are, in fact, few longitudinally tracked attitudes that have changed more in the United States over this time frame than has support for the right of the terminally ill to take their own lives. The largest increases in agreement with SUICIDE.ILL occurred between 1985 and 1986 (a 7.6 percentage point rise) and between 1989 and 1990 (a 9.3 percentage point increase). What pre-Kevorkian stories occurred during these periods to account for these sudden spurts? They were the deaths of Karen Ann Quinlan in 1985 and of Nancy Cruzan in 1990, two young(16) adult females whose brain-dead existences raised numerous moral questions in the popular media. There was also in 1985 the Paul Brophy story, who shared the women's fate and whose family, like Cruzan's, sought to halt the administration of food and water through a stomach tube. Several national surveys were conducted dealing with the withdrawal of life-sustaining treatment and the administration of lethal injections for those hopelessly ill, increasing public discourse and thought on the topic. "Harper's Index" began including numbers of Americans joining the Hemlock Society each month and CNN made a "factoid" of the number of Americans in persistent vegetative states.

Support for SUICIDE.ILL and EUTHANASIA generally decrease with age yet increase for all age groups over time. In the combined 1993-1994 surveys, for instance, 68% of those 18 to 29 and 40% of those 80 years of age and older agreed that persons with incurable diseases have the right to end their own life, equally increasing from 50% and 21%, respectively, in 1977-1978. Although the much greater support for the physician-assisted death question brings regression effects to the analysis (hence the relatively small increase in support among those 18 to 29, from 69% to 75% between 1977-1978 and 1993-1994), the longitudinal increase in agreement with EUTHANASIA was greatest for those aged 80 and older, rising from 31% to 55%.

Such longitudinal change in age-group agreement with these two items suggests cohort effects are at work. With few exceptions, the general pattern has been increasing approval for both means of ending life among all cohorts, particularly those born after 1920. Given the strong positive correlation between these questions and increasing education and diminishing religiosity, as more highly educated and less religious cohorts reach old age, we can expect increasing support for suicide and euthanasia among older individuals.(17)

There has been a consistent increase of support for suicide among all of these older groups over time. Less consistent has been their increasing approval for physician-assisted death. Although there was virtually no change between the first and last periods among White males and Black females, agreement with EUTHANASIA increased by three quarters for older Black males.

Those with the highest (White males) and lowest (Black females) suicide rates are most and least likely to agree with the right of the terminally ill to commit suicide. There is, however, a flip-flop between Black males and White females, with the latter—although having the lower suicide rate—being more likely to agree with SUICIDE.ILL.

Controlling for education and religiosity does not explain away the race-sex differences in support for suicide, although the sexual differences within each race is contracted.

Does the higher rate of support for suicide by the White males somehow reflect their lesser happiness in old age? Interestingly not. Over all of the survey years, it is the White male who is most likely to report being "very happy" (40%, compared with 35% of White females, 30% of Black females, and 25% of Black males). Further, it is not the case that personal unhappiness is more likely to lead White males to agree with SUICIDE.ILL—in fact, only for this group of older individuals is there no difference between the most and least happy in agreement that the terminally ill have the right to take their own lives. Such suggests that it is, indeed, philosophical matters of control and not emotional depression influencing their responses.

In sum, it seems that those most concerned with having (e.g., the most educated), experiencing (e.g., White males), or believing in (e.g., the least religious) personal control over one's own life are the most likely to endorse euthanasia and the right of the terminally ill to commit suicide.

Conclusion

For any cultural ethos to make sense, good lives must have good deaths. The ability of a society to allocate as many good deaths as possible to its members is a measure of its cultural adequacy. However, Americans are not very good at their goodbyes and social closures. Judging from the increasing legal involvements in the endings of our work careers (e.g., the mandatory retirement and downsizing controversies), family relations (e.g., divorce, disinheritances), and life itself (e.g., the controversies surrounding Jack Kevorkian and the right-to-die movements), where there is an absence of cultural consensus over exactly how endings should be conducted, others will take control. From our longitudinal analyses, however, there are clear signs that there is growing approval for the moral right of the terminally ill to have the options of euthanasia and suicide. As we have seen, support for these options is increasing among the more recent, more educated, and less religious cohorts.(18)

Americans are increasingly cognizant of the loss of control experienced by institutionalized terminally ill patients. Loss of control is increasingly viewed to lead to the loss of dignity; dying patients' basic human rights are seen to be violated when they lack the knowledge and power to make decisions (Levine & Scotch, 1970). Dying well

440

means having the right to know one's condition and the ability to choose or reject life-prolonging treatment regimens. But the fact remains that as the dying person deteriorates, others must take control of the life remaining. Hence the possibility of dying well also hinges on the relationship between the dying individual and caregivers. This becomes problematic in the case of the elderly, who are often perceived incapable of managing their own lives anyway. In fact, according to Kastenbaum and Aisenberg (1972, p. 121), rather than being provided with appropriate environment and care, the terminally ill elderly person is more likely to be rejected as a deviant and denied control in that being both old and dying is doubly stigmatizing. Thus abilities to die well are interwoven with opportunities to age well.

With superannuated lives, controversies surrounding the quantity versus the quality of existence will undoubtedly multiply in these increasingly budget-minded times.(19) The state euthanasia referendums occurred where they did (California, Washington, and Oregon) in the early 1990s because of the relatively low religiosity of the area and the relatively weak power of the Catholic Church. In 1994, *The New England Journal of Medicine* proposed the creation of a national policy for allowing physician-assisted suicide while outlining safeguards against abuses (Miller et al., 1994). In the same year, in a ruling striking down Washington state's 140-year-old ban on assisted suicide, U.S. District Court Judge Barbara Rothstein ruled that the Fourteenth Amendment clause against state infringement on individual liberty guarantees people not only the right to terminate pregnancies but also the right to end their own lives without government interference. Concurrently, with the perception that abortion was just the beginning of a slippery slope of the death ethic, opponents of the right-to-die are forging connections with powerful antiabortion groups in what may be the second phase of the prolife movement.

Will legitimating (or, at least, destigmatizing) the option of suicide(20) for the terminally ill, through measures such as allowing physicians to prescribe lethal doses of medication, lead to increasing suicide rates? I suggest not. In fact, simply having the option may enhance older persons' ability to age and die well.(21) When people believe they have the ability to control or cope with specific situations, self-confidence and self-efficacy are enhanced. By simply having the option to die when facing the challenges of disintegration and deterioration, future cohorts of increasingly educated older individuals may well devise new strategies and standards for aging well. And, as Americans will decreasingly be able to think of themselves as a nation of the young (with more than one in five projected to be 65 and older within half a century), these new models will undoubtedly receive greater publicity and receptivity.

Notes

1. The mother, Ida Rollin, was diagnosed as having ovarian cancer in 1981. After two bouts with chemotherapy for ovarian cancer, her mother lost her hair, control of her bowels, and ability to eat because of an intestinal blockage. When her doctors gave her 6 months to live, she told her daughter that she wanted to die. The daughter and her husband phoned physicians across the country attempting to find out what pills would enable her mother to commit suicide painlessly and with dignity. After considerable searching, they found one. Ida swallowed the pills in front of them.

2. At least one carried the suicide note left by a couple (Malcolm, 1984).

3. The book begins with the line, "This is the scenario: you are terminally ill, all medical treatments acceptable to you have been exhausted, and the suffering in its different forms is unbearable" (Humphry, 1991, p. 20).

4. Physicians, too, are often accomplices in this deception game. Studios reveal physicians often believing that the terminally ill really do not want to know about their condition and that to tell them destroys hope and accelerates death. Glaser and Strauss (1965) modeled this informational game in their elaborations of "awareness contexts," that takes into account the combination of what each actor knows about the identity of the other and his or her own identity in the eyes of the other. Because most terminally ill persons know they are dying, a typical game is one of mutual pretense awareness. Here the terminally ill patient, family, and staff are all fully aware of the forthcoming death but pretend that recovery is forthcoming.

5. For instance, consider the publicized discovery of Adele Gaboury in Worcester, Massachusetts in 1993. As the 73-year-old recluse lay dead on her kitchen floor for 4 years, neighbors continued to mow her lawn and postal carriers continued delivering her mail through a slot in the door. Even when police

searched the home 3 days prior to her discovery, responding to complaints about it being a health hazard, they missed her badly decomposed body in 6 feet of trash. And what of the hundreds of elderly Chicagoans who died in their non-air-conditioned homes during the brutal heat wave in the summer of 1995? Why wasn't there anyone who cared enough to check up on them?

6. Examples of such new standards and opportunities can he found in sports. Consider, for instance, the Special Olympics, the age-grading of track and field records, or golf's Senior Tour.

7. In 1994, the "End of Life: Issues and Implementation of Advanced Directives Under Health Care Reform" Congressional hearing was before the Senate Committee on Finance, not within a committee responsible for legal or moral deliberation (U.S. Senate Committee on Finance, 1994).

8. Following this logic, as Jennifer Solomon noted in reviewing an earlier draft of this article, Elvis is "alive" because he is still "producing" revenue; individuals in irreversible vegetative states are alive because they still are consumers of medical care.

9. In the same year, the Time/CNN "Beyond the Year 2000" poll (1992) revealed that 75% of Americans expected a cure for AIDS and 80% a cure for cancer.

10. The "social death" of President Ronald Reagan comes to mind. The disease is increasingly common with advancing years; of Americans aged 85 and older, approximately one third have Alzheimer's, compared with 5% at age 65 (Altman, 1994).

11. This 1992 figure of hospice patients is approximately one tenth the number of Americans who died that year.

12. An 1848 lithograph "The Life and Age of Man. Stages of a Man's Life from the Cradle to the Grave" (Baille, 1848; also quoted in Achenbaum & Kusnerz, 1978, p. 2) illustrates the span's zenith at age 50 with the following caption: Strength falls at fifty but with wit fox-like he helps to manage it. In the 1890s, a similar span-of-life depiction can he found in an advertisement of the Glastonbury Knitting Company, with the following stage labelings: 10 years Childhood 20 years Eager

& Earnest 30 years In the Thick of the Fight 40 years Full Manhood 50 years Prime of Life 60 years Retrospective 70 years Old Age 80 years Resigned 90 years 2nd Childhood

13. Making lesser persons of those most likely to die lessens the social readjustments necessitated by their disappearance. Thus there was the nonperson status of young children up until the eighteenth century in the West when they constituted the majority of all deaths (Aries, 1962) and the reason for greater emphasis on affectionate parent-child relationships in colonial America as child mortality rates lowered (Smith, 1980).

14. Over the past decade, for instance, I have been administering the *Psychology Today* "You and Death" questionnaire on the first day of class (Designed by E. Shneidman, with E. Parker & G. R. Funkhouser, this is a modification of a questionnaire that E. Shneidman developed with the assistance of four of his graduate assistants, C. Dowell, R. Goldstein, D. Goleman, & B. Smith; "Psychology Today Questionnaire," 1970) to those enrolled in my Death and Dying course (N = 341, 1985-1995). Even in this relatively homogeneous group (18-22 years of age, upper middle-class, Anglo) of undergraduates at a small Southwestern liberal arts college, there has been a clear absence of consensus.

Table 47.1. To the question, "If you had a choice, what kind of death would you prefer?" the responses broke down as follows (in percentages):

	Male	Female
Tragic, violent death	3	2
Sudden but not violent death	22	29
Quiet, dignified death	36	54
Death in the line of duty	4	0
Death after a great achievement	10	4
Suicide	4	.5
Homicidal victim	1	0
There is no "appropriate" kind of death	14	6
Other	5	5
Total (N)	110	225

15. This is not meant to imply that such models do not exist, but rather that owing to cultural ageism and death-denials, publicity is typically not given to them. In fact, the models receiving publicity are more typically negative, such as Kalish's "New Ageism," which "stereotypes the elderly in terms of the characteristics of the least capable, least healthy, and least alert of the elderly" (1979, p. 398). Research indicates that the vast majority of older persons hold the same ageist stereotypes as younger individuals and yet view themselves as exceptions, and that older individuals who feel that others are worse off than themselves have higher life satisfaction than those feeling others are as well off or better (Kearl, 1982). But for how long can standards for gauging the adequacy of one's aging and dying be based on negative reference groups and role models?

16. The fact that it was not the similar fate of an older individual that so dominated American attention is worth observing. Certainly a higher proportion (and number) of older persons exist in such limbo states. Is their social status so minimal, is old age so associated with death, that their stories do not provoke the ethical controversies as when younger adults find themselves in this plight?

17. To ascertain what percentage of these historical shifts in support for euthanasia and suicide were due to cohort effects as opposed to year effects, the Davis (1987) standardizing methodology for estimating the effects of newcomers, leavers, and year effects in longitudinal surveys was employed. In the case of SUICIDE.ILL, approximately 70% of the historical change was due to year (or period) effects; of the 30% attributed to cohort changes, 52% of the change was due to newcomers and 48% was due to the older cohorts dying out. For the oldest cohorts over this time frame, support increased by 12% for those born prior to 1911 (from 26.4% in 1977-1978 to 38.3% in 1993-1994), by 13.7% for those born between 1911 and 1919 (from 28.9% to 42.6%), and by 11.2% for those born during the 1920s (from 33.2% to 44.4%). In sum, the 60% increase over 17 years in Americans' approval of the terminally ill committing suicide is due more to changes in collective attitude than to cohort dynamics.

Cohort effects were, however, more dominant in the historical shift in euthanasia attitudes: Here only 22% of the attitude shift was due to year effects, with 55% of the cohort effect being due to newcomers and 45% due to leavers. Focusing on the attitudes of the three oldest cohorts (those born prior to 1911, 1911-1919, and 1920-1929), between 1977-1978 and 1993-1994, support for physician-assisted death increased by 4% among those born 1910 or earlier, decreased by 10.5% among those born between 1911 and 1919, and increased by 8.4% among those born during the 1920s. For these three cohorts, the educational effect (which is also highly correlated with survival rates) on attitudes is most pronounced, with those having 4 or more years of college experience being twice as likely to support suicide and 20% more likely to support euthanasia.

Pursuing further this positive influence of education on support for our two death questions coupled with the positive influence of decreasing religiosity, we find the two predictors to be additive in their effect. Among those 65 and older in the total sample, agreement with both questions consistently rises as education increases and religiosity decreases, with 94% of the most educated and religiously unaffiliated older persons agreeing with both SUICIDE.ILL and EUTHANASIA, compared to only 12% of the least educated and most religious.

18. In a personal communication with Derek Humphry (May 1995), he noted that the "typical Hemlock member is White, middle-aged, female, college-educated, and . . . not very religious, more often than not a Unitarian or a Congregationalist." However, since the beginning of the AIDS epidemic, membership is becoming more male and more youthful.

19. Total health spending has grown from less than 6% of the gross national product 3 decades ago to greater than 13% by the mid-1990s, with projections that it could reach 37% of GNP by 2030. Medicare disbursements alone will exceed 2.5% of the nation's gross domestic product in 1995, with perhaps as much as 30% of the total going to older individuals in their last 6 months of life.

20. There may be the need for a new word in the language for the suicides of the terminally ill who can no longer cope with the pains of existence. Ralph Miro, founder of Compassion in Dying, the group that spearheaded the Washington state euthanasia referendum, argues that the distinction between suicide

(the result of depression) and "hastened death" is analogous to the distinction between rape and love making (1994).

21. The reason is the "control button" attributional effect, based on Lefcourt's (1976, pp. 3-6) intriguing experiment. Two groups of adult subjects were given complex puzzles to solve and a proofreading task to perform. To make their jobs more challenging there was a loud, randomly occurring distracting noise that included "a combination of two people speaking Spanish, one speaking Armenian, a mimeograph machine running, a desk calculator, a typewriter, and street noise— producing a composite, nondistinguishable roar." The control group was simply told to work at the task, whereas members of the experimental group were given a button that they could push to turn off the noise. Although the button was never pushed, the second group solved 5 times the number of puzzles as the group without the button and made far fewer proofreading errors.

References

Altman, L. K. (1994, November 7). Reagan meant to raise awareness of Alzheimer's. *New York Times*, p. A13.

Achenbaum, W. A., & Kusnerz, P. A. (1978). *Images of old age in America 1790 to the present*. Ann Arbor, MI: Institute of Gerontology, University of Michigan-Wayne State University.

Aries, P. (1962). *Centuries of childhood: A social history of family life* (R. Baldick, Trans.). New York: Vintage.

Aries, P. (1974). *Western attitudes toward death: From the middle ages to the present*. Baltimore: Johns Hopkins University Press.

Aries, P. (1975). Death inside out. In P. Steinfels & R. Veatch (Eds.), *Death inside out: The Hastings Center report* (pp. 9-24). New York: Harper & Row.

Aries, P. (1981). *The hour of our death*. New York: Alfred A. Knopf.

Baffle, J. (1848). "The life and age of man. Stages of a man's life from the cradle to the grave" (lithograph, Library of Congress, Neg. No. LC-USZ62-2852).

Bauman, Z. (1992). *Mortality, immortality and other life strategies*. Stanford, CA: Stanford University Press.

Baumeister, R. (1991). *Meanings of life*. New York: Guilford.

Becker, E. (1973). *The denial of death*. New York: Free Press.

Belkin, L. (1991, January 10). As family protests, hospital seeks an end to woman's life support. *New York Times*, pp. A1, C20.

Belkin, L. (1992, March 2). Choosing death at home: Dignity with its own toll. *New York Times,* pp. A1, B12.

Brock, D. B., Holmes, M. B., Foley, D. J., & Holmes, D. (1992). Methodological issues in a survey of the last days of life. In R. B. Wallace & R. F. Woolson (Eds.), *The epidemiologic study of the elderly* (pp. 315-332). New York: Oxford University Press.

Butler, R. (1975). *Why survive? Being old in America*. New York: Harper & Row.

Callahan, D. (1987). *Setting limits: Medical goals in an aging society*. New York: Simon & Schuster.

Darrach, B. (1992). Aging. *Life*, 15(10), 32-45.

Davis, J. A. (1987). *Social differences in contemporary America*. New York: Harcourt Brace Jovanovich.

Davis, J. A., & Smith, T. W. (1994). *General social surveys, 1972-1994* (Machine-readable data file). Produced by the National Opinion Research Center, Chicago. Tape distributed by the Roper Public Opinion Research Center, Storrs, CT. Micro diskette and codebook prepared and distributed by MicroCase Corporation, Bellevue, WA.

de Beauvoir, S. (1972). *The coming of age* (P. O'Brian, Trans.). New York: G. P. Putnam.

Dempsey, D. (1977). *The way we die: An investigation of death and dying in America today*. New York: McGraw-Hill.

Dossey, L. (1982). *Space, time & medicine*. Boulder, CO: Shambhala.

Fairlie, H. (1988, March 28). Talkin' 'bout my generation. *New Republic*, pp. 19-22.

Fairlie, H. (1989, January 23). Fear of living. *New Republic*, pp. 14-19.

Feifel, H. (1959). *The meaning of death*. New York: McGraw-Hill.

Freidson, E. (1970). *The profession of medicine*. New York: Harper & Row.

Glaser, B. G., & Strauss, A. L. (1965). *Awareness of dying*. Chicago: Aldine.

Goffman, E. (1963). *Stigma: Notes on the management of spoiled identities*. Englewood Cliffs, NJ: Prentice Hall.

Gorer, G. (1965*). Death, grief and mourning*. New York: Doubleday Anchor.

Harrington, A. (1977*). The immortalist*. Millbrae, CA: Celestial Arts.

Harris, L. (1975). *The myth and reality of aging in America*. Washington, DC: National Council on the Aging.

Hochschild, A. (1973). *The unexpected community*. Englewood Cliffs, NJ: Prentice Hall.

Humphry, D. (1991*). Final exit: The practicalities of self-deliverance and assisted suicide for the dying*. Eugene, OR: Hemlock. (Distributed by Carol Publishing of Secaucus, NJ)

Illich, I. (1975). The political uses of natural death. In P. Steinfels & R. Veatch (Eds.), *Death inside out: The Hastings Center report* (pp. 25-42). New York: Harper & Row.

Illich, I. (1976). *Medical nemesis: The expropriation of health*. New York: Pantheon.

Johnson, T. F. (1995). Aging well in contemporary society: Introduction. *American Behavioral Scientist, 39*(2), 120-130.

Kalish, R. (1979). The new ageism and the failure models: A polemic. *Gerontologist, 19*, 398-402.

Kastenbaum, R. J., & Aisenberg, R. (1972). *The psychology of death*. New York: Springer.

Kearl, M. (1982). An inquiry into the positive personal and social effects of old age stereotypes among the elderly. *International Journal of Aging and Human Development, 14*(4), 277-290.

Kearl, M. (1985). The aged as pioneers in time: On temporal discontinuities, biographical closure, and the medicalization of old age. In C. Gaitz, G. Niederehe, & N. Wilson (Eds.), *Aging*

2000: Our health care destiny, Vol. II: Psychosocial and policy is-sues (pp. 43-59). New York: Springer-Verlag.

Kearl, M. (1989). *Endings: A sociology of death and dying*. New York: Oxford University Press.

Kearl, M. (1993). Dying American style: From moral to technologi-cal rite of passage. *American Journal of Ethics and Medicine*, 2(1), 12-18.

Kearl, M. (1995). Death and politics: A psychosocial perspective. In H. Wass & R. Neimeyer (Eds.), *Dying: Facing the facts* (pp. 3-23). Washington, DC: Taylor & Francis.

Kearl, M. (in press). You never have to die! On Mormons, mediums, cryonics, & the American immortalist ethos. In G. Howarth, A. Kellehear, & K. Charmaz (Eds.), *The unknown country: Death in the societies of Australia, Britain, and the USA*.

Kochanek, K. D., & Hudson, B. L. (1995). Advance report of final mortality statistics, 1992. *Monthly Vital Statistics Report*, 43(6S). Hyattsville, MD: National Center for Health Statistics.

Lefcourt, H. M. (1976). *Locus of control: Current trends in theory and research*. Hillsdale, NJ: Lawrence Erlbaum.

Lentzner, H. R., Pamuk, E. R., Rhodenhiser, E. P., Rothenberg, R., & Powell-Griner, E. (1992). The quality-of-life in the year before death. *American Journal of Public Health*, 82, 1093-1098.

Levine, S., & Scotch, N. A. (1970). Dying as an emerging social prob-lem. In O. G. Brim, H. E. Freeman, S. Levine, & N. E. Scotch (Eds.), *The dying patient* (pp. 211-224). New York: Russell Sage.

Mcintosh, J. L. (1985). Suicide among the elderly: Levels and trends. *American Journal of Orthopsychiatry*, 55(2), 288-293.

McMillan, A., Mentnech, R. M., Lubitz, J., McBean, A.M., & Russell, D. (1990). Trends and patterns in place of death for medicare enrollees. *Health Care Financing Review*, 12(1), 1-7.

Malcolm, A. (1984, September 24). Some elderly choose suicide over lonely, dependent life. *New York Times*, pp. 1, 13.

Meehan, P. J., Saltzman, L. E., & Sattin, R. W. (1991). Suicides among older United States residents: Epidemiologic characteris-tics and trends. *American Journal of Public Health*, 18, 1198-1200.

Miller, F. G, Quill, T. E., Brody, H., Fletcher, J. C., Gostin, L. O., & Meier, D. E. (1994). Sounding board: Regulating physician-assisted death. *The New England Journal of Medicine*, 331, 119-123.

Miro, R. (1994, October 13). *Compassion in dying*. Public talk presented at Trinity University, San Antonio, TX.

Morrison, R. S., Olson, E., Mertz, K. R., Meier, D. E. (1995). The inaccessibility of advance directives on transfer from ambulatory to acute care settings. *Journal of the American Medical Association*, 274(6), 478-487.

Nationline: Grim numbers on elderly, suicide. (1992, December 11). *USA Today*, p. 12A.

Platt, M. (1980). Would human life he better without death? *Soundings: An Interdisciplinary Journal*, 63(3), 321-338.

A Psychology Today questionnaire: You & death. (1970, August). *Psychology Today*, pp. 67-72.

Riley, J. (1983). Dying and the meanings of death: Sociological inquiries. *Annual Review of Sociology*, 9, 191-216.

Rollin, B. (1985). *Last wish*. New York: Linden/Simon & Schuster.

Rosenblatt, A., Greenberg, J., Solomon, S., Pyszczynski, T., & Lyon, D. (1989). Evidence for terror management theory: I. The effects of mortality salience on reactions to those who violate or uphold cultural values. *Journal of Personality and Social Psychology*, 57(4), 681-690.

Rothenberg, R., Lentzner, H. R., & Parker, R. A. (1991). Population aging patterns: The expansion of mortality. *Journal of Gerontology*, 46, S66-S70.

Shneidman, E. (Ed.). (1980). *Death: Current perspectives* (2nd ed.). Palo Alto, CA: Mayfield.

Smith, D. E. (1980*). Inside the great house: Planter family life in eighteenth-century* Chesapeake society. Ithaca, NY: Cornell University Press.

Solomon, M. Z., O'Donnell, L., Jennings, B., Guilfoy, V., Wolf, S. M., Nolan, K., Jackson, R., Koch-Weser, D., & Donnelley, S. (1993). Decisions near the end of life: Professional views on life-sustaining treatments. *American Journal of Public Health*, 83, 14-23.

Time/CNN Poll conducted by Yankelovich. (1992). *Beyond the year 2000* [Special issue]. 140(27), 12-13.

U.S. Bureau of the Census. (1992). *Statistical abstract of the United States: 1993*. Washington, DC: U.S. Government Printing Office.

U.S. House Select Committee on Aging. (1987). *Exploding the myths: Caregiving in America* (Comm. Pub. No. 99-611). Washington, DC: U.S. Government Printing Office.

U.S. Senate Committee on Finance. (1994). *End of life: Issues and implementation of advanced directives under health care reform* (Comm. Pub. No. 103:1008). Washington, DC: U.S. Government Printing Office.

Walter, T. (1993). Sociologists never die: British sociology and death. In D. Clark (Ed.), *The sociology of death* (pp. 264-295). Oxford, UK: Blackwell/The Sociological Review.

Weisman, A. (1972). *On dying and denying*. New York: Behavioral Publications.

Weisman, A. (1978). An appropriate death. In R. Fulton, E. Markusen, G. Owen, & J. L. Scheiber (Eds.), *Death and identity: Challenge and change* (pp. 193-194). Reading, MA: Addison-Wesley.

—by Michael C. Kearl

Michael C. Kearl is a professor of sociology at Trinity University in San Antonio, Texas. He teaches and publishes in the areas of social gerontology, death and dying, generations, social psychology, knowledge, and the sociology of time. He is author of *Endings: A Sociology of Death and Dying* and coauthor with Chad Gordon of *Social Psychology: Shaping Identity, Thought, and Conduct*. During the 1980s he served as a public member of the Texas State Board of Morticians and served on the advisory board of St. Benedict's Hospice. He is currently working on *The American Mind: Social Connections & Mental Processes*, a CHIPendale-based workbook for analyzing causal models, and *The Times of our Lives*, a collection of essays regarding time's role in everyday life.

Part Seven

Additional Help
and Information

Chapter 48

Glossary

adult foster care: Involves a family caring for a dependent person

caloric restriction: An experimental approach to studying longevity in which life spans of laboratory animals have been extended by reducing calories while the necessary level of nutrients is maintained.

cell senescence: The stage at which a cell has stopped dividing permanently.

chromosomes: Structures in the cell's nucleus, made up of protein and DNA, that contain the genes.

cytokines: Proteins that are secreted by cells and regulate the behavior of other nearby cells through signals. Cytokine signals trigger activity in some types of immune cells, and cause changes in many different types of cells throughout the body.

DHEA (dehydroepiandrosterone): A chemical made by the adrenal glands, which sit on top of each kidney. Although it is not known whether DHEA itself causes hormonal effects, the body breaks DHEA down into two hormones that are known to affect us in many ways: estrogen and testosterone.

Excerpted from Elder Action: Action Ideas for Older Persons and Their Families, *In Search of the Secrets of Aging*, National Institute of Aging "Age Pages," NIH Pub. No. 93-2756, Second Edition 1996, National Institute on Aging (NIA), NIH Pub. No. 94-3452, NIH Pub. No. 93-3256, and *Talking with Your Doctor: A Guide for Older People*, December 1994.

DNA (deoxyribonucleic acid): A large molecule that carries the genetic information necessary for all cellular functions, including the building of proteins.

diagnosis: The identification of a disease or physical problem. The doctor makes a diagnosis based on the symptoms the patient is experiencing and on the results of his or her examination, laboratory work, and other tests.

estrogen: The female hormone estrogen is used in hormone replacement therapy to relieve discomforts of menopause. Produced mainly, by the ovaries, it shoes the bone thinning that accompanies aging and may help prevent frailty and disability. repaired may help determine the rate of aging.

free radicals: Molecules with unpaired electrons that react readily with other molecules. Oxygen free radicals, produced during metabolism, damage cells and may be responsible for aging in tissues and organs.

gene: A segment of DNA that contains the "code" for a specific protein or other product.

gene expression: The process by which genes are transcribed and translated into proteins. Age-related changes in gene expression may account for some of the phenomena of aging.

glycation: The process by which glucose links with proteins and causes them to bind together, thus stiffening tissues and leading to the complications of diabetes and perhaps some of the physiologic problems associated with aging.

group homes: Provide independent, private living in a house shared by several senior citizens who split the cost of rent, housekeeping services, utilities, and meals.

guaiac stool test: This stool test is sometimes called a "fecal" or "stool" occult test or "hemoccult" test. This test can find unseen blood in stool samples. Your doctor can give you a simple kit to collect stool samples at home. Or, your doctor can do the test as part of a rectal exam.

Hayflick limit: The finite number of divisions of which a cell is capable.

human growth hormone: A chemical made by the pituitary gland, just under the brain, and important for normal development and maintenance of our tissues and organs. It is especially important for normal growth in children

independent retirement housing: Providing meals, activities, house-keeping and maintenance to more active seniors.

interleukins: A type of cytokine. The amount present in the body varies with age.

insomnia: Taking a long time to fall asleep (more than 30 to 45 minutes), waking up many times each night, or waking up early and being unable to get back to sleep.

lymphocytes: Small white blood cells that are important to the immune system. A decline in lymphocyte function with advancing age is being studied for insights into aging and disease.

mammogram: An x-ray of the breast

maximum life span: The greatest age reached by any member of a given species.

melatonin: This hormone from the pineal gland responds to light and seems to regulate sleep onset, timing of sleep-wake phases, and seasonal changes in the body.

mitochondria: Cell organelles that metabolize sugars into energy. Mitochondria also contain DNA, which is damaged by the high level of free radicals produced in the mitochondria.

pap smear: A test usually done at the same time as the pelvic exam. During this test, the doctor removes a few cells from the cervix with a swab. The cells then are checked under a microscope.

pelvic exam: A test where the doctor feels the internal sex organs, bladder, and rectum for any changes in size or shape.

photoaging: The process initiated by sunlight through which the skin becomes drier and loses elasticity. Photoaging is being studied for clues to aging because it has the same effect as normal aging on certain skin cells.

proliferative genes: Genes that promote cell division or proliferation; also known as oncogenes.

prostate-specific antigen test (PSA): This test measures the level of a specific protein in a man's blood. The protein seems to increase in cases of prostate cancer and other prostate diseases.

proteins: Molecules made up of amino acids arranged in a specific order determined by the genetic code. Proteins are essential for all life processes. Certain ones, such as the enzymes that protect against free radicals and the lymphokines produced in the immune system, are being studied extensively by gerontologists.

rectal exam: In this test, the doctor gently feels for any bumps or irregular areas on the rectum.

sigmoidoscopy or "procto": The doctor looks for cancer in the colon and rectum with a thin, lighted instrument called a sigmoidoscope.

sleep apnea: A common problem that causes breathing to stop for periods of up to 2 minutes, many times each night. Central sleep apnea happens when the respiratory muscles do not function as they should; obstructive sleep apnea happens when something blocks the flow of air through the neck passage.

symptom: Evidence of a disease or disorder in the body. Examples of symptoms include pain, fever, unexplained weight loss or gain, or disrupted sleep.

telomeres: Repeated DNA sequences found at the ends of chromosomes; telomeres shorten each time a cell divides.

testosterone: The male hormone testosterone is produced in the testes and may decline with age, though less frequently or, significantly than estrogen in women.

transrectal ultrasound (TRUS): A test which detects cancer by using sound waves produced by an instrument inserted into the rectum. The waves bounce off the prostate, and the pattern of the echoes made by the waves is converted to a picture by computer. TRUS is not a routine test. The doctor will use this exam to help diagnose a man's problem.

trophic factors: Substances that help control the growth and repair of our tissues and organs throughout our lives. Some trophic factors are considered hormones. Researchers are studying them to find out if decreasing levels of these factors are responsible, at least in part, for the diseases and disabilities seen in aging.

tumor suppressor genes: Genes that inhibit cell division or proliferation.

Chapter 49

Additional Reading

Depression, Grief, and Loss

How To Survive the Loss of a Love, Melba Colgrove, Los Angeles; Prelude Press, 1991.

Principles of Geriatric Medicine and Gerontology: Third Edition, Hazzard WR, ed., New York: McGraw-Hill, Inc., 1994, pp 1103-1110.

Growing Old

A Consumer's Guide to Aging, Dr. David H. Solomon, et al., Baltimore: The Johns Hopkins University Press, 1992.

Enjoy Old Age: A Program of Self Management, B.F.Skinner & M.E. Vaughan, NYC: Norton, 1983.

Old Age Is Not For Sissies, Art Linkletter, New York: Penguin Books 1988.

The Second 50 Years: Reference Manual for Senior Citizens, Walter J. Cheney, William J. Diehm, Frank E. Seeley, New York: Athena Books, 1992.

Memory

Don't Forget: Easy Exercises for a Better Memory at Any Age, D.C. Lapp, NYC: McGraw Hill, 1987.

Memory, B. Gordon, New York: Master Media, 1995.

Memory Fitness Over Forty, R. West, Gainesville, Fla: Triad, 1985.

Memory Loss in Later Life, Nancy L. Mace and Peter V. Rabins, M.D., Baltimore: The Johns Hopkins University Press, 1991.

Super Memory, D.J. Herrmann, Emmaus, PA: Rodale, 1990.

Your Memory. (2nd. edition), K.L. Higbee, Englewood Cliffs, N.J.: Prentice Hall, 1988.

Women and Aging

The Change: Women, Aging and the Menopause, Germaine Greer, New York: Knopf Random House, 1992.

Choice Years, Judith Paige and Pamela Gordon. New York: Villard Books, 1991.

Managing Your Menopause, Wulf H. Utian, M.D., Ph.D., and Ruth S. Jacobowitz. New York: Fireside/Simon & Schuster, 1990.

*The Menopause, Hormone Therapy, and Women's Health —
Background Paper*. Congress of the United States, Office of Technology Assessment, May 1992.

Menopause and Midlife Health, Morris Notelovitz and Diana Tonnesen, New York: St. Martin's Press, 1994.

Menopause News, ed. Judy Askew, 2074 Union St., San Francisco, CA 94123.

The Menopause Self-Help Book, Susan M. Lark, M.D. Berkeley: Celestial Arts, 1990.

The New Ourselves Growing Older, Paula Brown Doress and Diane Laskin Siegal. New York: Simon and Schuster, 1994 (in cooperation with the Boston Women's Health Book Collective).

The Silent Passage: Menopause, Gail Sheehy, New York: Random House, 1991.

Who, What, Where? Resources for Women's Health & Aging, National Institute on Aging, March 1992.

Grandparenting

The Grandparents' Guide is available free of charge from the Consumer Information Center (Item 606E), Pueblo, Colorado 81009

Retirement

The Only Retirement Guide You'll Ever Need, Kathryn and Ross Petras, Simon & Schuster.

Retire Smart, David and Virginia Cleary, Allworth Press.

Chapter 50

Who Cares: Sources of Information about Health Care Products and Services

Introduction

Every day, millions of senior citizens face questions about health-related products and services they see in the marketplace, get in the mail, read about in the newspaper, and hear about on radio and television. Unfortunately, it can be difficult for consumers to tell the difference between facts and fiction when it comes to selecting a health care product or service.

The Federal Trade Commission and your state Attorney General, as well as other agencies and organizations, can help you see through misleading or deceptive claims and protect your consumer rights.

The FTC and your state Attorney General have written this article to help you learn how to spot misleading or deceptive claims and where to get information; whether you're managing your own health care or that of a family member or a friend. We hope it will encourage you to ask questions and speak out if your instincts tell you that something about a health care product or service may not measure up to its promise.

Hearing Aids

"My hearing aid doesn't work too well. The dealer won't repair it to my satisfaction, even though his advertisement said the hearing aid was guaranteed. He hasn't given me a refund either. What can I do?"

A publication from the Federal Trade Commission and the National Association of Attorneys General, undated.

More than 24 million Americans have some type of hearing impairment. Many people can benefit from a hearing aid, but not everyone. How will you know? The process begins with a careful fitting by a qualified audiologist or seller. Be sure to ask about a trial period when you can test the aid for free. Ask about guarantees and warranties, too. It's important to get these in writing.

Regulations that cover many important aspects of hearing aid sales for consumers are enforced by the U.S. Food and Drug Administration. One regulation requires that you are told about the need for a medical evaluation by a physician before you buy an aid; another requires that aids come with instruction books covering use, maintenance, and repair.

Who Cares:

State Attorney General

Federal Trade Commission
Division of Marketing Practices
6th Street and Pennsylvania Ave., NW
Washington, D.C 20580 202-326-3128

Food and Drug Administration
Consumer Affairs Information Line
1-800-532-4440 (toll-free)

American Speech-Language-Hearing Association
Consumer Hot Line 1-800-638-8255 (toll-free)

National Institute On Deafness and Other Communication Disorders
Information Clearinghouse
1-800-241-1044 (toll-free/voice)

Switching Prescriptions

"I've been taking a prescription drug that really helps control a chronic problem. The pharmacist just called to say that my doctor switched me to a different drug. He says the switch will save me money because it will cost my drug-benefit plan less. But I don't know why I should switch. The new drug might not work as well. Am I giving up quality just to save the drug plan a few cents? Can I talk to my drug man about refusing the switch?"

In the past few years, many prescription drug companies have formed business relationships with pharmacy groups and insurance companies that handle drug-benefit plans. In some cases, pharmacies and insurers receive rebates or other financial incentives when they convince a plan member to switch to a different drug made by a "partner" manufacturer.

If you are uncomfortable about making a switch, call the Food and Drug Administration, your local Department of Health, or your local Board of Pharmacy. They can help you decide whether it makes sense to change your medication.

Meantime, you may want to ask your pharmacist or physician a few important questions: Will the new drug work as well for your condition? Are there different side effects or risks? Are the dosage levels the same? Is there a business connection between the pharmacist and the drug manufacturer? Will the switch save you or your benefit plan money or cost you money?

Who Cares:

State Attorney General
Federal Trade Commission
Division of Service Industry Practices
6th Street and Pennsylvania Ave., NW
Washington, D.C. 20580 202-326-3305

Food and Drug Administration
Consumer Affairs Information Line
1-800-532-4440 (toll-free)

National Institute on Aging Information Center
1-800-222-2225 (toll-free/voice)
1-800-222-4225 (toll-free TTY)

Local Board of Health

Local Board of Pharmacy

American Pharmaceutical Association
Patient Information 1-800-237-2742 (toll-free)

U.S. Pharmacopoeia
1-800-488-2665 (toll-free)

American Association of Retired Persons
601 E Street, NW
Washington, D.C. 20049
202-434-2277

Nursing Facilities

"My father is in a nursing facility. I'm really worried about him. He's losing weight. He seems disoriented. I hope he is receiving decent care. But how can I find out? Who can I talk to? What can I do?"

Every nursing home should have a complaint procedure policy. If you have concerns or complaints, ask about the policy and follow the organization's procedures. You also may want to ask the nurse in charge to review your family member's care plan. If you still are uncomfortable with the situation, speak to the director of nursing, the social worker, or the administrator or check to see if the nursing home has a family council, a group of advocates who try to improve the quality of life in the home.

Often, nursing homes operated by large corporations have toll-free telephone numbers you can use to speak to a regional supervisor.

Who Cares:

State Ombudsman

State Department of Licensing and Certificate

State or local Office on Aging

State Health or Welfare Department

State Attorney General

U.S. Administration on Aging
Eldercare Locator 1-800-677-1116 (toll-free)

American Association of Homes and Services for the Aging
1-800-508-9442 (toll-free)

National Citizens Coalition for Nursing Home Reform
1424 16th Street, NW, Suite 202
Washington, D.C 20036-2211
202-332-2275

Alternative Medicines

"My brother has been diagnosed with cancer. He wants to find out about alternative medicine as a possible treatment. He has seen ads for a clinic that claims to have an amazing success rate using unconventional approaches to cure many forms of cancer and other serious ailments. Should he believe them?"

Many unconventional treatments for cancer and other diseases are on the market. A few have undergone rigorous scientific testing for their curative value. Many that have been tested don't show effectiveness. Still, some forms of alternative therapy are recognized as helpful in caring for patients and helping them cope with some illnesses.

Usually, a primary care physician is the best source of information about alternative medicine as a supplement to conventional treatments. If someone tries to sell you an alternative treatment by promising that it is effective, ask for a copy of the studies that prove it. Then ask your primary care physician or family doctor to review the studies to determine their credibility.

If you think you've been misled by advertisements for either alternative medicine or conventional treatments, be cautious and complain.

Who Cares:

State Attorney General

Federal Trade Commission
Division of Service Industry Practices
6th Street and Pennsylvania Ave., NW
Washington, D.C. 20580
202-326-3305

Food and Drug Administration
Consumer Affairs Information Line
1-800-532-4440 (toll-free)

National Cancer Institute
Cancer Information Service
1-800-422-6237 (toll-free)

American Cancer Society
1-800-227-2345 (toll-free)

Cataract Surgery

"My vision is getting worse. Things look pretty foggy. It's hard for me to drive at night because headlights really bother me. Today's newspaper had an ad about a large medical center that specializes in cataract surgery. The ad says the surgery is simple and has no risks. The center guarantees that patients will be able to see perfectly after surgery. I don't know what to do."

Cataracts are a normal part of aging; they usually develop over time and don't have to be removed immediately. You generally can wait to have the surgery until your vision begins to bother you.

If your doctor tells you that you have a cataract, ask whether you need surgery right away, what your risks are based on your general health, and what type of surgery may be appropriate for you, should you choose it.

Be suspicious of any promotion promising completely successful, risk-free cataract surgery. Cataract surgery has a very high success rate, but no surgery is free from risk. Serious complications are rare, but when they do occur, they could result in loss of vision.

Who Cares

State Attorney General

Federal Trade Commission
Division of Service Industry Practices
Street and Pennsylvania Ave., NW
Washington, D.C. 20580
326-3305

National Eye Institute
Bethshda, MD 20892
301-496-5248

National Society to Prevent Blindness
1-800-331-2020 (toll-free)

American Academy of Ophthalmology
National Eye Care Project Helpline
1-800-222-3937 (toll-free)

National Center for Vision and Aging
1-800-334-5497 (toll-free)

Prevent Blindness America
1-800-331-2020 (toll-free)

Arthritis Cure

"I saw an ad in the paper that said, 'CURE YOUR ARTHRITIS WITHOUT DRUGS WITH THIS ALL-NATURAL, GOVERNMENT-APPROVED REMEDY.' The idea of a 'natural' remedy appeals to me and I'm impressed that the ad says the product is 'approved' by a government agency. But I think these so-called cures sometimes promise more than they can deliver. How can I get more information about products like this?"

The U.S. Department of Health and Human Services' National Health Information Center can help you get in touch with public and private groups that have information about traditional and alternative therapies for arthritis and other conditions. Your public library also may have a computer link to provide you with direct access to the National Health Information Center.

To check on whether a product is "government approved," to learn more about an over-the-counter drug, prescription drug, cosmetic, or medical device, or to report an adverse reaction to any of these products, call the Food and Drug Administration's Consumer Affairs Information Line.

For the latest information on vitamins and nutritional supplements, call the FDA's Center for Food Safety and Applied Nutrition.

Who Cares:

State Attorney General

Federal Trade Commission
Division of Advertising Practices
6th Street and Pennsylvania Ave., NW
Washington, DC 20580
202-326-3131

U.S. Department of Health and Human Services
National Health Information Center
1-800-336-4797 (toll-free)

Food and Drug Administration
Consumer Affairs Information Line
1-800-532-4440 (toll-free)

Food and Drug Administration
Center for Food Safety and Applied Nutrition
1-800-332-4010 (toll-free)

Direct-Mail Schemes

"Someone sent me a newspaper clipping with a product that's supposed to reverse the effects of aging. On the article was a handwrit-
ten note that said, 'Try this. It works! R.' I don't know who R is. Is
this product on the level? What should I do?"

Some direct-mail marketers advertise their products through ads
disguised as "clippings" sent by unnamed "friends." The fact is that
R doesn't exist. The company got your name from a mailing list and
sent the note from R to you and thousands of other consumers.

Other popular tricks are to design the envelope to look like a check
or letter from a government agency, or to mimic the style of urgent
overnight mail deliveries.

If a company uses a deceptive tactic on the outside of an envelope,
be skeptical about what's inside, too. Report any questionable solici-
tation you receive in the mail to your local Postmaster or Postal Inspector.

Check the phone book for the phone number.

Who Cares:

Chief Postal Inspector
United States Postal Service
Washington, D.C.
202-268-4298

State Attorney General

Federal Trade Commission
Division of Advertising Practices
6th Street and Pennsylvania Ave., NW
Washington, D.C. 20580
202-326-3131

National Institute on Aging
Information Center
1-800-222-2225 (toll-free/voice)
1-800-222-4225 (toll-free/TTY)

Abusive Care-Givers

"I have a home health aide who cooks for me because I live alone and I can't cook for myself anymore. Her cooking is so bad that sometimes I can't eat what she makes. She hits me. I'm afraid to tell anyone because the agency never does anything about it when my friends complain about their aides. I'm afraid no one will believe me. If I report her and she finds out, she'll hurt me more. I don't know what to do."

No one should be abused-physically or verbally-by anyone, including family members or care-givers. Everyone has the right to feel safe and secure in their own home. If you or someone you know is being abused in any way, report it. Everyone has the right to be protected.

Who Cares:

Local Police, Sheriff's Office, or State Attorney General

State Department of Aging

U.S. Administration On Aging
Eldercare Locator
1-800-677-1116 (toll-free)

Who to Contact if You are Deceived

Think you've been mislead or deceived by an advertisement for a health care product or service or a medical procedure? Contact your state Attorney General, or the Federal Trade Commission in Washington, DC or at one of the 10 FTC regional offices:

1718 Peachtree Street, NW, Suite 1000
Atlanta, GA 30367
404-347-4836

101 Merrimac Street, Suite 810
Boston, MA 02114
617-424-5960

55 East Monroe Street, Suite 810
Chicago, IL 60603
312-353-4423

668 Euclid Avenue, Suite 520-A
Cleveland, OH 44114
216-522-4207

1999 Bryan Street, Suite 2150
Dallas, TX 75201
214-979-0213

1961 Stout Street, Suite 1523
Denver, CO 80294
303-844-2271

11000 Wilshire Boulevard, Suite 13209
Los Angeles, CA 90024
310-235-4000

150 William Street, Suite 1300
New York, NY 10038
212-264-1207

901 Market Street, Suite 570
San Francisco, CA 94103
415-356-5270

2806 Federal Building
915 Second Avenue
Seattle, WA 98174
206-220-6363

Federal Trade Commission
6th Street & Pennsylvania Ave., NW
Room 403
Washington, D.C. 20580
World Wide Web Site at: http:\ \www.ftc.gov

State Attorney General
Office of Consumer Protection for Your State Capital

(Many Attorneys General have toll-free consumer hotlines. Check with
your local directory assistance.)

Chapter 51

Who's Who in Healthcare

In many cases, the family doctor is no longer the sole provider of medical care and advice for older Americans. Older people are treated not only by doctors and nurses, but by technicians, medical assistants, and therapists. With this variety of health providers, it is important to understand which professionals can offer the best and least costly care for a specific problem and which services normally will be paid by Medicare.

The following definitions cover some, but not all, of the medical practitioners frequently seen by older people.

Doctors of medicine (M.D.) use all accepted methods of medical care. They treat disease and injuries, provide preventive care, do routine checkups, prescribe drugs, and do some surgery. M.D.'s complete medical school plus 3 to 7 years of graduate medical education. They must be licensed by the state in which they practice.

Doctors of osteopathic medicine (D.O.) provide general health care to individuals and families. The training osteopaths receive is similar to that of an M.D. In addition to treating patients with drugs, surgery, and other treatments, a D.O. may emphasize movement in treating problems of muscles, bones, and joints.

Family practitioners are M.D.'s or D.O.'s who specialize in providing comprehensive, continuous health care for all family members, regardless of age or sex.

A National Institute on Aging "Age Page," 1991.

Geriatricians are physicians with special training in the diagnosis, treatment, and prevention of disorder in older people. Geriatric medicine recognizes aging as a normal process, not a disease state.

Internists (M.D. or D.O.) specialize in the diagnosis and medical treatment of diseases in adults. Internists do not deliver babies.

Surgeons treat diseases, injuries, and deformities by operating on the body. A general surgeon is qualified to perform many common operations, but many specialize in one area of the body. For example, neurosurgeons treat disorders relating to the nervous system, spinal cord, and brain; orthopedic surgeons treat disorders of the bones, joints, muscle, ligaments, and tendons; and thoracic surgeons treat disorders to the chest.

The above physicians may refer patients to the following specialists:

- Cardiologist—a heart specialist
- Dermatologist—a skin specialist
- Endocrinologist—a specialist in disorders of the glands of internal secretion, such as diabetes
- Gastroenterologist—a specialist in diseases of the digestive tract
- Gynecologist—a specialist in the female reproductive system
- Hematologist—a specialist in disorders of the blood
- Nephrologist—a specialist in the function and diseases of the kidneys
- Neurologist—a specialist in disorders of the nervous system
- Oncologist—a specialist in cancer
- Ophthalmologist—an eye specialist
- Otolaryngologist—a specialist in diseases of the ear, nose, and throat
- Physiatrist—a specialist in physical medicine and rehabilitation
- Psychiatrist—a specialist in mental, emotional, and behavioral disorders
- Pulmonary specialist—a physician who treats disorders of the lungs and chest
- Rheumatologist—a specialist in arthritis and rheumatism

- Urologist—a specialist in the urinary system in both sexes and the male reproductive system.

Most of the services of M.D.'s and D.O.'s are covered by Medicare.

Dental Care

Dentists (D.D.S. or D.M.D.) treat oral conditions such as gum disease and tooth decay. They give regular checkups and routine dental and preventive care, fill cavities, remove teeth, provide dentures, and check for cancers in the mouth. Dentists can prescribe medication and perform oral surgery. A general Dentist might refer patients to a specialist such as an oral surgeon, who does difficult tooth removals and surgery on the jaw; an endodontist, who is an expert on root canals; a periodontist, who is knowledgeable about gum diseases; or a dentist who specializes in geriatrics. Medicare will not pay for any dental care except for surgery on the jaw or facial bones.

Eye Care

Ophthalmologists (M.D. or D.O.) specialize in the diagnosis and treatment of eye diseases. They also prescribe eyeglasses and contact lenses. Ophthalmologists can prescribe drugs and perform surgery. They often treat older people who have glaucoma and cataracts. Medicare helps pay for all medically necessary surgery or treatment of eye diseases and for exams and eyeglasses to correct vision after cataract surgery. But it will not pay for a routine exam, eyeglasses, or contact lenses.

Optometrists (O.D.) generally have a bachelor's degree plus 4 years of graduate training in a school of optometry. They are trained to diagnose eye abnormalities and prescribe, supply, and adjust eyeglasses and contact lenses. In most states optometrists can use drugs to diagnose eye disorders. An optometrist may refer patients to an ophthalmologist or other medical specialist in cases requiring medication or surgery. Medicare pays for only a limited number of optometric services.

Opticians fit, supply, and adjust eyeglasses and contact lenses which have been prescribed by an ophthalmologist or optometrist. They cannot examine or test the eyes, or prescribe glasses or drugs. Opticians are licensed in 22 states and may have formal training. Traditionally, most opticians are trained on the job.

Mental Health Care

Psychiatrists (M.D. or D.O.) treat people with mental and emotional difficulties. They can prescribe medication and counsel patients, as well as perform diagnostic tests to determine if there are physical problems. Medicare will pay for a portion of both inpatient and outpatient psychiatric costs.

Psychologists (Ph.D., Psy.D., Ed.D., or M.A.) are health care professionals trained and licensed to assess, diagnose, and treat people with mental, emotional, or behavioral disorders. Psychologists counsel people through individual, group, or family therapy. Medicare will pay for a portion of psychologists' counseling services when performed in connection with the services of a psychiatrist or other physician.

Nursing Care

Registered nurses (R.N.) may have 2, 3, or 4 years of education in a nursing school. In addition to giving medicine, administering treatments, and educating patients, R.N.'s also work in doctors' offices, clinics, and community health agencies. Medicare does not cover private duty nursing. It helps pay for general nursing services by reimbursing hospitals, skilled nursing facilities, and home health agencies for part of the nurses' salaries.

Nurse practitioners (R.N. or N.P.) are registered nurses with training beyond basic nursing education. They perform physical examinations and diagnostic tests, counsel patients, and develop treatments programs. Nurse practitioners may work independently, such as in rural clinics, or may be staff members at hospitals and other health facilities. They are educated in a number of specialties, including gerontological nursing. Medicare will help pay for services performed under the supervision of a doctor.

Licensed practical nurses (L.P.N.) have from 12 to 18 months of training and are most frequently found in hospitals and long term care facilities where they provide much of the routine patient care. They also assist physicians and registered nurses.

Rehabilitative Care

Occupational therapists (O.T.) assist those whose ability to function has been impaired by accident, illness, or other disability.

They increase or restore independence in feeding, bathing, dressing, homemaking, and social experiences through specialized activities designed to improve function. Occupational therapy services are paid by Medicare if the patient is in a hospital or a skilled nursing facility or is receiving home health care. Coverage is also available for services provided in physicians' offices or to hospital outpatients, O.T.'s have either a bachelor's or master's degree with special training in occupational therapy.

Physical therapists (P.T.) help people whose strength, ability to move, or sensation is impaired. They may use exercise; heat, cold, or water therapy; or other treatments to control pain, strengthen muscles, and improve coordination. All P.T.'s complete a bachelor's degree and some receive further postgraduate training. Patients are usually referred to a physical therapist by a doctor, and Medicare pays some of the costs of outpatient treatments. Physical therapy performed in a hospital or skilled nursing facility is covered by Medicare.

Speech-language pathologists are concerned with speech and language problems. Audiologists are concerned with hearing disorders. Both specialists test and evaluate patients and provide treatment to restore as much normal function as possible. Many speech-language pathologists work with stroke victims, people who have had their vocal cords removed, or those who have developmental speech and language disorders. Audiologists work with people who have difficulty hearing. They recommend and sometimes dispense hearing aids. Speech-language pathologists and audiologists have at least a master's degree. Most are licensed by the state in which they practice. Medicare generally will cover the diagnostic services of speech-language pathologists and audiologists; it will not cover routine hearing evaluations or hearing aid services.

General Care

Pharmacists are knowledgeable about the chemical makeup and correct use of medicines—the names, ingredients, side effects, and uses in the treatment of medical problems. Pharmacists have legal authority to dispense drugs according to formal instructions issued by physicians, dentists, or podiatrists. They also can provide information on nonprescription products sold in pharmacies. Pharmacists must complete 5 or 6 years of college, fulfill a practical experience requirement, and pass a state licensing examination to practice.

477

Physician assistants (P.A.) usually work in hospital's or doctor's offices and do some of the tasks traditionally performed by doctors, such as taking medical histories and doing physical examination. Education for a P.A. includes 2 to 4 years of college followed by a 2-year period of specialized training. P.A.'s must always be under the supervision of a doctor. Medicare will pay for the services provided by a P.A. only if they are performed in a hospital or doctor's office under the supervision of a physician.

Podiatrists (D.P.M.) diagnose, treat, and prevent diseases and injuries of the foot. They may do surgery, make devices to correct or prevent foot problems, provide toenail care, and prescribe certain drugs. A podiatrist completes 4 years of professional school and is licensed. Medicare will cover the cost of their services except routine foot care. (However, routine foot care is covered if it is necessary because of diabetic complications.)

Registered dietitians (R.D.) provide nutrition care services and dietary counseling in health and disease. Most work in hospitals, public health agencies, or doctors' offices, but some are in private practice. R.D.'s complete a bachelor's or a graduate degree with a program in dietetics/nutrition and complete an approved program in dietetic practice such as an internship. Medicare generally will not pay for dietitian services; however, it does reimburse hospitals and skilled nursing facilities for a portion of dietitian's salaries.

"Nutritionist" is a broad term. Currently, practitioners who wish to call themselves nutritionists need not fulfill a licensing or certification requirement. The title may be used by a wide range of people, including R.D.'s, those who take a correspondence or other short-term course in nutrition, or even people who are self-taught. Before seeking the advice of a health practitioner in nutrition, it is a good idea to ask what kind of training and practical experience the person has received.

Social workers in health care settings go after community services for patients, provide counseling when necessary, and help patients and their families handle problems related to physical and mental illness and disability. They frequently coordinate the multiple aspects of care related to illness, including discharge planning from hospitals. A social worker's education ranges from a bachelor's degree to a doctorate. Most have a master's degree (M.S.W.). Medicare covers services provided by social workers if they work in such settings as hospitals, home health care agencies, hospices, and health maintenance organizations.

These and other health professionals are especially important to older adults, some of whom require a great deal of medical attention. Ideally, all health professionals will work together to provide older people with care that is comprehensive, cost-effective, and compassionate.

For additional resources on health and aging, write to the National Institute on Aging Information Center, P.O. Box 8057, Gaithersburg, MD 20898-8057.

Chapter 52

Resources

Administration on Aging's Elder Care Locator
800-677-1116

Agency for Health Care Policy and Research (AHCPR)
P.O. Box 8547
Silver Spring, MD 20907
800-358-9295; 888-586-6340 (hearing impaired)
E-mail: info@ahcpr.gov
Internet: http://www.ahcpr.gov/consumer/

Alzheimer's Association
Suite 1000, 919 North Michigan Avenue
Chicago, IL 60611
800-272-3900; 312-335-1110
Fax: 312-335-1110
E-mail: info@alz.org
Internet: http://www.alz.org

Alzheimer's Disease Education and Referral (ADEAR) Center
P.O. Box 8250
Silver Spring, MD 20907-8250
800-438-4380; Fax: 301-495-3334
E-mail: adear@alzheimers.org
Internet: http://www.alzheimers.org

American Association of Nurse Anesthetists (AANA)
222 S. Prospect Avenue
Park Ridge, IL 60068-4001
847-692-7050.
Fax: 847-692-6968
E-mail: info@aana.com
Internet: http://www.aana.com

AARP (American Association of Retired Persons)
601 E. St. N.W.
Washington, DC 20049
800-424-3410
E-mail: member@aarp.org
Internet: http://www.aarp.org/

AARP Pharmacy
PO Box 883
Libertyville, IL 60048
800-424-3410
Internet: http://www.inetport.com/~gra/aarpp.htm

American College of Sports Medicine
P.O. Box 1440
Indianapolis, IN 46206-1440
317-637-9200
Fax: 317-634-7817
E-mail: devacsm@acsm.org
Internet: http://acsm.org

American College of Surgeons
633 North Saint Clair Street
Chicago, IL 60611
312-202-5000
Fax: 312-202-5001
E-mail: postmaster@facs.org
Internet: http://www.facs.org

American Heart Association
National Center
Public Information Department
7272 Greenville Avenue
Dallas, TX 75231-4596
214-373-6300
E-mail: ncrp@heart.org
Internet: http://www.amhrt.org

American Society of Anesthesiologists (ASA)
520 North Northwest Highway
Park Ridge, IL 60068
847-825-5586
Fax: 847-825-1692
E-mail: mail@ASAhq.org
Internet: http://www.asahq.org

Cancer Information Service (CIS)
800-4-CANCER

Children of Aging Parents
Suite 302-A 1609 Woodbourne Road
Levittown, PA 19057-1511
215-945-6900

Choice in Dying
1035 30th Street, NW
Washington, DC 20007
202-338-9790
Fax: 202-338-0242
E-mail: CID@choices.org
Internet: http://www.choices.org

Council of Better Business Bureaus, Inc
4200 Wilson Boulevard
Suite 800
Arlington, VA 22203
703-276-0100
Fax: 703-525-8277
Internet: http://www.bbb.org/council.htm

Eldercare Locator Service
Suite 100, 1112 16th Street NW
Washington, DC 20036
800-677-1116
Internet: http://www.ageinfo.org/naicweb/elderloc/elderloc.html

Federal Trade Commission
600 Pennsylvania Avenue, NW
Washington, DC 20580
202-382-4357
Internet: http://www.ftc.gov

Food and Drug Administration
HFE-88
5600 Fishers Lane
Rockville, MD 20857
800-532-4440
Internet: http://www.fda.gov

Health Care Financing Administration
7500 Security Blvd.
Baltimore, Maryland 21244-1850
410-786-3000
Internet: http://www.hcfa.gov/

Help for Incontinent People (HIP)
P.O. Box 544
Union, SC 29379
803-579-7900
800-252-3337
Fax: 803-579-7902
E-mail: hwinfo@healthy.net
Internet: http://www.healthy.net/pan/cso/cioi/HIP.HTM

National Arthritis, Musculoskeletal and Skin Diseases Information Clearinghouse (NIAMS)
1 AMS Circle
Bethesda, MD 20892
301-495-4484
Fax: 301-587-4352
Internet: http://www.nih.gov/niams/healthinfo/info.htm

National Association of Insurance Commissioners
120 West Twelfth St., Suite 1100
Kansas City, MO 64105-1925
816-842-3600
Fax: 816-471-7004
Internet: http://www.naic.org

Office of Cancer Communications
National Cancer Institute, Building 31, Room 10A 18
Bethesda, Md. 20892
800-4-CANCER

National Center for Nutrition and Dietetics Consumer Nutrition Hotline
800-366-1655
900-225-5267

National Center on Elder Abuse
Suite 500, 810 First Street NE
Washington, DC 20002
202-682-2470

National Council on Patient Information and Education
202-347-6711

The National Council on the Aging
409 Third Street, SW
Washington, DC 20024
202-479-1200
800-424-9046
Fax: 202-479-0735
E-mail: info@ncoa.org
Internet: www.ncoa.org

National Heart, Lung, and Blood Institute Information Center
P.O. Box 30105
Bethesda, MD 20824-0105
Fax: 301-251-1223
E-mail: NHLBIIC@dgsys.com
Internet: http://guidetohealth.com/lnk/link6.html

National Hospice Organization
Suite 901, 1901 North Moore Street
Arlington, VA 22209
703-243-5900
Fax: 703-525-5762
Internet: http://www.nho.org

NIMH Depression Awareness, Recognition and Treatment Program
Room 10c-03, 5600 Fishers Lane
Rockville, MD 20857
800-421-4211

The National Institute on Aging (NIA)
Building 31, Room 5C27
31 Center Drive, MSC 2292
Bethesda, MD 20892-2292
800-222-2225
800-222-4225 (TTY)
E-mail: niainfo@access.digex.net
Internet: http://www.nih.gov/nia/health/health.htm

National Organization for Victim Assistance (NOVA)
1757 Park Rd., NW
Washington, D.C. 20010
202-232-6682
NOVA's 24 hour hotline is 1-800-TRY-NOVA
Fax: 202-462-2255
E-mail: nova@try-nova.org
Internet: http://www.try-nova.org/

National Sleep Foundation
729 Fifteenth Street, NW, Fourth Floor
Washington, DC 20005
E-mail: natsleep@aerols.com
Internet: http://www.sleepfoundation.org/default.html

National Stroke Association
96 Inverness Drive East, Suite I
Englewood, CO 80112-5112
649-9299
800-787-6537
Fax-649-1328
Internet: http://www.stroke.org

Sexuality Information and Education Council of the United States
Suite 2500, 130 West 42nd Street
New York, NY 10036
212-819-9770
Fax: 212-819-9776
E-mail: siecus@siecus.org
Internet: http://www.siecus.org/

The Simon Foundation
P.O. Box 835
Wilmette, IL 60091
800-237-4666
847-864-3913
Fax: 847-864-9758
E-mail: simoninfo@simonfoundation.org
Internet: http://www.simonfoundation.org/html/f/f.htm

United Seniors Health Cooperative (USHC)
409 Third Street, SW, Second Floor
Washington, D.C. 20045
202-479-6973
Fax: 202-479-6660
E-mail: 103707.140@compuserve.com
Internet: http://www.ushc-online.org

The U.S. Consumer Product Safety Commission (CPSC)
301-504-0990
800-638-2772
800-638-8270 (hearing impared)
Fax: 301-504-0124
Internet: http://www.cpsc.gov

U.S. Postal Service
Office of Criminal Investigation
Washington, DC 20260-2166

Weight-control Information Network
1 Win Way
Bethesda, MD 20892-3665
301-984-7378
800-WIN-8098
Fax: 301-984-7196
E-mail: win@info.niddk.nih.gov
Internet: http://www.niddk.nih.gov/health/nutrit/win.htm

USDA's Meat and Poultry Hotline
800-535-4555
202-720-3333

New Website for Seniors

Access America for Seniors—Home Page
Internet: http://www.seniors.gov

Chapter 53

State Agencies on Aging

Designated by the Governor and State Legislature, State Agencies on Aging provide leadership and guidance to the agencies and organizations serving the elderly within their State. Serving as advocates for older people, the agencies oversee a complex, statewide service system designed to complement other human service systems. State Agencies on Aging foster the expansion of community-based services and provide policy direction and technical assistance to the Area Agencies on Aging within their States. To learn more about the State aging network, contact your State Agency on Aging.

Alabama

Alabama Commission on Aging
RSA Plaza, Suite 470
770 Washington Avenue
Montgomery, AL 36130
(334) 242-5743
(334) 242-5594 fax
e-mail: mbeck@coa.state.al.us
http://webserver.dsmd.state.al.us/coa

Alaska

Alaska Commission on Aging
Division of Senior Services
Department of Administration
P.O. Box 110209
Juneau, AK 99811-0209
(907) 465-3250
(907) 465-4716 fax
http://www.state.ak.us/local/akpages/ADMIN/dss/homess.htm

Excerpted from *Resource Directory for Older People*, National Institute on Aging, NIH Pub. No. 95-738, March 1996; contact information verified and updated in 1998.

Arizona

Aging and Adult Administration
Department of Economic Security
1789 W. Jefferson, Site Code 950A
Phoenix, AZ 85007
(602) 542-4446
(602) 542-6575 fax

Arkansas

Div. of Aging and Adult Services
Arkansas Dept. of Human Services
P.O. Box 1437, Slot 1412
1417 Donaghey Plaza
South Little Rock, AR 72203-1437
(501) 682-2441
(501) 682-8155 fax
http://ww.dhs.com

California

California Department of Aging
1600 K Street
Sacramento, CA 95814
(916) 322-5290
(916) 324-1903 fax
http://www.aging.state.ca.us

Colorado

Aging and Adult Services
Department of Human Services
110 16th Street, Suite 200
Denver, CO 80202
(303) 620-4147
(303) 620-4191 fax

Connecticut

Community Services Division of
 Elderly Services
25 Sigourney Street
Hartford, CT 06106-5033
(860) 424-5277
(203) 424-4966 fax
e-mail: adultserv.dss@po.state.ct.us
http://ww.dss.state.ct.us

Delaware

Delaware Department of
 Health and Social Services
Division of Services for Aging
 and Adults with Physical
 Disabilities
Second Floor Annex
1901 North DuPont Highway
New Castle, DE 19720
(302) 577-4791
or (800) 223-9074
(302) 577-4793 fax

District of Columbia

District of Columbia Office on
 Aging
441 4th Street NW
Suite 900 South
Washington, DC 20001
(202) 724-5622
(202) 724-4979 fax
http://www.ci.washington.dc.us

Florida

Department of Elder Affairs
4040 Esplanade Way, Suite 152
Tallahassee, FL 32399-7000
(850) 414-2000
(850) 414-6216 fax
http://www.state.fl.us/doea/doea.
 html

Georgia

Division of Aging Services
Dept. of Human Resources
Thirty Sixth Floor
2 Peachtree Street, NW
Atlanta, GA 30303
(404) 657-5258
(404) 657-5285 fax

Idaho

Idaho Commission on Aging
700 W. Jefferson, Room 108
P.O. Box 83720
Boise, ID 83720
(208) 334-3833
(208) 334-3033 fax

Illinois

Illinois Department on Aging
421 E. Capitol Avenue, Suite 100
Springfield, IL 62701-1789
(217) 785-2870
(312) 814-2630 Chicago Office
(217) 785-4477 fax

Indiana

Division of Disability, Aging and
  Rehabilitative Services
Br. of Aging and In-Home Services
402 West Washington Street
Indianapolis, IN 46207-7083
(317) 232-7122 or
toll free in-state (800) 545-7763
(317) 232-7867 fax

Iowa

Department of Elder Affairs
200 Tent Street, 3rd Floor
Des Moines, IA 50309-3609
(515) 281-5187 or
complaint hotline (800) 532-3213
(515) 281-4036 fax

Kansas

Department on Aging
New England Building
503 S. Kansas
Topeka, KS 66603-3404
(913) 296-4986
(785) 296-0256 fax

Kentucky

Kentucky Office of Aging
Cabinet for Families & Children
275 E. Main Street, 5th Floor W.
Frankfort, KY 40621
(502) 564-6930
(502) 564-4595 fax

Louisiana

Governor's Office of Elderly
  Affairs
P.O. Box 80374
Baton Rouge, LA 70898-0374
(504) 342-7100
(504) 342-7133 fax

Maine

Bureau of Elder and Adult
  Services
Department of Human Services
219 Capitol Street
State House, Station 11
Augusta, ME 04333-0011
(207) 624-8060
(207) 624-8124 fax

Maryland

Maryland Office on Aging
State Office Building, Rm 1007
301 West Preston Street
Baltimore, MD 21201-2374
(410) 767-1102
(410) 333-7943 fax

Massachusetts

Massachusetts Executive Office
  of Elder Affairs
One Ashburton Place, 5th Floor
Boston, MA 02108
(617) 727-7750
(617) 727-9368 fax

Michigan

Office of Services to the Aging
P.O. Box 30676
Lansing, MI 48909
(517) 373-8230
(517) 373-7876 Director
(517) 373-4092 fax

Minnesota

Minnesota Board on Aging
444 Lafayette Road
St. Paul, MN 55155-3843
(612) 296-2770 or (800) 882-6262
(612) 297-7855 fax
http://www.dhs.state.mn.us

Mississippi

Div. of Aging and Adult Services
750 North State Street
Jackson, MS 39202
(601) 359-4925
(601) 359-4370 fax
e-mail: elanderson@mdhs.state.
  ms.us
http://www.mdhs.state.ms.us

Missouri

Division on Aging
Department of Social Services
P.O. Box 1337
615 Howerton Court
Jefferson City, MO 65102-1337
(573) 751-3082
(573) 751-8687 fax

Montana

Office on Aging
Department of Family Services
P.O. Box 8005
Helena, MT 59604-8005
(406) 444-5900 or (800) 332-2272
(406) 444-5956 fax

Nebraska

Department on Aging
P.O. Box 95044
301 Centennial Mall
South Lincoln, NE 68509-5044
(402) 471-2307
(402) 471-4619 fax
http://www.hhs.state.ne.us

Nevada

Nevada Div. for Aging Services
340 North 11th Street, Suite 203
Las Vegas, NV 89101
(702) 486-3545
(702) 486-3572 fax

New Hampshire

Div. of Elderly and Adult Services
State Office Park South
115 Pleasant St. Annex Bldg. #1
Concord, NH 03301-3843
(603) 271-4680
(603) 271-4643 fax
http://www.nhworks.state.nh.us

New Jersey

New Jersey Division on Aging
Dept. of Community Affairs
12 Quakerbridge Plaza
Trenton, NJ 08625-0807
(800) 729-8820 or (609) 558-3139
(609) 633-6609 fax

New Mexico

State Agency on Aging
La Villa Rivera Building,
  Ground Floor
228 East Palace Avenue
Santa Fe, NM 87501
(505) 827-7640
(505) 827-7649 fax

New York
NY State Office for the Aging
2 Empire State Plaza
Albany, NY 12223-1251
(800) 342-9871 or (518) 474-8388
(518) 474-0608 fax
e-mail: feedback@aging.state.ny.us
http://www.aging.state.ny.us/
nysofa

North Carolina
Division of Aging
Taylor Hall, Dorothea Dix
Hospital Campus
693 Palmer Drive
Raleigh, NC 27603
(919) 733-3983
(919) 733-0443 fax

North Dakota
Department of Human Services
Aging Services Division
600 South 2nd St., Suite 1C
Bismarck, ND 58504-5729
(701) 328-8910
(701) 328-8989 fax

Ohio
Ohio Department of Aging
50 West Broad Street, 9th Floor
Columbus, OH 43215-5928
(614) 644-7967
(614) 466-5741 fax

Oklahoma
Services for the Aging
Department of Human Services
P.O. Box 25352
Oklahoma City, OK 73125
(405) 521-2281 or 521-2327
(405) 521-2086 fax

Oregon
Senior and Disabled Services
Division
500 Summer Street NE, 2nd Floor
Salem, OR 97310-1015
(503) 945-5811
(503) 373-7823 fax
http://www.sdsd.hr.state.or.us

Pennsylvania
Pennsylvania Dept. of Aging
555 Walnut Street, 5th Floor
Harrisburg, PA 17101-1919
(717) 783-1550
(717) 783-6842 fax

Puerto Rico
Commonwealth of Puerto Rico
Governor's Office of Elderly
Affairs
P.O. Box 50063, Old San Juan
Station
San Juan, PR 00902
(787) 721-4560
(787) 721-6510 fax

Rhode Island
Department of Elderly Affairs
160 Pine Street
Providence, RI 02903-3708
(401) 222-2858

South Carolina
Department of Health and
Human Services
Office on Aging
1801 Main Street
Columbia, SC 29203-8206
(803) 253-6177
(803) 253-4173 fax

South Dakota

Office of Adult Services and
  Aging
Richard F. Kneip Building
700 Governors Drive
Pierre, SD 57501-2291
(605) 773-3656
(605) 773-6834 fax

Tennessee

Commission on Aging
Andrew Jackson Building
500 Deaderick Street
9th Floor
Nashville, TN 37243-0860
(615) 741-2056
(615) 741-3309 fax

Texas

Department on Aging
P.O. Box 12786 Capitol Station
Austin, TX 78711
(512) 424-6840
(512) 424-6890 fax
e-mail: mail@pdoa.state.tx.us
http://www.pdoa.state.tx.us

Utah

Division of Aging and Adult
  Services
Box 45500
120 North 200 West
Salt Lake City, UT 84145-0500
(801) 538-3910
(801) 538-4395 fax
e-mail:
  helengoddard@email.state.
  ut.us

Vermont

Vermont Department of Aging
  and Disabilities
Dept. of Licensing and Protection
Waterbury Complex
103 South Main Street
Waterbury, VT 05671
(802) 241-2345
(802) 241-2358 fax
e-mail: dad@vt.us
http://www.state.vt.us

Virginia

Virginia Dept. for the Aging
1600 Forest Avenue
Suite 102, Preston Bldg.
Richmond, VA 23229
(804) 662-9333
(804) 662-9354 fax
http://www.aging.state.va.us

Virgin Islands

Virgin Islands Department of
  Human Services
Knud Hansen Complex
Building A
1303 Hospital Ground
Charlotte Amalie, VI 00802
(809) 774-1166
(809) 774-3466 fax

Washington

Aging and Adult Services
  Administration
Department of Social and
  Health Services
P.O. Box 45600, M/S 45600
Olympia, WA 98504-5600
(425) 493-2500
(306) 438-8633 fax

West Virginia

West Virginia Commission on
  Aging
Holly Grove, State Capitol
1900 Kanawha Boulevard East
Charleston, WV 25305-0160
(304) 558-3317
(304) 558-0004 fax
e-mail: hollygrove@juno.com

Wisconsin

Bureau of Aging and Long Term
  Care Resources (BALTCR)
Suite 300
217 South Hamilton
Madison, WI 53703
(608) 266-2536
(608) 267-3203 fax

Wyoming

Department of Health
Division on Aging
Hathaway Building, 1st Floor
2300 Capital Avenue
Cheyenne, WY 82002-0480
(307) 777-7986
(307) 777-5340 fax
e-mail:
  wmilto@missc.state.wy.us

Index

Index

Contagious & Non-Contagious Infectious Diseases Sourcebook

Basic Information about Contagious Diseases like Measles, Polio, Hepatitis B, and Infectious Mononucleosis, and Non-Contagious Infectious Diseases like Tetanus and Toxic Shock Syndrome, and Diseases Occurring as Secondary Infections Such as Shingles and Reye Syndrome, Along with Vaccination, Prevention, and Treatment Information, and a Section Describing Emerging Infectious Disease Threats

Edited by Karen Bellenir and Peter D. Dresser. 566 pages. 1996. 0-7808-0075-3. $78.

Death & Dying Sourcebook

Basic Information for the Layperson about End-of-Life Care and Related Ethical and Legal Issues, Including Chief Causes of Death, Autopsies, Pain Management for the Terminally Ill, Life Support Systems, Coma, Euthanasia, Assisted Suicide, Hospice Programs, Living Wills, Near-Death Experiences, Counseling, Mourning, Organ Donation, Cryogenics and Physician Training and Liability, Along with Statistical Data, a Glossary, and Listings of Sources for Additional Help and Information

Edited by Annemarie Muth. 600 pages. 1999. 0-7808-0230-6. $78.

Diabetes Sourcebook, 1st Edition

Basic Information about Insulin-Dependent and Noninsulin-Dependent Diabetes Mellitus, Gestational Diabetes, and Diabetic Complications, Symptoms, Treatment, and Research Results, Including Statistics on Prevalence, Morbidity, and Mortality, Along with Source Listings for Further Help and Information

Edited by Karen Bellenir and Peter D. Dresser. 827 pages. 1994. 1-55888-751-2. $78.

"...very informative and understandable for the layperson without being simplistic. It provides a comprehensive overview for laypersons who want a general understanding of the disease or who want to focus on various aspects of the disease." — *Bulletin of the MLA, Jan '96*

Diabetes Sourcebook, 2nd Edition

Basic Consumer Health Information about Type 1 Diabetes (Insulin-Dependent or Juvenile-Onset Diabetes), Type 2 (Noninsulin-Dependent or Adult-Onset Diabetes), Gestational Diabetes, and Related Disorders, Including Diabetes Prevalence Data, Management Issues, the Role of Diet and Exercise in Controlling Diabetes, Insulin and Other Diabetes Medicines, and Complications of Diabetes Such as Eye Diseases, Periodontal Disease, Amputation, and End-Stage Renal Disease; Along with Reports on Current Research Initiatives, a Glossary, and Resource Listings for Further Help and Information

Edited by Karen Bellenir. 725 pages. 1998. 0-7808-0224-1. $78.

Diet & Nutrition Sourcebook, 1st Edition

Basic Information about Nutrition, Including the Dietary Guidelines for Americans, the Food Guide Pyramid, and Their Applications in Daily Diet, Nutritional Advice for Specific Age Groups, Current Nutritional Issues and Controversies, the New Food Label and How to Use It to Promote Healthy Eating, and Recent Developments in Nutritional Research

Edited by Dan R. Harris. 662 pages. 1996. 0-7808-0084-2. $78.

"Useful reference as a food and nutrition sourcebook for the general consumer."
— *Booklist Health Sciences Supplement, Oct '97*

"Recommended for public libraries and medical libraries that receive general information requests on nutrition. It is readable and will appeal to those interested in learning more about healthy dietary practices."
— *Medical Reference Services Quarterly, Fall '97*

"With dozens of questionable diet books on the market, it is so refreshing to find a reliable and factual reference book. Recommended to aspiring professionals, librarians, and others seeking and giving reliable dietary advice. An excellent compilation." — *Choice, Feb '97*

Diet & Nutrition Sourcebook, 2nd Edition

Basic Consumer Health Information about Dietary Guidelines, Recommended Daily Intake Values, Vitamins, Minerals, Fiber, Fat, Weight Control, Dietary Supplements, and Food Additives; Along with Special Sections on Nutrition Needs throughout Life and Nutrition for People with Such Specific Medical Concerns as Allergies, High Blood Cholesterol, Hypertension, Diabetes, Celiac Disease, Seizure Disorders, Phenylketonuria (PKU), Cancer, and Eating Disorders, and Including Reports on Current Nutrition Research and Source Listings for Additional Help and Information

Edited by Karen Bellenir. 600 pages. 1999. 0-7808-0228-4. $78.

Domestic Violence Sourcebook

Basic Information about the Physical, Emotional and Sexual Abuse of Partners, Children, and Elders, Including Information about Hotlines, Safe Houses, Safety Plans, Resources for Support and Assistance, Community Initiatives, and Reports on Current Directions in Research and Treatment; Along with a Glossary, Sources for Further Reading, and Listings of Governmental and Non-Governmental Organizations

Edited by Helene Henderson. 600 pages. 1999. 0-7808-0235-7. $78.

Ear, Nose & Throat Disorders Sourcebook

Basic Information about Disorders of the Ears, Nose, Sinus Cavities, Pharynx, and Larynx, Including Ear Infections, Tinnitus, Vestibular Disorders, Allergic and Non-Allergic Rhinitis, Sore Throats, Tonsillitis, and Cancers That Affect the Ears, Nose, Sinuses, and Throat, Along with Reports on Current Research Initiatives, a Glossary of Related Medical Terms, and a Directory of Sources for Further Help and Information

Edited by Karen Bellenir and Linda M. Shin. 592 pages. 1998. 0-7808-0206-3. $78.

Endocrine & Metabolic Disorders Sourcebook

Basic Information for the Layperson about Pancreatic and Insulin-Related Disorders Such as Pancreatitis, Diabetes, and Hypoglycemia; Adrenal Gland Disorders Such as Cushing's Syndrome, Addison's Disease, and Congenital Adrenal Hyperplasia; Pituitary Gland Disorders Such as Growth Hormone Deficiency, Acromegaly, and Pituitary Tumors; Thyroid Disorders Such as Hypothyroidism, Graves' Disease, Hashimoto's Disease, and Goiter; Hyperparathyroidism; and Other Diseases and Syndromes of Hormone Imbalance or Metabolic Dysfunction, Along with Reports on Current Research Initiatives

Edited by Linda M. Shin. 632 pages. 1998. 0-7808-0207-1. $78.

Environmentally Induced Disorders Sourcebook

Basic Information about Diseases and Syndromes Linked to Exposure to Pollutants and Other Substances in Outdoor and Indoor Environments Such as Lead, Asbestos, Formaldehyde, Mercury, Emissions, Noise, and More

Edited by Allan R. Cook. 620 pages. 1997. 0-7808-0083-4. $78.

"... a good survey of numerous environmentally induced physical disorders ... a useful addition to anyone's library."
— *Doody's Health Science Book Reviews, Jan '98*

"... provide[s] introductory information from the best authorities around. Since this volume covers topics that potentially affect everyone, it will surely be one of the most frequently consulted volumes in the *Health Reference Series*." — *Rettig on Reference, Nov '97*

"Recommended reference source."
— *Booklist, Oct '97*

Ethical Issues in Medicine Sourcebook

Basic Information about Controversial Treatment Issues, Genetic Research, Reproductive Technologies, and End-of-Life Decisions, Including Topics Such as Cloning, Abortion, Fertility Management, Organ Transplantation, Health Care Rationing, Advance Directives, Living Wills, Physician-Assisted Suicide, Euthanasia, and More; Along with a Glossary and Resources for Additional Information

Edited by Helene Henderson. 600 pages. 1999. 0-7808-0237-3. $78.

Fitness & Exercise Sourcebook

Basic Information on Fitness and Exercise, Including Fitness Activities for Specific Age Groups, Exercise for People with Specific Medical Conditions, How to Begin a Fitness Program in Running, Walking, Swimming, Cycling, and Other Athletic Activities, and Recent Research in Fitness and Exercise

Edited by Dan R. Harris. 663 pages. 1996. 0-7808-0186-5. $78.

"A good resource for general readers."
— *Choice, Nov '97*

"The perennial popularity of the topic ... make this an appealing selection for public libraries."
— *Rettig on Reference, Jun/Jul '97*

Food & Animal Borne Diseases Sourcebook

Basic Information about Diseases That Can Be Spread to Humans through the Ingestion of Contaminated Food or Water or by Contact with Infected Animals and Insects, Such as Botulism, E. Coli, Hepatitis A, Trichinosis, Lyme Disease, and Rabies, Along with Information Regarding Prevention and Treatment Methods, and a Special Section for International Travelers Describing Diseases Such as Cholera, Malaria, Travelers' Diarrhea, and Yellow Fever, and Offering Recommendations for Avoiding Illness

Edited by Karen Bellenir and Peter D. Dresser. 535 pages. 1995. 0-7808-0033-8. $78.

"Targeting general readers and providing them with a single, comprehensive source of information on selected topics, this book continues, with the excellent caliber of its predecessors, to catalog topical information on health matters of general interest. Readable and thorough, this valuable resource is highly recommended for all libraries."
— *Academic Library Book Review, Summer '96*

"A comprehensive collection of authoritative information." — *Emergency Medical Services, Oct '95*

Continues next page

Gastrointestinal Diseases & Disorders Sourcebook

Basic Information about Gastroesophageal Reflux Disease (Heartburn), Ulcers, Diverticulosis, Irritable Bowel Syndrome, Crohn's Disease, Ulcerative Colitis, Diarrhea, Constipation, Lactose Intolerance, Hemorrhoids, Hepatitis, Cirrhosis, and Other Digestive Problems, Featuring Statistics, Descriptions of Symptoms, and Current Treatment Methods of Interest for Persons Living with Upper and Lower Gastrointestinal Maladies

Edited by Linda M. Ross. 413 pages. 1996. 0-7808-0078-8. $78.

"... very readable form. The successful editorial work that brought this material together into a useful and understandable reference makes accessible to all readers information that can help them more effectively understand and obtain help for digestive tract problems." — *Choice, Feb '97*

Genetic Disorders Sourcebook

Basic Information about Heritable Diseases and Disorders Such as Down Syndrome, PKU, Hemophilia, Von Willebrand Disease, Gaucher Disease, Tay-Sachs Disease, and Sickle-Cell Disease, Along with Information about Genetic Screening, Gene Therapy, Home Care, and Including Source Listings for Further Help and Information on More Than 300 Disorders

Edited by Karen Bellenir. 642 pages. 1996. 0-7808-0034-6. $78.

"Provides essential medical information to both the general public and those diagnosed with a serious or fatal genetic disease or disorder." — *Choice, Jan '97*

"Geared toward the lay public. It would be well placed in all public libraries and in those hospital and medical libraries in which access to genetic references is limited." — *Doody's Health Sciences Book Review, Oct '96*

Head Trauma Sourcebook

Basic Information for the Layperson about Open-Head and Closed-Head Injuries, Treatment Advances, Recovery, and Rehabilitation, Along with Reports on Current Research Initiatives

Edited by Karen Bellenir. 414 pages. 1997. 0-7808-0208-X. $78.

Health Insurance Sourcebook

Basic Information about Managed Care Organizations, Traditional Fee-for-Service Insurance, Insurance Portability and Pre-Existing Conditions Clauses, Medicare, Medicaid, Social Security, and Military Health Care, Along with Information about Insurance Fraud

Edited by Wendy Wilcox. 530 pages. 1997. 0-7808-0222-5. $78.

"The layout of the book is particularly helpful as it provides easy access to reference material. A most useful addition to the vast amount of information about health insurance. The use of data from U.S. government agencies is most commendable. Useful in a library or learning center for healthcare professional students." — *Doody's Health Sciences Book Reviews, Nov '97*

Healthy Aging Sourcebook

Basic Consumer Health Information about Maintaining Health through the Aging Process, Including Advice on Nutrition, Exercise, and Sleep, Along with Help in Making Decisions about Midlife Issues and Retirement, Practical and Informed Choices in Health Consumerism, and Data Concerning the Theories of Aging, Aging Now, and Aging in the Future, Including a Glossary and Practical Resource Directory

Edited by Jenifer Swanson. 500 pages. 1999. 0-7808-0390-6. $78.

Immune System Disorders Sourcebook

Basic Information about Lupus, Multiple Sclerosis, Guillain-Barré Syndrome, Chronic Granulomatous Disease, and More, Along with Statistical and Demographic Data and Reports on Current Research Initiatives

Edited by Allan R. Cook. 608 pages. 1997. 0-7808-0209-8. $78.

Kidney & Urinary Tract Diseases & Disorders Sourcebook

Basic Information about Kidney Stones, Urinary Incontinence, Bladder Disease, End Stage Renal Disease, Dialysis, and More, Along with Statistical and Demographic Data and Reports on Current Research Initiatives

Edited by Linda M. Ross. 602 pages. 1997. 0-7808-0079-6. $78.

Learning Disabilities Sourcebook

Basic Information about Disorders Such as Dyslexia, Visual and Auditory Processing Deficits, Attention Deficit/Hyperactivity Disorder, and Autism, Along with Statistical and Demographic Data, Reports on Current Research Initiatives, an Explanation of the Assessment Process, and a Special Section for Adults with Learning Disabilities

Edited by Linda M. Shin. 579 pages. 1998. 0-7808-0210-1. $78.

Medical Tests Sourcebook

Basic Consumer Health Information about Medical Tests, Including Periodic Health Exams, General Screening Tests, X-ray and Radiology Tests, Electrical Tests, Tests of Body Fluids and Tissues, Scope Tests, Lung Tests, Gene Tests, Pregnancy Tests, Newborn Screening Tests, Sexually Transmitted Disease Tests, and Computer Aided Diagnoses; Along with a Section on Paying for Medical Tests, a Glossary, and Resource Listings

Edited by Joyce B. Shannon. 600 pages. 1999. 0-7808-0243-8. $78.

Men's Health Concerns Sourcebook

Basic Information about Health Issues That Affect Men, Featuring Facts about the Top Causes of Death in Men, Including Heart Disease, Stroke, Cancers, Prostate Disorders, Chronic Obstructive Pulmonary Disease, Pneumonia and Influenza, Human Immunodeficiency Virus and Acquired Immune Deficiency Syndrome, Diabetes Mellitus, Stress, Suicide, Accidents and Homicides; and Facts about Common Concerns for Men, Including Impotence, Contraception, Circumcision, Sleep Disorders, Snoring, Hair Loss, Diet, Nutrition, Exercise, Kidney and Urological Disorders, and Backaches

Edited by Allan R. Cook. 760 pages. 1998. 0-7808-0212-8. $78.

Mental Health Disorders Sourcebook

Basic Information about Schizophrenia, Depression, Bipolar Disorder, Panic Disorder, Obsessive-Compulsive Disorder, Phobias and Other Anxiety Disorders, Paranoia and Other Personality Disorders, Eating Disorders, and Sleep Disorders, Along with Information about Treatment and Therapies

Edited by Karen Bellenir. 548 pages. 1995. 0-7808-0040-0. $78.

"This is an excellent new book . . . written in easy-to-understand language."
— *Booklist Health Science Supplement, Oct '97*

". . . useful for public and academic libraries and consumer health collections."
— *Medical Reference Services Quarterly, Spring '97*

"The great strengths of the book are its readability and its inclusion of places to find more information. Especially recommended." — *RQ, Winter '96*

". . . a good resource for a consumer health library."
— *Bulletin of the MLA, Oct '96*

"The information is data-based and couched in brief, concise language that avoids jargon. . . . a useful reference source." — *Readings, Sept '96*

"The text is well organized and adequately written for its target audience." — *Choice, Jun '96*

". . . provides information on a wide range of mental disorders, presented in nontechnical language."
— *Exceptional Child Education Resources, Spring '96*

"Recommended for public and academic libraries."
— *Reference Book Review, '96*

Ophthalmic Disorders Sourcebook

Basic Information about Glaucoma, Cataracts, Macular Degeneration, Strabismus, Refractive Disorders, and More, Along with Statistical and Demographic Data and Reports on Current Research Initiatives

Edited by Linda M. Ross. 631 pages. 1996. 0-7808-0081-8. $78.

Oral Health Sourcebook

Basic Information about Diseases and Conditions Affecting Oral Health, Including Cavities, Gum Disease, Dry Mouth, Oral Cancers, Fever Blisters, Canker Sores, Oral Thrush, Bad Breath, Temporomandibular Disorders, and other Craniofacial Syndromes, Along with Statistical Data on the Oral Health of Americans, Oral Hygiene, Emergency First Aid, Information on Treatment Procedures and Methods of Replacing Lost Teeth

Edited by Allan R. Cook. 558 pages. 1997. 0-7808-0082-6. $78.

"Recommended reference source." — *Booklist, Dec '97*

Pain Sourcebook

Basic Information about Specific Forms of Acute and Chronic Pain, Including Headaches, Back Pain, Muscular Pain, Neuralgia, Surgical Pain, and Cancer Pain, Along with Pain Relief Options Such as Analgesics, Narcotics, Nerve Blocks, Transcutaneous Nerve Stimulation, and Alternative Forms of Pain Control, Including Biofeedback, Imaging, Behavior Modification, and Relaxation Techniques

Edited by Allan R. Cook. 667 pages. 1997. 0-7808-0213-6. $78.

"The information is basic in terms of scholarship and is appropriate for general readers. Written in journalistic style . . . intended for non-professionals. Quite thorough in its coverage of different pain conditions and summarizes the latest clinical information regarding pain treatment." — *Choice, Jun '98*

"Recommended reference source."
— *Booklist, Mar '98*

Continues next page

Physical & Mental Issues in Aging Sourcebook

Basic Consumer Health Information on Physical and Mental Disorders Associated with the Aging Process, Including Concerns about Cardiovascular Disease, Pulmonary Disease, Oral Health, Digestive Disorders, Musculoskeletal and Skin Disorders, Metabolic Changes, Sexual and Reproductive Issues, and Changes in Vision, Hearing, and Other Senses; Along with Data about Longevity and Causes of Death, Information on Acute and Chronic Pain, Descriptions of Mental Concerns, a Glossary of Terms, and Resource Listings for Additional Help

Edited by Heather E. Aldred. 625 pages. 1999. 0-7808-0233-0. $78.

Pregnancy & Birth Sourcebook

Basic Information about Planning for Pregnancy, Maternal Health, Fetal Growth and Development, Labor and Delivery, Postpartum and Perinatal Care, Pregnancy in Mothers with Special Concerns, and Disorders of Pregnancy, Including Genetic Counseling, Nutrition and Exercise, Obstetrical Tests, Pregnancy Discomfort, Multiple Births, Cesarean Sections, Medical Testing of Newborns, Breastfeeding, Gestational Diabetes, and Ectopic Pregnancy

Edited by Heather E. Aldred. 737 pages. 1997. 0-7808-0216-0. $78.

". . . for the layperson. A well-organized handbook. Recommended for college libraries . . . general readers."
— Choice, Apr '98

"Recommended reference source."
— Booklist, Mar '98

"This resource is recommended for public libraries to have on hand."
— American Reference Books Annual, '98

Public Health Sourcebook

Basic Information about Government Health Agencies, Including National Health Statistics and Trends, Healthy People 2000 Program Goals and Objectives, the Centers for Disease Control and Prevention, the Food and Drug Administration, and the National Institutes of Health, Along with Full Contact Information for Each Agency

Edited by Wendy Wilcox. 698 pages. 1998. 0-7808-0220-9. $78.

Rehabilitation Sourcebook

Basic Information for the Layperson about Physical Medicine (Physiatry) and Rehabilitative Therapies, Including Physical, Occupational, Recreational, Speech, and Vocational Therapy; Along with Descriptions of Devices and Equipment Such as Orthotics, Gait Aids, Prostheses, and Adaptive Systems Used during Rehabilitation and for Activities of Daily Living, and Featuring a Glossary and Source Listings for Further Help and Information

Edited by Theresa K. Murray. 600 pages. 1999. 0-7808-0236-5. $78.

Respiratory Diseases & Disorders Sourcebook

Basic Information about Respiratory Diseases and Disorders, Including Asthma, Cystic Fibrosis, Pneumonia, the Common Cold, Influenza, and Others, Featuring Facts about the Respiratory System, Statistical and Demographic Data, Treatments, Self-Help Management Suggestions, and Current Research Initiatives

Edited by Allan R. Cook and Peter D. Dresser. 771 pages. 1995. 0-7808-0037-0. $78.

"Designed for the layperson and for patients and their families coping with respiratory illness. . . . an extensive array of information on diagnosis, treatment, management, and prevention of respiratory illnesses for the general reader."
— Choice, Jun '96

"A highly recommended text for all collections. It is a comforting reminder of the power of knowledge that good books carry between their covers."
— Academic Library Book Review, Spring '96

"This sourcebook offers a comprehensive collection of authoritative information presented in a nontechnical, humanitarian style for patients, families, and caregivers."
— Association of Operating Room Nurses, Sept/Oct '95

Sexually Transmitted Diseases Sourcebook

Basic Information about Herpes, Chlamydia, Gonorrhea, Hepatitis, Nongonoccocal Urethritis, Pelvic Inflammatory Disease, Syphilis, AIDS, and More, Along with Current Data on Treatments and Preventions

Edited by Linda M. Ross. 550 pages. 1997. 0-7808-0217-9. $78.